# THE CARDIOVASCULAR MRI TUTORIAL

## LECTURES AND LEARNING

# THE CARDIOVASCULAR MRI TUTORIAL

## LECTURES AND LEARNING

## Robert W. W. Biederman, MD, FACC, FASA
*Director, Cardiovascular Magnetic Resonance Imaging*
*Associate Professor of Medicine*
*Drexel University College of Medicine*
*Center for Cardiovascular Magnetic Resonance Imaging*
*The Gerald McGinnis Cardiovascular Institute*
*Allegheny Singer Research Institute*
*Allegheny General Hospital*
*Pittsburgh, Pennsylvania*

## Mark Doyle, PhD
*Professor of Medicine*
*Drexel University College of Medicine*
*Center for Cardiovascular Magnetic Resonance Imaging*
*The Gerald McGinnis Cardiovascular Institute*
*Allegheny Singer Research Institute*
*Allegheny General Hospital*
*Pittsburgh, Pennsylvania*

## June Yamrozik, BS, RT (R)(MR)
*Cardiovascular Magnetic Resonance Imaging Technologist*
*Center for Cardiovascular Magnetic Resonance Imaging*
*The Gerald McGinnis Cardiovascular Institute*
*Allegheny Singer Research Institute*
*Allegheny General Hospital*
*Pittsburgh, Pennsylvania*

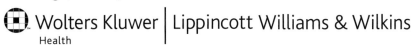

Wolters Kluwer | Lippincott Williams & Wilkins
Health

Philadelphia · Baltimore · New York · London
Buenos Aires · Hong Kong · Sydney · Tokyo

*Acquisitions Editor:* Frances R. DeStefano
*Managing Editor:* Chris Potash
*Project Manager:* Jennifer Harper
*Manufacturing Manager:* Benjamin Rivera
*Marketing Manager:* Kimberly Schonberger
*Design Coordinator:* Terry Mallon
*Production Services:* Laserwords Private Limited, Chennai, India

---

**Library of Congress Cataloging-in-Publication Data**

Biederman, Robert W. W.
  The cardiovascular MRI tutorial : lectures and learning / Robert W. W. Biederman, Mark Doyle, June Yamrozik.
    p. ; cm.
  Includes bibliographical references and index.
  ISBN 978-0-7817-7216-7 (alk. paper)
  1. Cardiovascular system—Magnetic resonance imaging—Programmed instruction. I. Doyle, Mark, 1959- II. Yamrozik, June. III. Title.
  [DNLM: 1. Cardiovascular Diseases—diagnosis. 2. Diagnostic Techniques, Cardiovascular. 3. Magnetic Resonance Imaging—methods. WG 141.5.M2 B585c 2008]
  RC670.5.M33B54 2008
  616.1'07548—dc22

                                                                    2007030622

---

*To Mark and June, my esteemed coauthors, I most gratefully thank them for their indomitable spirit, ideas, and willingness to tackle our project with such zeal, probably always wondering if I would make my deadline. This treatise was accomplished with assistance and endless energy of Ron Williams. I neither asked for nor would have taken 'time off' for this labor such that it occurred at odd hours of the day and night. I thank my lovely wife, Kimberly, for without her indefatigable support and love this book could never have occurred. To Brittani, Addison, and Caroline who endured those long nights, weekends, and holidays, especially Christmas 2006, with their Dad hovered over the laptop, go my heartfelt thanks for their understanding and patience. To the patients, colleagues, coworkers, and friends who contributed in their own special way toward making this endeavor possible. To James Magovern, MD who was and continues to epitomize the life of a true gentleman and inspiring clinical researcher. To Fran at LWW who took our fledgling idea and ran with it. And finally, to my parents, especially to my Dad, a fellow scientist, for instilling in me the inquisitive nature of discovery from which much of these pages are derived.*

Robert W. W. Biederman, Pittsburgh, May 2007

*I have attempted to express ideas and concepts in my own manner, but obviously I am indebted to the MRI community at large where these ideas have originated and were developed. Many of the illustrations were prepared using Mathlab software (The Mathworks, Natick, MA).*

*This work is dedicated to my mother, father, wife, and children, Abby and Andrew.*

Mark Doyle, Pittsburgh, May 2007

*I'd like to thank Dr. Robert Biederman and Dr. Mark Doyle for believing in me and providing me with this opportunity to showcase my talents. Dr. Vikas Rathi was my mentor and friend always providing me with the answers that I needed to my numerous questions. My mom and sister, Carol are my support system and encouraged me throughout this endeavor. Many thanks go out to the staff of LWW for making this book a reality.*

*This book is dedicated to my father who would be very proud of this undertaking.*

June Yamrozik, Pittsburgh, May 2007

# CONTENTS

# FOREWORD

Over the years I have had the pleasure of writing forewords for a number of books that I considered to be timely and to fulfill important objectives. Without hesitation I would say that *Cardiovascular MRI Tutorial: Lectures and Learning*, by Robert Biederman, M.D., in collaboration with Mark Doyle, Ph.D., and June Yamrozik, RT, is perhaps the most outstanding book for which I have had the pleasure to write a foreword. Why?

This is not just a textbook; this is an extraordinary educational tool on a rapidly evolving technology in the cardiovascular field: Cardiac Magnetic Resonance (CMR). To my knowledge this is the first CMR book that is not only succinct, informative, and thorough but also includes an accompanying DVD with more than 500 video clips that permits the user to customize his/her own series of didactic modifiable lectures. In fact this book contains the largest series of CMR images compiled—more than 1,000—along with 37 complete "lectures" and 200 stand-alone cases interweaved within text that, for the first time, is aimed at the clinician, the physicist, and the CMR technologist, as it is written by an expert in each one of those capacities. With almost 40 hours of teaching material provided, one may think that the claim to succinctness is unfounded, but on the contrary, by treating each topic area separately and in detail, the authors rapidly get to the core of the subject matter and no time is wasted on preambles. Material is presented concretely (even k-space) and at an appropriate level of depth, well beyond the superficial format found in many introductory texts but without falling into the trap of being so all-inclusive as to become abstract. Whether you read the book from cover to cover, view the DVD as a series of PowerPoint presentations, or delve into chapters at will, you will undoubtedly come away with a firm grasp of CMR essentials. *Cardiovascular MRI Tutorial* is sure to become a classic.

This work is most fitting; the CMR technique deservedly has taken center stage for those interested in interrogating the cardiovascular system with tools that have been honed in the last 5 years to a precise degree, in some cases by this team. I have watched this burgeoning field develop with keen interest over the last few decades and have come to view CMR as *the* modality with the current capability and future promise to systematically employ a myriad of techniques to evaluate the heart and related vasculatures. The ability of CMR to divine anatomy and physiology in the form of structure, function, blood flow, valve assessment, myocardial perfusion, and viability as well as the unique ability to characterize tissue, I believe, places it as the imaging standard for many of the clinical (and research) uses required in this day and age. I am particularly fond of the images representing plaque characterization using the capability of CMR to noninvasively and without either contrast or radiation define what I believe are cardinal features delineating the "high-risk" plaque for what will likely become the "missing link" for demonstrating future adverse prognostic features within those plaques.

This book is a tribute to the skill of the three authors, now working out of the Center for Cardiovascular Magnetic Resonance Imaging at the Allegheny Singer Research Institute in Pittsburgh, representing their nearly total 50-year perspective. And so it is with great pleasure that I pen these words to relate my enthusiasm for this work as a remarkable addition to the field of imaging. It is obviously a work that comes directly from their heart—the heart of a clinician, a physicist, and a technologist—as the authors peer into your patient's heart and, most importantly for you, into the hearts of their readers, for whom this work was aimed.

VALENTIN FUSTER, MD, PhD
*Professor of Medicine/Cardiology*
*Mount Sinai School of Medicine*
*Past President American Heart Association*
*Past President World Heart Association*

# PREFACE

The field of cardiovascular magnetic resonance (CMR) imaging has grown at an almost exponential rate, producing a technology that is mature enough to address clinical questions ranging from the routine through the highly complex. This makes CMR an ideal imaging modality: noninvasive, rapid, and safe. With the capability of addressing nearly every cardiovascular condition known, it has become the modality of choice for many routine indications.

To the uninitiated, CMR's technological wizardry may appear to be almost unassailable and it was our intention to present this fascinating and multifaceted topic in a practical, logical, and understandable manner to allow mastery and demystification of the technology. Charged with this lofty mandate, we quickly realized that this could not be easily accomplished using a single format or approach.

The unique format that we chose to present the material combined the cohesive narrative form of the written word, in a generously illustrated book, with a lecture type format of PowerPoint presentations, providing a dimension that "brings to life" the many dynamic aspects of CMR with illustrative animations and cine presentations.

The intended audience for this multimedia treatise consists of physicians, physicists, technologists, and teachers. The material is presented succinctly, but thoroughly, which serves the novice, who is rapidly introduced to key concepts, the clinician who can quickly locate the relevant CMR views needed, the technologist who needs to navigate to the correct view, as well as the advanced user who wants to optimize the clinical experience for the patient.

The book contains 37 chapters with more than 500 images and line art illustrations, with each chapter having a corresponding PowerPoint presentation that elaborates upon the written material and is suitable for self-study or presentation in a lecture format. Inevitably in such a broad and complex topic there is a danger that, by accommodating the needs of the novice through the advanced user, the material is treated either superficially or as a seeming interminable drudge of laborious and exhaustive detail. We addressed this by dividing the material into three distinct sections: Imaging Basics (1–3), Clinical Applications (4–16), and Advanced Training (17–37). This structure is designed to allow the novice to follow the material in sequential chapter order, whereas those more familiar with CMR can delve into specialized topic areas as needed, because each is presented in an essentially stand-alone manner. For example, the clinician can read the clinical application sections in an environment protected from parenthetical or repetitive descriptions of the physical principles involved, while having full access to the physical principles in clearly delineated chapters. However, in such a technologically rich modality, it is inevitable that a deep and thorough understanding can only be gained by considering the advanced aspects of the technology. In the Advanced Training section we present this material, not as a weapon to induce blunt instrument trauma to the reader, but in a manner designed to educate, inform, and empower.

The CD contains 37 dynamic PowerPoint presentations, designed to accompany each book chapter, and contains movies illustrating basic and advanced cardiac and cardiovascular images and concepts, with more than 1,500 illustrations and animations, distilling in a comprehensive manner the clinical practice and scientific research experience of more than two decades.

Each PowerPoint presentation has been crafted and modified to present material in an understandable manner based on years of feedback from medical students, residents, fellows, and cardiologists/radiologists (to whom we are very grateful). As an educational tool, the PowerPoint format allows us to present a higher level of detailed illustration than is conventionally incorporated in a printed book. However, the bulleted format of the PowerPoint does not lend itself to unaided understanding, and the printed book provides the full context for each presentation, effectively unlocking the information contained in the PowerPoint presentations. Importantly, each chapter in the CD can be used either in a stand-alone manner or with user modification to supplement their presentations of didactic material and we hope that this material will aid in wide dissemination of knowledge.

Our philosophy in presenting the material is to quickly introduce each topic, and then to creatively revisit the material throughout the chapter. In this way, the reader is not initially overburdened with meticulous detail but after completing the book and CD, will have been exposed to a thorough treatment concerning the practice and technology of CMR. In our extensive field-testing of the material, we have designed presentations of general and highly specialized topics in a comprehensive manner that does not necessarily require exposure to earlier topics, because each concept is explained sufficiently for the needs of each chapter. For instance, in evaluating any book dealing with magnetic resonance imaging (MRI), the section dealing with k-space, which is the ubiquitously referenced CMR signal space, is often referred to and forms a *litmus test* for other material: Is the treatment superficial, overly mathematical, disjointed, or plain unintelligible? We hope that our treatment passes this inspection, and also serves to illustrate the philosophy with which other topics are presented.

Chapter 1, presenting an overview, quickly introduces the topic of k-space sufficient for the novice to appreciate its central importance and relationship to gradients and images. Chapter 21 is a treatment of applied k-space, showing the relationship between imaging parameters selected at the console and the manner in which k-space data are acquired, exposing the user to the "hands-on" experience of k-space. Chapter 24 is a formal treatment of k-space, where its mathematical and physical origins are developed, and given the background established in earlier chapters, the reader could now appreciate this mathematical treatment. Chapter 34 will not let the matter rest, and presents a less formal,

but highly illustrative description of k-space. These specific chapters are not the only treatment given to k-space, the properties of which permeate through the material ranging from topics as diverse as artifacts to Z-gradients.

To complete the appreciation of this material, a perspective concerning the authors is warranted. With only three authors contributing to the direct writing of material, our goal as a small group of experts (with more than 50 years of combined experience in CMR) who have a close working relationship was to compile and arrange the material in logical order with a minimum of repetition, speaking with one voice. We have largely tried to limit discussion of broader research topics, and mainly focused on the experiences gained at our laboratory representing both academic- and community-based imaging experiences. We hope that this book and CD comprehensively provide the reader with usable knowledge concerning this advancing technology, to benefit their scientific and clinical applications of CMR, and provide a basis for others to build upon as the discipline matures.

www.AGHCardiacMRI.org

# THE CARDIOVASCULAR MRI TUTORIAL

## LECTURES AND LEARNING

# PART I

# Imaging Basics

# CHAPTER 1

# Overview of Cardiovascular Magnetic Resonance Imaging

Mark Doyle

There are several important conceptual elements required to understand magnetic resonance imaging (MRI), and this broad overview seeks to introduce these and establish a framework for further in-depth studies. The topics summarized here are as follows:

- Signal source
- Signal characteristics
- Magnetic gradients
- K-space
- Gradient echo
- Spin echo
- Hardware

## SIGNAL SOURCE

Unlike most imaging modalities MR has several conceptual difficulties:

- The origin of the signal for MR is not intuitively obvious.
- The means of forming an image is not intuitively obvious.
- Image contrast depends on many factors.

To address these we will begin with basic principles to develop an initial understanding before proceeding in later chapters into more in-depth treatments. At the most basic level, the human body is composed of approximately 70% water, which in turn is made up of an oxygen atom and two hydrogen atoms. The hydrogen atom is composed of a single proton, which has the nuclear property of spin (see Fig. 1-1). Conceptually, we can imagine the nucleus spinning just like a spinning top. Owing to the property of spin and due to the electrical charge contained within the nucleus, the proton generates a magnetic field, that is, a *magnetic dipole*. Because the nuclear spinning action was responsible for this property, the magnetic dipole is

referred to as a *spin*. The property that is imaged in MRI is the distribution of spins. If a spinning top is tipped over, it will precess (i.e., slowly wobble). The wobbling action is slow relative to its spinning frequency. In summary, the physical properties required to cause a spin to precess are:

- Spin
- Force field (e.g., gravity)
- Tipping action

This principle can be directly applied to magnetic spins in that protons are directly analogous to spinning tops. If they can be tipped over with respect to the magnetic (force) field, then they will precess. Of interest to cardiovascular magnetic resonance (CMR) is the fact that a precessing proton, due to its magnetic property, will emit an electromagnetic signal, which can be

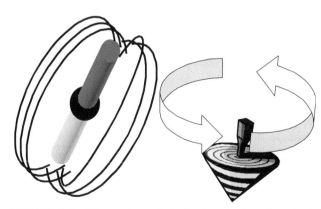

FIGURE 1-1   The nucleus of the hydrogen atom is a single proton. It behaves as if it were a bar magnet (a magnetic dipole) with north and south poles. The proton has the additional property that it spins on its axis, just like a spinning top. The combined properties of magnetism and spinning action are summed into the all-encompassing term, *spin*. Mapping the distribution of spins is the process of imaging.

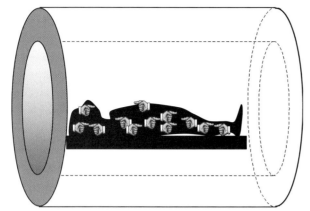

**FIGURE 1-2**   When a body is placed inside a strong magnetic field (represented by the cylindrical structure), some spins align with the main magnetic field (low energy state), and an almost equal number of spins fall into antialignment. These two opposing spin systems tend to cancel each other, and only a very small net magnetic field is set up in the body.

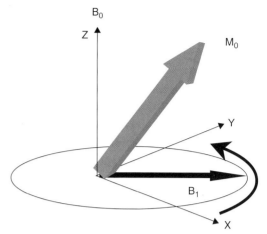

**FIGURE 1-3**   The direction of the main magnetic field formed by the scanner system is, by convention, referred to as the "Z" axis, or longitudinal direction. The plane transverse to the Z direction contains the "X" and "Y" axes. The net magnetization from the body is referred to as $M_0$, and can be thought of as initially pointing along the "Z" a xis. To tip the $M_0$ magnetization from alignment with the main magnetic field $B_0$, a small rotating magnetic field, $B_1$, is applied in the transverse plane. $B_1$ is applied at the resonance frequency of the system, and consequently exerts a strong influence on $M_0$, easily tipping it into the transverse plane.

detected and ultimately imaged. For protons the precessional frequency ($\omega$) is in the radio frequency (RF) range, hence the sample emits an RF signal. Signal detection is accomplished by placing an electrical conductor in the vicinity of the precessing proton, which in turn induces a voltage in the conductor. This voltage is known as the *electromotive force* (EMF). Thereby, a conducting coil acts as the receiver for the CMR signal.

When considering magnetism and the human body, intuition does not serve us well. Intuitively, one might expect all the spins in the body (which effectively act as bar magnets) to align with an externally applied magnetic field. However, this is not the case. Quantum mechanical laws prohibit all the spins from occupying the lowest energy state (i.e., aligning with the magnetic field) (see Fig. 1-2). In essence, the body's heat acts as an energy source that allows the spins to resist alignment with the magnetic field, and therefore the body only becomes very weakly magnetized. Further, after positioning the body in the magnet, there is still no detectable signal given off by the body. Therefore, the only thing accomplished by placing the patient in the magnet is the generation of a net magnetization vector, $M_0$. To generate a detectable signal, $M_0$ must be made to precess, and when precessing, it will emit an RF signal. To make $M_0$ precess, it must be tipped from alignment with the main magnetic field $B_0$. A key point to address now is, how to tip over the magnetization vector, $M_0$. The magnetization vector can be tipped into the "transverse" plane by applying a small, rotating magnetic field, $B_1$ (see Fig. 1-3). The $B_1$ field is applied at the natural precession frequency of the spins ($\omega$) and exploits the resonance phenomena to exert a large influence on the spin system with

the expenditure of relatively little energy. The rotating $B_1$ field is referred to as an *RF pulse* and has several properties:

- It is applied in the transverse plane.
- It is applied at the resonance frequency.
- The resonance frequency is in the RF range.

At the resonance frequency, the $B_1$ field only has to be applied for a very short duration (~1 ms) and consequently is referred to as the *excitation RF pulse*.

## SIGNAL CHARACTERISTICS

There are a few more aspects of the spin system to understand before the basics of MRI can be appreciated. The net magnetization vector, $M_0$, is composed of many individual spins and the body can be regarded as an environment with energy, collectively known as the *lattice*. Each spin is in a constant state of energy exchange with the lattice and with other spins. Owing to these interactions, the spin system undergoes a process known as *spin relaxation*. In terms of the spin system, relaxation is the process whereby the system returns to its lowest energy configuration. There are two relaxation time scales referred to as *T*1 and *T*2. To illustrate these, consider a magnetization vector, $M_0$, tipped over by 90 degrees (i.e., into the so-called transverse plane). The T1 relaxation process describes the process of realignment with the main magnetization vector, $\mathbf{B}_0$, and is referred to as *spin-lattice relaxation*. Similarly, the T2 relaxation describes the process of loss of coherence between individual spins, and is referred to as *spin–spin relaxation*. Both the T1 and T2 relaxation processes express the rate of energy exchange of individual spins, which are governed by random events and are quantized. Therefore, T1 and T2 decay curves are exponential (i.e., similar to radioactive decay). The T1 of myocardium is approximately 900 ms and its T2 is approximately 70 ms at field strength of 1.5 T. The T2 decay process is a characteristic of the material, and pure materials such as cerebrospinal fluid (CSF) tend to have long T2 values. These are essentially the values obtained under "laboratory conditions" and in practice the observed T2 decay is also dependent on the characteristics of the scanner system, such as the degree of nonuniformity of the magnetic field, which results in an apparent reduction in T2. In reality, the observed T2 is always lower than the material's actual T2, and this reduced value is termed $T2^*$ (pronounced "T2 star"). The MR signal that ultimately is generated is referred to as a *free induction decay* or (FID):

- *F*ree, because it is generated by natural precession rather than forced precession by application of an RF pulse.
- *I*nduction, because it is sensed by electromagnetic induction in a receiver coil.
- *D*ecay, because it decays due to T1 and T2 processes.

## MAGNETIC GRADIENTS

It is not sufficient to generate an FID and spatial information must be encoded into the FID signal. The key element to encoding this information is the application of magnetic gradients. Gradients are used in two key processes:

- Slice selection
- Image formation

A magnetic gradient can be applied along the body, which is graphically represented by a sloped line, but physically represents a 3-D variation of magnetic field across the body. The first element of slice selection is to apply a linear gradient perpendicular to the desired slice orientation (see Fig. 1-4). From the Larmor equation, this imposes a range of resonance frequencies along the body. The gradient effectively differentiates planes of tissue with respect to their resonance frequency. If only a single frequency were excited, then an infinitely thin slice would be selected. Therefore, the next step is to selectively excite a narrow range of frequencies to achieve slice selection.

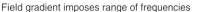

Field gradient imposes range of frequencies

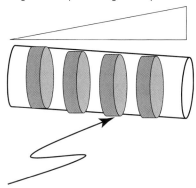

Apply RF at frequency to select this slice

**FIGURE 1-4**    The first element of slice selection is to apply a linear magnetic gradient along the length of the body in a direction perpendicular to the desired slice selection. The linear gradient sets up a linear range of resonance frequencies in the body. Each unique resonance frequency describes an infinitely thin slice within the body. Applying a radio frequency (RF) pulse at that unique resonance frequency excites the spins only in that infinitely thin plane.

To appreciate how a "narrow band" of frequencies can be excited, a mathematic detour must be taken to introduce Fourier theory. Fourier theory and Fourier transforms (FTs) are used ubiquitously in MRI. Fourier theory states that any line shape or waveform can be made by adding sine and cosine waves of various amplitudes and frequencies. The FT of the original waveform produces the amplitudes of the sine and cosine waves corresponding to each component frequency. Further, the original waveform is a function in one domain, and the Fourier coefficients (i.e., the amplitudes of the sine and cosine waves) form a function in the inverse domain. For example, a shape in the time domain has Fourier coefficients in the frequency domain. In this MRI example, the FT of a square function generates Fourier coefficients in the shape of a "sinc function" (a sinc function is a decaying sine wave). Therefore, to achieve slice selection we require the RF pulse, which is applied in the time domain, to be modified in shape by a sinc function, whereas gradients applied to the body cause the body's spins to resonate at a continuum of frequencies (i.e frequency domain) ranging from low frequencies in low gradients to high frequencies in high gradients. To excite a narrow range of frequencies with a square cross-section, the gradient is applied to impose a frequency range and the RF pulse is shaped like a sinc function (see Fig. 1-5). The slice orientation can be controlled by changing the gradient direction and the slice thickness can be selected by altering the width excited by the RF pulse, which can be accomplished by either adjusting the gradient strength or adjusting the RF sinc function characteristics.

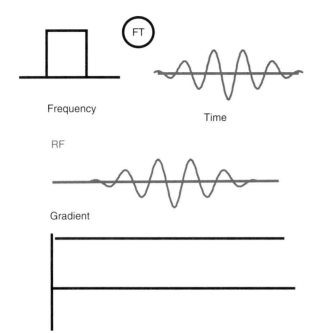

**FIGURE 1-5** The selection of a slice of finite thickness involves modifying the radio frequency (RF) pulse with a special shape. Fourier theory gives us the shape of this pulse. The desired slice profile is a square function, i.e., across the thickness of the slice, all spins are excited equally, and outside of the slice, the spins are not excited. This a represented by the ideal square slice profile. Fourier theory tells us that the fourier transform (FT) of this function is a decaying since function. Therefore, the RF pulse must be shaped in the form of this decaying sine wave. Slice selection is then achieved by applying the linear magnetic gradient along the body, at the same time that a modulated RF pulse is applied.

Imaging can be succinctly described as the encoding of spatial information. In a similar manner to slice selection, which was achieved by application of a gradient to differentiate regions of the body with respect to their resonance frequency, spatial encoding can also be accomplished. Application of a gradient to the selected slice will result in selection of columns of spins with the same frequency. The FID signal acquired in the presence of this gradient contains a range of frequency information. To extract the amplitudes of these frequencies, an FT is applied to the time domain signal to yield the frequency domain information. It can be appreciated that this frequency domain information directly relates to a projection of the object in a direction perpendicular to the applied gradient (see Fig. 1-6). By successively applying the gradient in a range of directions, a series of projections can be built up. One imaging technique that can be applied using these projections is that of projection reconstruction (PR). The PR method is used in computed tomography (CT) and single photon emission computed tomography (SPECT)

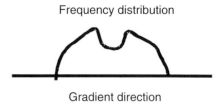

**FIGURE 1-6** The elements of spatial encoding within the selected slice are illustrated. By applying a linear gradient across the slice in the left to right direction, a series of perpendicular columns of spins are set up, each column is characterized by a unique resonance frequency. The signal that is sampled in the presence of this gradient contains these frequencies. To determine the frequency distribution, a Fourier transform of the signal is taken, which forms a projection of the spin signal along the vertical direction. An image may be formed by obtaining a series of such projections, each obtained in a different direction, achieved by applying the imaging gradient in a series of different orientations around the slice.

imaging and can also be used in MRI. By acquiring multiple projections around the object spanning 180 degrees, MR signals can be formulated to generate PR images. However, it is possible to go beyond PR and an alternative reconstruction method was developed to overcome the disadvantages of PR, which include the "star" artifact and uneven resolution (lower toward periphery).

## K-SPACE

Any image can be represented in Fourier space by performing a 2-D FT on the image. In MRI terminology, this Fourier space representation is referred to as *k-space*. Because the properties of k-space are central to understanding many aspects of MRI, its properties will be dealt with throughout further chapters. However, in this overview, it is sufficient to point out that there is a relationship between k-space and the MRI signal (see Fig. 1-7). The reasoning is as follows:

- The MRI gradients impose a frequency distribution across the body.
- The FT relates time domain signal to the frequency domain signal.
- The MRI signal is acquired in time.

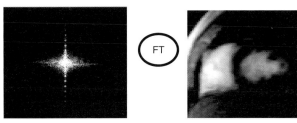

**FIGURE 1-7** The principles of k-space are illustrated. By formatting the series of magnetic resonance (MR) signals acquired in the presence of multiple, but successively applied, imaging gradients, the signal data can be formed in to k-space, as shown here on the left. By applying a fourier transform (FT) to this k-space data, an image of the object will be directly formed. One advantage of the k-space representation of data is that image generation is a one-step process. There are other advantages that make this an attractive process.

- The time signal sampled in MRI has the potential to be assembled in the order required by k-space.

When the signal is arranged in the special order required by k-space, it can be directly related to an image by performing the FT operation. In most imaging sequences it is convenient to represent k-space as a rectangular matrix. Most MR sequences fill this matrix one line at a time and k-space is commonly represented as a series of organized lines arranged in a rectangular grid. In this format, it is convenient to think of k-space requiring encoding in the X and Y directions, each applied separately. To encode separate X and Y data in k-space, the spatial encoding gradients must be applied at different points in time (i.e only X or only Y), not simultaneously. Consequently, a time delay is required between slice excitation and signal read out to encode the k-space information. Although this delay may be as short as 1 ms, it nevertheless requires special treatment in that it requires an "echo". For an example from nature, when we shout at a mountain, we get an echo, which is not the original signal but a delayed (and distorted) copy of the original. Here we introduce the gradient echo and spin echo procedures.

## GRADIENT ECHO

One type of echo is the gradient echo. Immediately upon excitation, all spins are in phase (corresponding to the original signal). Application of a magnetic gradient will dephase spins due to the spatial distribution of spins and the range of frequencies imposed by the gradient. By reversing the gradient at some point later in time, the spins will refocus and form a signal echo. The signal detected during a gradient echo consists of an increasing signal, up to an echo peak, followed by a decaying signal, as spins dephase in the opposite direction. The echo

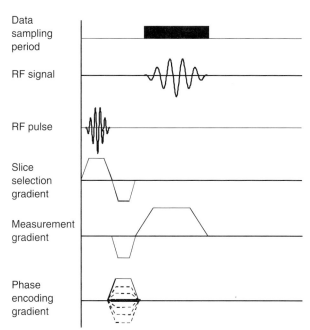

**FIGURE 1-8** The gradient echo imaging sequence is illustrated. The top two lines represent where signal is sampled, showing the form of the signal. The data-sampling period coincides with the gradient echo signal, which is digitally sampled and stored in the system's computer. The shaped radio frequency (RF) pulse is applied in the presence of the slice selection gradient. The measurement gradient is applied as a bipolar shape (e.g., negative lobe followed by a positive lobe), which forms the signal echo. The phase encoding gradient is applied as a series of progressively incrementing gradients (*dotted lines*), to encode data in the format required for k-space.

time (TE) is defined as the time from signal origination to the echo peak. In gradient-recalled echo (GRE) imaging, the multiple lines of k-space are encoded by repeated application of a stepped "phase encoding gradient" while each line of k-space is acquired by application of a "measurement" or "frequency encoding gradient" which forms the echo signal (see Fig. 1-8).

## SPIN ECHO

Another type of echo is termed the *spin echo*. Consider the net magnetization vector, $\mathbf{M_0}$, being tipped by a 90 degree RF pulse. Once excited, the continuum of spins will dephase due to a variety of causes including, T2 relaxation and inhomogeneities in the main magnetic field (the $\mathbf{B_0}$ field). After dephasing has occurred for several milliseconds, a second RF pulse of strength 180 degrees is applied. This pulse has the effect of flipping the spin system like a pancake. Because the spins are physically in the same spatial location, they will continue to evolve under the influence

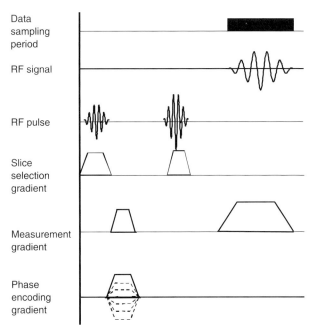

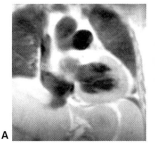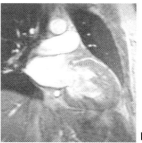

A                                                                    B

**FIGURE 1-10** Spin echo **(A)** and gradient echo **(B)** images are compared. The spin echo image shows blood pool signal as a region of low signal (black blood), whereas the gradient echo signal shows blood as a high signal (bright blood).

**FIGURE 1-9** The spin echo imaging sequence is illustrated. The top line represents the data-sampling period, which coincides with the echo signal (radio frequency [RF] signal, second line), which is digitally sampled and stored in the system's computer. The shaped RF pulse is applied in the presence of the slice selection gradient. In this sequence, two RF pulses are applied; the second one recalls the signal as an echo of the first RF pulse. The measurement gradient is applied as a pair of positive lobes, each applied on either side of the second RF pulse. The phase encoding gradient is applied as a series of progressively incrementing gradients (*dotted lines*), to encode data in the format required for k-space.

moving spins may only receive one or the other pulses (see Fig. 1-10). Both imaging sequences can be applied with additional contrast pulses, such as the inversion recovery (IR) pulse.

## HARDWARE

Although scanners come in different configurations there are several unifying elements. The main magnetic field ($B_0$) is typically generated by electromagnetic coils, wound on a cylindrical surface. The magnetic gradients and RF fields are also generated by electromagnetic coils wound on a cylindrical surface. Therefore, the main magnet, gradient coils, and RF coils are compactly housed in the same unit. The power units for these components are housed in a separate room, and the control unit is housed in an adjacent room, typically with a window, allowing visual contact with the patient in the scanner.

## SUMMARY

MR has a unique, versatile, and abundant signal source, which is the body itself. Controllable RF and gradients are required to achieve slice selection and encode image in formation. Substantial hardware and software control are required to manage the gradients, harness the signal, and convert it into an image.

of the local inhomogeneities, and, due to the pancake flip, will come back into focus (less T2 effects). The spin echo imaging sequence requires application of two RF pulses for the encoding of each k-space line. Consequently, TEs are typically longer than for GRE sequences, being in excess of 20 ms (see Fig. 1-9). In general terms, GRE and spin echo are primarily different in the way in which blood is imaged. In GRE imaging, flowing blood generates a bright signal (flow refreshment effect) whereas in spin echo imaging, flow is generally absent, because spins must receive both RF pulses to contribute to the image and thus

# CHAPTER 2

# Cardiovascular Magnetic Resonance Imaging Equipment

Mark Doyle

## OVERVIEW

Cardiovascular magnetic resonance (CMR) utilizes a great deal of hardware. The major equipment systems for a CMR facility are as follows:

- Magnet
- Gradients
- Radio frequency (RF)
- Scanner room
- Patient monitoring
- Scan controller
- Peripheral equipment

## MAGNETIC RESONANCE IMAGING SYSTEM

Currently, the CMR environment is organized around a suite of rooms, with one room devoted to the main system, one to power equipment, and one to scan control (see Fig. 2-1). Typically, other ancillary rooms that are common to any imaging facility are required and include patient reception, changing rooms, preparation, and interview areas. The heart of the magnetic resonance imaging (MRI) system is the main magnet. Commonly this is of a superconducting design, with the gradients and RF coils housed within it, with the whole assembly located in the scanner room. Accompanying the MRI unit are the power and control systems required to generate the imaging waveforms and to drive current through the gradient and RF systems. These are located in a power room, which has special cooling requirements to deal with the heat dissipation that is required. The third main area is devoted to scanner control and monitoring, and is usually referred to as the *control room*. Typically, the control room is arranged to provide a direct line of sight between the scanner operator and the patient in the scanner.

## MAGNET

The most efficient magnet design is of the electromagnetic type, with the electrical windings wound on a cylindrical former. The coil windings are cooled to liquid helium temperature ($4^\circ$K) allowing them to become superconducting, that is, current will continue to flow even after the power source is removed. To keep the magnet at $4^\circ$K requires isolating the system thermally. This is accomplished by surrounding the windings in a vacuum chamber and filling the cavity with liquid helium. Under normal operating conditions, helium will boil off and escape from the system. In order to conserve helium, a helium reliquefying system is typically integrated into the system; limiting "top-up" fills to greater than 1-year intervals. The chirping sound often heard in the scanner room is associated with the reliquification pump. In regions of the world where liquid helium cannot be easily obtained, it is possible to use nonsuperconducting

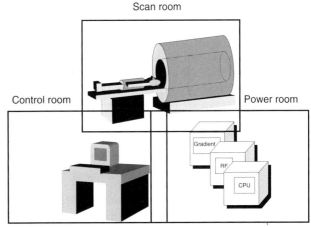

**FIGURE 2-1** The three main rooms associated with the magnetic resonance imaging (MRI) system are the scan room, the control room, and the power room. They are arranged in a contiguous manner for optimum utility.

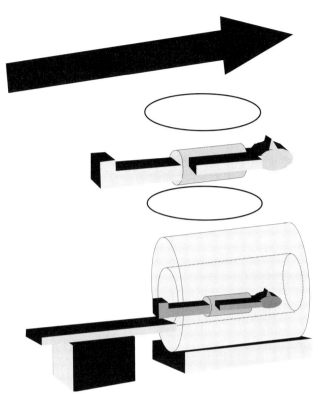

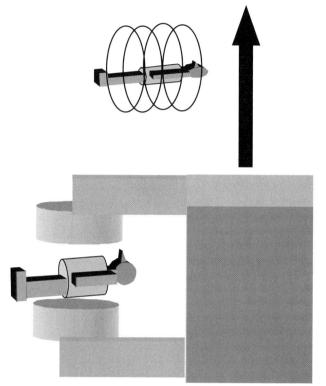

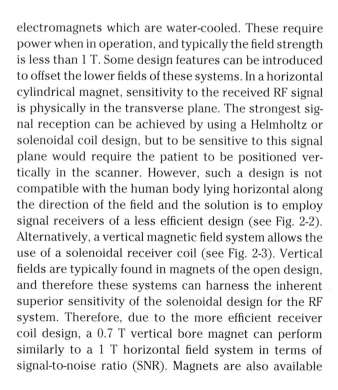

**FIGURE 2-2** A cylindrical design of magnet with the patient lying horizontally is shown. The main direction of the field is indicated by the arrow and the radio frequency (RF) receiver coils that are arranged in the horizontal plane are sensitive to magnetization in the vertical (i.e., transverse) plane. Although this design is common, signal reception is suboptimal.

**FIGURE 2-3** A vertical bore magnet system with the patient lying horizontally is shown. In this configuration a solenoidal receiver coil can be used, with sensitivity to radio frequency (RF) in the horizontal plane. This orientation of receiver coil is optimal, which, to some extent, may compensate for the lower field strength typical of this design.

electromagnets which are water-cooled. These require power when in operation, and typically the field strength is less than 1 T. Some design features can be introduced to offset the lower fields of these systems. In a horizontal cylindrical magnet, sensitivity to the received RF signal is physically in the transverse plane. The strongest signal reception can be achieved by using a Helmholtz or solenoidal coil design, but to be sensitive to this signal plane would require the patient to be positioned vertically in the scanner. However, such a design is not compatible with the human body lying horizontal along the direction of the field and the solution is to employ signal receivers of a less efficient design (see Fig. 2-2). Alternatively, a vertical magnetic field system allows the use of a solenoidal receiver coil (see Fig. 2-3). Vertical fields are typically found in magnets of the open design, and therefore these systems can harness the inherent superior sensitivity of the solenoidal design for the RF system. Therefore, due to the more efficient receiver coil design, a 0.7 T vertical bore magnet can perform similarly to a 1 T horizontal field system in terms of signal-to-noise ratio (SNR). Magnets are also available

of a permanent design, which do not required power to generate a field, but typically their strength is limited to a maximum of 0.3 T.

## GRADIENT SYSTEM

Three strong electromagnetic gradients built into the scanner system constitute the primary gradients. They are activated when current is passed through them and are driven by powerful amplifiers. Typically, the gradients are designed to allow the maximum access for the patient, and in the case of the horizontal bore cylindrical system, the gradients are wound on a cylindrical former, which is located in the magnet bore. To appreciate the gradient design, it is important to note some salient properties of each gradient:

- The magnetic field from each gradient varies in only one spatial direction.
- The field from each gradient is applied to the body over a volume.

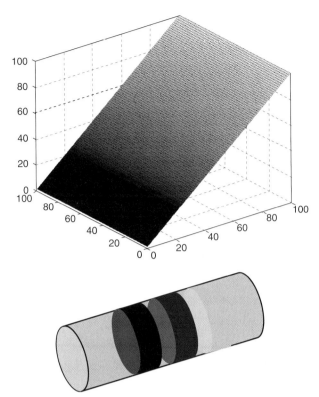

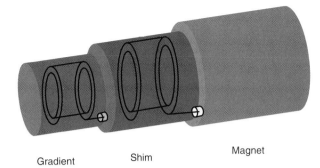

**FIGURE 2-5**  A telescoped view of three magnetic systems: main magnet, shim magnet (to correct for field inhomogeneities), and the primary gradients (X, Y, and Z). In the assembled system, the gradient and shim coils would be slid into the magnet in a symmetric manner.

**FIGURE 2-4**  The three dimensionality of the gradient field is indicated. The gradient establishes parallel planes of spins that experience a uniform magnetic field strength. Three such planes are indicated.

• The direction of the field is always aligned with the main field direction.

The result of applying a gradient in this manner is that parallel planes within the body are established, each plane being at a uniform, but unique magnetic field strength (see Fig. 2-4). The field strength imposed on the body by a gradient is key to the imaging process. It is necessary to encode information in three orthogonal directions, which requires application of up to three imaging gradients. It should be noted that when two gradients are simultaneously applied, only a single gradient is realized, formed by the vector sum of the two component gradients. Therefore, two gradients applied simultaneously produce only a single gradient at an angle to the original two. In this case, the combined gradients simply change the orientation of the parallel planes of uniform magnetic field within the body. The primary gradients are very powerful, and generally require cooling by circulating chilled water thought the system. A water chiller located in the power room is required. Adequate removal of heat from the gradients allows them to perform at a high duty cycle. The power supplies for each of the electromagnetic gradients are housed in the power room. Usually the cables and coolant are passed through a "penetration panel" into the scanner system. The penetration panel filters out RF noise and signal that would otherwise contaminate images.

## SHIM GRADIENT COILS

Static imperfections in the magnetic field (i.e., inhomogeneities) can be removed by applying shim gradients. These are a combination of linear and nonlinear gradients that are located outside of the primary gradients (see Fig. 2-5). They are powered using low-level static current supplies. Some scans are highly sensitive to $B_0$ homogeneities, as follows:

• Those requiring spectral suppression of the fat or water signals
• Those that require steady-state conditions
• Those employing long echo times

These scans may require improved homogeneity for the local body region being imaged, that is, they require dynamic shimming. The body introduces inhomogeneities in $B_0$, and the scanner can typically perform a limited amount of dynamic shimming automatically to overcome this. Manual override is permitted in the shimming process, but may be time consuming to apply.

## RADIO FREQUENCY COILS

Two primary RF coils used in the CMR system are as follows:

• Transmit
• Receive

The body RF coil is built into the scanner unit and is used to transmit RF in a relatively uniform manner to the patient. However, in most cases the body coil is

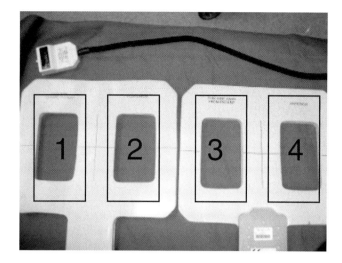

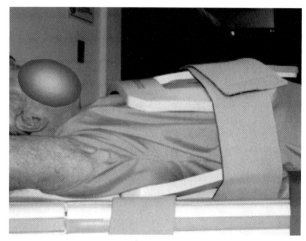

**FIGURE 2-6** The two halves of a phased array receiver coil are shown, with four individual coil elements indicated. The patient is positioned on top of the lower coil, and the upper coil is placed on the patient's chest. The whole assembly is held together with a wide velcro strap for stability.

generally considered too poor to receive an adequate signal. To improve signal reception, phased array coils are used. These exploit the observation that signal reception is improved if the receiver coil is placed in close proximity to the body region being imaged. In this case a number of coil elements, each positioned over a specific body region, can be combined to improve the overall SNR and simultaneously achieve extended coverage of the body (see Fig. 2-6). However, this is accomplished at the loss of signal uniformity. Phased array coils are typically configured with 4, 8, 16, or 32 elements. Each coil element primarily receives a signal from a very localized region of the body and requires its own receiver channel in the scanner electronics. The advantage of using an array of small receiver coils is the high SNR realized for each region. However, this

has to be balanced by the depth sensitivity of each coil element. As a general rule, the maximum usable penetration depth of each coil is approximately equal to the coil's radius.

## RADIO FREQUENCY-FREE ROOM

The scanner has to be screened from all sources of electromagnetic radiation that would interfere with signal detection. Because the signal is in the RF range, these sources of signal are plentiful, and to prevent this form of interference, the scanner is housed in a Faraday cage. A Faraday cage is constructed by forming a double layer wall of conducting material such as copper (see Fig. 2-7). Even the windows and doors form a part of the screen, and a copper mesh permeates any windows in the room. The door and doorframe are specially designed to form a continuous electrical conducting surface, and the whole system is securely grounded at a single point. Normally, the copper screening material is hidden from view, giving the appearance of a perfectly ordinary, perfectly normal room. Because the scanner is housed in an electromagnetic-free room, all signals and current entering or leaving have to pass through a panel where they are filtered to avoid introducing frequencies that would affect the MRI signal. To accomplish this a penetration panel is used, which incorporates filters designed for each line that enters or exits the scanner room. Further, to allow some limited access for IV lines that cannot be filtered in this way, a wave-guide is provided. This is a metal tube approximately 2 ft in length, which rapidly attenuates any RF signal entering it.

## PATIENT MONITORING

Patient monitoring is a crucial safety issue, and includes the following:

- Voice contact—microphone
- Visual contact—line of sight and/or video
- Echocardiography (ECG)
- Pulse oximetry
- Blood pressure (BP)
- MR images used directly

Given that it is important to create an environment in which the patient feels comfortable, music of the patient's choice is often fed in to the scanner. However, this should not interfere with the ability to communicate with the patient. Therefore, a unit that allows the scan operator to interrupt the music is essential to permit clear two-way communication. This is typically accomplished using a switch-activated microphone, which, when activated, interrupts the music signal.

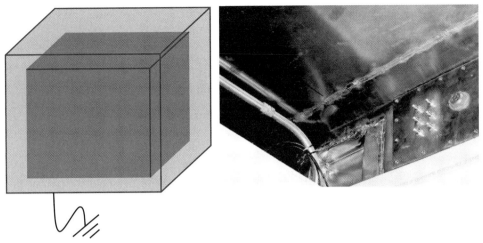

**FIGURE 2-7**    The scan room is isolated from radiofrequency interference by constructing a Faraday cage. In this design, a double-walled structure is constructed of conducting material (such as copper sheeting). The structure is grounded at a single point to avoid ground loops. Electromagnetic radiation is attenuated in the skin of the cage material and does not enter the scan environment. In the second panel a section of the scan room ceiling is exposed to show the copper sheeting underneath. Notice the seam soldering that has been performed to join sheets along their edges.

The ECG signal is used to monitor the patient and register the scans to the patient's heart rhythm. Most commonly, ECG electrode pads are attached to the patient's chest and the ECG leads built into the scanner are used (see Fig. 2-8). The ECG signal cannot be used to monitor the ECG T wave due to electrical interference caused by the magnet. The T wave occurs at a time of rapid blood movement out of the heart. Because blood is a conducting fluid, this generates an electrical signal due to interaction with the main magnetic field, which is the origin of the T wave distortion. However, vector ECG approaches, which process the ECG signal may overcome this limitation to some extent.

Respiratory monitoring can be achieved by attaching a bellows-type belt around the patient's waist. As the bellows expands and contracts with the patient's breathing, a signal is fed into the scanner system. This

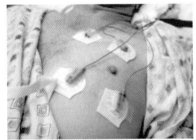
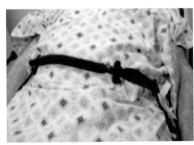
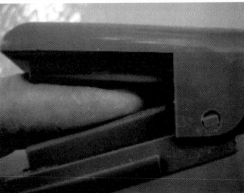
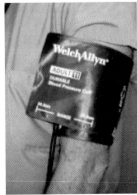

**FIGURE 2-8**    Four commonly used patient monitoring devices are shown, top left and clockwise: echocardiography (ECG) pads, respiratory monitoring belt and bellows, inflatable blood pressure cuff, and pulse oximetry finger probe. The signal from these devices is typically converted to an optical signal for transmission to remote telemetry devices, thereby avoiding radio frequency (RF) transmissions within the scan room.

signal allows compliance with breathing instructions to be observed. Also, the respiratory signal can be used directly by the scanner to perform respiratory gating. The respiratory signal can be analyzed by the scanner's computer to estimate the position within the respiratory cycle, and used directly to control when data are taken, thereby eliminating the need for breath-holding. Typically, respiratory-gated scans take approximately 50% longer than breath-hold scans but scan quality is generally higher with breath-hold scans. However, some 3D sequences are only feasible with respiratory gating. The respiratory and cardiac monitoring signals will typically be displayed near the operator console. The appearance of these signals can generally be controlled from the console.

A video camera in the scan room allows the patient to be seen even if line of sight vision is obstructed. The camera works in the high field due to its charged coupled device (CCD) design.

BP is monitored using a standard arm cuff, and can typically be inflated when manually triggered or at predetermined time intervals. The BP is monitored on a console separate from the operator's console.

Pulse oximetry can be measured using a device that fits over the finger. By monitoring changes in light intensity that pass through the skin, blood oxygenation levels can be monitored on a beat-to-beat basis.

## SCAN CONTROL

The control console allows a number of tasks essential to successful imaging to be accomplished, including the following:

- Planning of scans
- Reviewing of data
- Measurement and quantification of image features
- Archiving
- Filming

During scanning, several processes are being performed, including the following:

- Issuing patient instruction and receiving feedback
- Planning future scans
- Acquiring images with specialized views and contrast
- Interactive identification of patient features

The ease with which these tasks are performed, in large part, determines how the scan will proceed. There are multiple variables that control scan duration and quality. These have to be balanced to keep scan times within reasonable limits as well as acquire the required information. Typically, a scan session lasts 45 minuets. Scan efficiency is dependent on the availability and ease

of use of scanner options and features, including the following:

- Real-time mode
- Parallel imaging utility
- Respiratory monitoring

Currently, the typical CMR scan is approximately 50% efficient, in that time spent on activities such as planning future scans and allowing the patient to recover from each breath-hold takes up approximately 50% of the total scan session (see Fig. 2-9). Real-time scan options allow the scanner to run continuously, using sequences such as the following:

- Spirals
- Echo planar imaging (EPI)
- Multiple echo train approaches

These sequences tend to be very loud and can be unnerving for patient and even for the scanner operator. These conditions compromise the ability to communicate with the patient. It is useful to consider things from the patient's perspective, in that it may be their first time in the scanner, and all the attendant commotion and noise may be unsettling for them. Further, real-time scan quality is generally too low to be of widespread diagnostic value, with the notable exception of real-time perfusion imaging. Apart from this use, real-time imaging is primarily used to plan views, which will be acquired at higher resolution in a non–real-time mode. However, as scan quality and the interface improve, real-time imaging is likely to increase in utility.

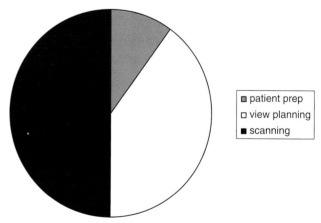

- patient prep
- view planning
- scanning

**FIGURE 2-9** An indication of usage of "patient time" in the scanner. For a typical scan session lasting 45 minutes, perhaps only 50% will be used in acquiring magnetic resonance (MR) data; the other 50% will be split between activities such as planning of views and patient preparation and instruction. Obviously, scanner efficiency may improve as technology advances.

Before scanning, the scanner performs operations to optimize scan performance. These series of operations are collectively termed *prescanning*, and accomplish the following:

- Determination of the correct RF power level
- Adjustment of the receiver signal gain
- Determination of the correct resonance frequency

Prescanning is performed automatically. However, there is an ability to manually override the prescan determined settings. Sometimes this is necessary if the patient has metallic implants that disrupt the prescan signals.

## PERIPHERAL EQUIPMENT

All equipment that is to be used in the scanner room must be established to be MR compatible. Typically, safety stickers identify these items, and it is imperative that all personnel adhere to safety regulations at all times.

The patient bed may be detachable to allow for patient preparation and treatment outside of the scanner room. The sliding table can usually be manually moved or motor driven when engaged with the scanner. Some sites find it useful to have two beds.

Contrast agent is rapidly administered as a bolus using a power injector. A dual syringe system is used to deliver two agents, such as the following:

- Contrast agent
- Saline flush

Each syringe is controlled remotely using a computer unit located in the control room. The system has several flexible programmable modes and safety limitations and pressure sensors allow for safe operation. An infusion pump that is programmable can be useful to deliver medication or a stress agent.

Wheelchair access to the scanner room is convenient, but not indispensable. For additional safety, remove the chair before placing the patient in the scanner. It is possible that a nonmagnetic chair, or attachment has made its way into the scan room, and if let loose, would accelerate toward the scanner bore. By removing the chair before the patient enters the bore, an accident may be circumvented.

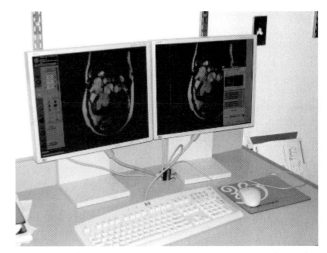

**FIGURE 2-10** A computer workstation separate from the main scanning console allows advanced processing of images to be performed without disrupting the scanning operation.

CMR involves performing multiple measurements on the image data, and these are generally performed on a workstation that is separate from the scan console (see Fig. 2-10). Processing performed on remote workstations includes the following:

- Volumetric measurements such as ejection fraction (EF), end-diastolic volume (EDV), end-systolic volume (ESV)
- Angiographic rendering
- Flow quantification
- Tag analysis

## SUMMARY

Although MR technology continues to evolve, there are fixed components such as the following:

- Magnet
- Gradients
- RF
- Computer control

For optimum efficiency and safety, these should be arranged to form an integrated whole.

# CHAPTER 3

# Imaging Methods

Mark Doyle

## OVERVIEW

To examine the inner workings of imaging, the following topics are covered here:

- Slice selection
- Encoding of spatial information
- Gradient echo
- Spin echo
- Stimulated echo
- Steady state free precession (SSFP)

These will be dealt with here in sufficient detail to form a basic foundation, in preparation for more in-depth coverage later in specialized chapters.

## SLICE SELECTION

### Slice Selection Basics

Slice selection is achieved by applying a linear magnetic field gradient to the body, which sets up a continuous and linear distribution of resonance frequencies across the body, in a direction that is perpendicular to the gradient. In conjunction with this gradient, a radio frequency (RF) pulse is applied at the central resonance frequency, which is designed to excite a range of frequencies corresponding to the slice width. The width of the excited band of frequencies is measured in Hertz (Hz), and is referred to as the *bandwidth* (BW). The Fourier relationship relates actions in the time domain to those in the frequency domain. Therefore, to excite a square BW of frequencies (i.e., frequency domain operation) we need to know how the RF pulse should be modulated, and this can be achieved by using the Fourier transform (FT). The FT of a square pulse is a shape termed a *sinc function* (similar to a decaying sine wave). Therefore, the time domain modulation shape of the RF pulse is exactly that of a sinc function. The BW of

the RF pulse is inversely proportional to the duration of the pulse:

- Short pulse—wide BW
- Long pulse—narrow BW

In magnetic resonance imaging (MRI), time is generally the most valuable commodity, and consequently, short RF pulses are preferred. Short pulses lead directly to short echo times (TEs), which yield better sensitivity to flow and provide further immunity from artifacts. Therefore, by the inverse relationship that exists between RF pulse duration and BW, short pulses necessarily excite a wide BW of frequencies. Consequently, because a short RF pulse excites a wide BW, a strong gradient is required to produce a thin slice. Therefore, there is a relationship established between four variables:

- Time of application of RF pulse
- Frequency BW excited
- Gradient strength required
- Physical slice thickness achieved

The nature of these relationships is illustrated in Fig. 3-1.

### Spin Dephasing and Slice Selection

Since the slice selective RF pulse is applied at the same time as the linear gradient, spins with a component in the transverse plane will become dephased. Therefore, spins throughout the thickness of the slice are effectively rotated relative to each other, covering a range of different phases. This range of phases (termed *spin phase dispersion*) results in reducing the signal strength. This particular form of phase dispersion is very organized, with the phase spread being incremental between adjacent spins, forming a linear progression of phase values across the slice thickness. Fortunately, a uniform phase distribution (i.e., a phase gradient) can

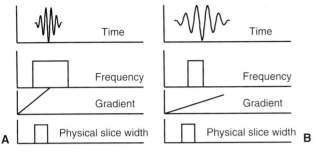

**FIGURE 3-1**    Relationships between time domain, frequency domain, gradients, and slice width are illustrated. In **(A)**, the time domain shows a short radio frequency (RF) pulse, applied to excite a wide frequency range, which in conjunction with a strong gradient produces a slice with the desired physical width. In contrast, in **(B)**, a long RF pulse is applied to excite a narrow frequency range, which in the presence of a weak gradient will excite the same physical slice width as in **(A)**.

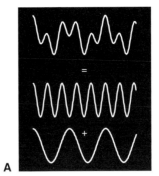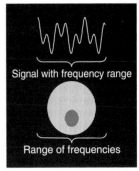

**FIGURE 3-2**    The principal of encoding frequency information is illustrated. In **(A)** a complex signal waveform is seen, and below it are shown the two primary (pure) frequencies that make up the signal. In this case, the addition of two distinct primary frequencies makes up a relatively complex signal waveform. In **(B)**, a physical object is represented with a gradient applied across it. The gradient imposes a range of (pure) frequencies across the object. The top panel shows the composite signal, which is composed of many distinct frequencies that are emitted by the selected slice of the object.

be undone by application of a uniform gradient with an opposite polarity compared to the slice selection gradient. This reversed gradient, applied following slice selection, will therefore "refocus" or "rewind" the phase dispersion. The refocusing gradient is applied at a level and duration such that it equals half the area of the primary slice selection gradient.

Each aspect of slice selection can be controlled by adjusting the slice selection gradient, including orientation, which is realized by changing the gradient direction, and slice thickness, which is adjusted by selecting the BW of the RF pulse in conjunction with appropriate selection of the gradient strength.

## SPATIAL ENCODING

A magnetic gradient applied to the body differentiates regions within the slice with respect to their resonance frequency. At one end of the body, the gradient subtracts from the main magnetic field, and at the other end of the body the gradient adds to the main magnetic field. Therefore, the spins ranging from one end of the body to the other resonate at a number of frequencies. These spins generate a signal that contains a continuum of frequencies when the gradient is applied. Although the net signal may look complex, it is simply composed of a sum of sine and cosine waves, each at a discrete and separate frequency (see Fig. 3-2). The FT is a mathematical operation that allows the complex waveform to be analyzed into its component frequencies. The output of the FT routine is the amplitude of each component frequency. By Fourier transforming the signal acquired when a gradient is applied, this allows the amplitude of the individual frequencies to be determined. It can be appreciated

that the amplitude of each frequency component when arranged in ascending order corresponds to a projection through the body in a direction perpendicular to the applied gradient.

If the sample were one-dimensional, then a single FT would be sufficient to image it, i.e. to find the amplitude corresponding to each point along the sample. However, most imaging situations are at least 2D, and sometimes 3D. To image a 2D sample, a 2D treatment of the signal must be applied. To see how this is achieved, consider a gradient applied for a period of time as being deconstructed into a series of gradients, each applied for a short time duration, e.g. a single gradient applied for 7 ms is equivalent to seven gradients of equal magnitude applied for 1 ms duration, each applied in a contiguous manner. Therefore, conceptually, it is possible to "split up" the sampling of signal in the presence of a gradient into a series of separately applied gradients, each applied for a short duration. Such an approach is used to encode a 2D image (see Fig. 3-3).

In the 2D signal encoding situation, one dimension is acquired during the application of a single, long duration, gradient (i.e., achieving one dimension of spatial encoding); whereas the second dimension is acquired by application of a series of short duration gradients, each gradient applied orthogonal to the initial spatial encoding gradient, Fig. 3-3. The resulting 2D signal distribution is termed *k-space*, or *phase space*. K-space has many properties of interest to MRI and these will be dealt with in greater detail in subsequent chapters. The main point to be made here is that,

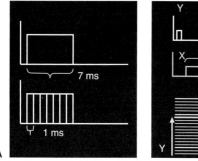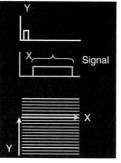

**FIGURE 3-3** The anatomy of a gradient is illustrated. In **(A)**, the top figure represents a gradient applied for duration 7 ms with a uniform amplitude. In the lower panel, the same gradient is represented as seven separate gradients, each applied for duration 1 ms, and arranged in a contiguous manner. This illustrates that a continuously applied gradient can be split into several subgradients. In **(B)**, two gradients are applied to encode one line of k-space. In this case, a short (phase encoding) gradient is applied before the longer (read-out) gradient. The longer gradient is responsible for reading out the signal associated with one line of k-space, and is applied in the same manner for each line. The shorter gradient is applied in an incremental manner such that it results in reading out successive lines. In effect, multiple applications of a series of short gradients are equivalent to a single long gradient, with each gradient applied in an orthogonal direction.

conventionally, each line of k-space requires application of two gradients:

- A short duration gradient, applied to prepare the signal, termed the *phase encoding gradient.*
- A longer duration gradient, applied as the signal is digitally sampled, termed the *measurement, or read gradient.*

## SIGNAL ECHO

To encode data in k-space, the free induction decay (FID) signal must be prepared (i.e., by application of the short duration gradient) before sampling a line of k-space (i.e., using the longer read out gradient). This requires delaying the signal acquisition from the start of the FID, which is generally timed from the middle of the slice selection process. Delaying the signal in MR (magnetic resonance) is achieved by recalling the signal at a later time as an "echo." By means of an echo, the required signal delay can be achieved and imaging (i.e., spatial encoding of data) can be accomplished. There are three types of echo, as follows:

- Gradient echo
- Spin echo
- Stimulated echo

Each echo has a distinct set of properties that dramatically affect the contrast achieved in MRI.

## GRADIENT ECHO

Application of a gradient to the spin system will dephase spins due to the spatial distribution of frequencies imposed by the gradient, that is, because all the spins are precessing at different rates they rapidly lose phase coherence and the signal is observed to decay. At some point later in time, when the spins have reached a certain degree of spin dephasing, the polarity of the gradient is reversed and applied at a constant level (see Fig. 3-4). Under the influence of this reversed gradient, spins at each location experience a reversal of their relative frequencies and they come back into focus. As spins come into phase alignment the signal increases in amplitude; this is the so-called echo signal. When the reverse polarity gradient has been applied for a period of time equal to the initial dephasing gradient the spins are at their highest level of refocusing, corresponding to the echo peak. As the reverse polarity gradient is left on for a further time period, the spins go past their focus condition, and continue to dephase, but in the opposite direction to their initial dephasing pattern. Therefore, application of the reverse gradient results in signal growth (to the echo peak) followed by signal decay. This symmetric rise, peak, and decay of signal constitute the echo signal.

By convention, the "leading" and "trailing" spins are represented diagrammatically with the understanding that, in between these two extremes, there exists a continuum of spin phases, Fig. 3-4. In Fig. 3-4, at the start of the gradient echo process, the leading and trailing spins are represented as precessing clockwise and counterclockwise, respectively, representing the relative precession due to the applied gradient. At the end of the initial gradient application period, the relative phases of the leading and trailing spins are shown in Fig. 3-4, indicating the condition of spin dephasing; complete dephasing is not shown, although in reality, the spins typically undergo many complete revolutions relative to each other. Note that the relative direction of spin precession at the end of the initial gradient period is the same as at the start of the initial gradient period, that is, the leading and trailing spins are represented as precessing clockwise and counterclockwise, respectively. Immediately upon reversal of the gradient polarity, the relative position of the leading and trailing spins remain unchanged, but it is the direction of precession that changes. Owing to this change of direction, the spins gradually come closer together in phase until at the echo peak they reach the point where they are the closest to fully rephrased.

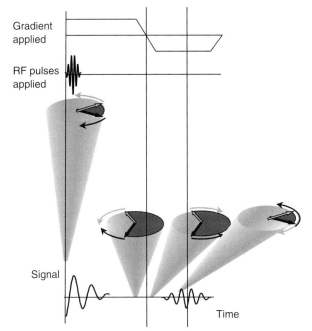

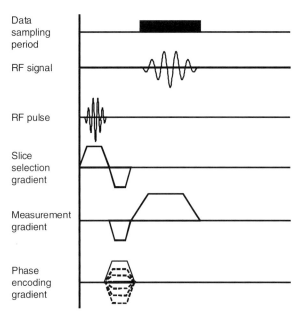

**FIGURE 3-4** The state of the spin system at key points in the gradient echo procedure is illustrated. At the start of the sequence all spins start off in phase, and in the presence of a gradient, spins precess with a range of frequencies. Relative to the central frequency, some spins appear to precess counter-clockwise, whereas some spins precess clockwise. As the gradient continues to be applied the spins continue to dephase and the signal decreases. At the point where the gradient is reversed, the spins are physically in the same positions as they were immediately before the gradient reversal (i.e., a high degree of dephasing). However, at this point the relative direction of precession is reversed for the representative spins shown. Consequently, as the gradient continues to be applied the phase of the spins gradually comes back into focus (forming the echo peak). Following the echo peak the gradient is still applied and the spins continue to dephase, resulting in echo decay.

**FIGURE 3-5** The gradient echo pulse sequence is illustrated. For each axis, the horizontal direction represents time, and each separate axis represents an activity that takes place during the gradient recalled echo (GRE) sequence. The top two lines represent when the radio frequency (RF) signal is sampled and how the signal appears. The slice selection RF pulse (transmitted to the body) is shown in combination with the slice selection gradient. The primary read-out or measurement gradient is responsible for forming the gradient echo signal. The phase encoding gradient is represented as a series of dashed lines, indicating that the gradient is applied at varying amplitudes, each applied during a separate application of the basic sequence, with each phase encoding step corresponding to one line of k-space.

We note that they will never fully rephase, due to the random effects of T2 relaxation. If the second, reverse polarity gradient is continued past the echo peak, the spins continue to dephase relative to each other, and the signal decays accordingly.

A gradient-recalled echo (GRE) "pulse sequence" is shown in Fig. 3-5. The pulse sequence is a diagrammatic representation of the gradients and RF, with strength, polarity and timing shown, that are required to acquire a line (or lines) of k-space. Each line of the pulse sequence represents an individual component: the RF pulse is applied by the scanner, while the echo signal is emitted by the body; the gradients: slice, measurement, and phase are shown; and the digital sampling window, when data are acquired for assembly into k-space, is indicated. Generally, the slice, measurement, and phase encoding gradients are orthogonal to each other. The combination of RF and slice selection gradient achieves the slice selection procedure; the measurement gradient generates the GRE; and the phase encoding gradient, represented as being applied multiple times, is used to encode each line of k-space. Therefore, the basic GRE sequence must be applied repeatedly to obtain each line of k-space. Data are acquired when the echo is forming, up to the echo peak, and through the echo decay. Note that gradients can overlap as long as no RF or data sampling is taking place. This allows some degree of compacting of the sequence. Also, note that multiple gradient switches are required for each application of the basic sequence, and that gradients are represented as not switching instantaneously, but have a trapezoidal transition. The trapezoidal shape is an important practical feature, and it can be appreciated that steeper slopes (i.e., faster gradient switching) can dramatically influence the duration of the GRE sequence. This is largely influenced by the

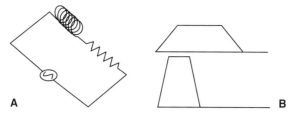

**FIGURE 3-6** Gradients and Inductance. Electrically, the imaging gradients are primarily represented as large inductors with a small resistance and powered by a voltage source. The large inductor resists the current from changing, which occurs either during establishing the gradient or switching the gradient off. In **(B)** two gradients are represented, the top one has a low amplitude, but is applied for a long duration; whereas in the lower panel, the gradient is applied for a short duration but at a higher amplitude. The area enclosed by each gradient is equivalent, and it is a key feature for imaging. It is apparent that the steeper gradient requires a higher voltage source to achieve imaging in a faster time.

properties of the gradient coil and current driving amplifiers.

## Gradient Coil Properties

The magnetic gradients are generated by electromagnetic coils (specially designed to provide the required linear gradients), and the polarity and strength of the gradient is determined by the direction and amount of current driven through each coil (see Fig. 3-6). One of the key properties that determines how easy (or hard) it is for the current to be driven through the coil is the coil's inductance. Inductance is similar to resistance, and is measured in Henries, with the symbol "L". However, unlike resistance, inductance only opposes establishing a current during a period of active change: the voltage (V) across a coil when a current (I) is being established is given by

$$V = dI/dt \times L$$

Therefore, for a given fixed voltage, the rate of change of current is determined by the inductance; that is, inductors impede the establishment of a current, but once established, inductors do not offer any resistance to current. Therefore, the most critical phase for a gradient is when it is changed: for example, turned on, off, or switched. To accomplish rapid gradient switching, powerful gradient amplifiers are required. The combination of gradient strength and the speed with which the gradient is established is described by the property of "slew rate". In general, rapidly switching the gradient translates to a shorter GRE sequence. Further, strong gradients can accomplish the required area

under the curve (i.e., gradient amplitude intergraded over time) and this turns out to be an important determinant in imaging speed and image quality (see Fig. 3-6). However, there is a physiologic constraint to the upper limit of slew rate; when this is reached a neuromuscular stimulation is activated, causing the patient to visibly twitch. While regulations governing these limits vary, the generally accepted threshold is 200 mT/m/second. Over the years, as MR systems have been developing, the slew rate has increased from approximately 1 to 150 mT/m/s.

## Echo Planar Imaging

Echo planar imaging (EPI) is a gradient echo technique that employs a train of echoes, with each separate echo encoding a complete line of k-space (see Fig. 3-7). EPI can produce an image in approximately 50 ms. To be effective, the train of echoes has to be compact, and therefore EPI requires high performance gradients due to the many gradient switches that are required. Owing to the long read out time associated with EPI, short T2 components tend to be blurred, due to progressive signal loss as the sequence progresses. A single-shot EPI image is generally of low resolution, with matrices of $64^2$ to $128^2$ being common, and the major application of

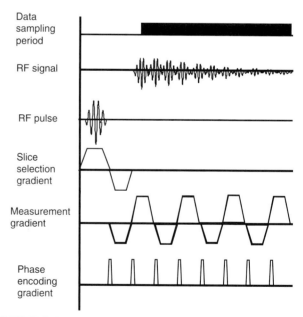

**FIGURE 3-7** Illustrated is the echo planar imaging sequence with the data sampling period, the train of gradient echo signals emitted from the body; the transmitted radio frequency (RF) pulse and slice selection gradient; the primary gradient echo, in which a series of echoes are recalled, and the train of phase encoding gradients.

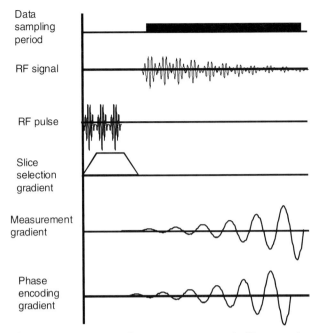

Data sampling period

RF signal

RF pulse

Slice selection gradient

Measurement gradient

Phase encoding gradient

**FIGURE 3-8**    The spiral imaging sequence is illustrated showing the data sampling period, received signal, the applied radio frequency (RF) pulse and gradient for slice selection. In this case the RF excitation pulse achieves slice selection in conjunction with the slice selection gradient, and simultaneously achieves selection of just the water signal by incorporating a spectrally selective pulse; the measurement and phase encoding gradients are represented as sinusoidal and cosinusoidal gradient trains, respectively, in which a series of echoes are recalled.

EPI to date is in functional brain imaging. However, EPI has some application to myocardial perfusion imaging.

## Spiral Scanning

Spiral scanning (and its variants) accomplish rapid imaging in a manner similar to EPI (i.e., the signal is recalled as a series of echoes), as shown in Fig. 3-8. However, in the case of spiral scanning, k-space is not mapped out in a rectilinear manner, but instead it is covered by a spiral trajectory. To accomplish this, gradually increasing sinusoidal and cosinusoidal gradients are used. In principle a spiral scan could be obtained in a single shot, but more commonly, multiple interleaved shots are used. In the interleaved version, each spiral arm is approximately 20 ms long, which is shorter than the 50 to 100 ms required for a single-shot scan, but is nevertheless still quite long when considering short T2 components, and may still result in blurring of some features. The spiral data requires regridding to accommodate the regular k-space matrix.

## Multishot Echo Planar Imaging or Multiple Echo Gradient Echo?

Although GRE requires multiple applications of the basic sequence to build up the required multiple lines of k-space it allows short TEs. Conversely, EPI images are rapidly acquired but its TE is generally too long for most cardiac applications. Consequently, a hybrid of the two has evolved, which acquires several lines of k-space for each application of the basic pulse sequence. Whether this is regarded as a multiecho GRE or as a multipass EPI sequence is open to debate. However, this hybrid scan may have some application to functional and perfusion imaging.

## SPIN ECHO

Thus far, all of the imaging sequences considered have been based on the gradient echo approach. Moving on from this, we note that there is a widely applied class of imaging sequences based on the spin echo approach. In a spin echo, the spin system is initially excited and spins proceed to dephase due to T2, $B_0$ inhomogeneities, and directly applied imaging gradients. As the spins dephase, the observed signal decays to zero. Following this occurrence, a second RF pulse is applied, which achieves spin refocusing in the form of a spin echo. The optimal strength of the second RF pulse is 180 degrees, which effectively flips the spin system like a pancake (see Fig. 3-9). Since the spins are physically in the same spatial location and in this case in the same physical gradient and $B_0$ conditions, they will continue to evolve under the influence of the applied gradient and local inhomogeneities etc. However, because the spins have undergone a 180 degrees flip they effectively precess in the opposite direction to which they started, and will therefore eventually come into focus (less T2 effects), as shown in Fig. 3-9.

For optimal performance, the excitation pulse strength should be 90 degrees, whereas the refocusing pulse should be 180 degrees. The echo refocuses at a time equal to the spacing between the 90 degrees and 180 degrees pulses (see Fig. 3-10). While the effects of T2 cannot be undone by a spin echo, the static effects of $B_0$ inhomogeneities can be undone. Therefore, spin echo sequences can be robustly applied in situations where high inhomogeneities are found. In a spin echo sequence, each line of k-space requires a single application of the basic sequence, and TEs are typically in excess of 20 ms.

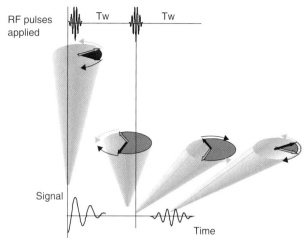

**FIGURE 3-9** For the spin echo sequence, the relative position of the "leading" and "trailing" spins are shown relative to the signal and radio frequency (RF) pulses. The initial RF pulse brings spins into the transverse plane where they immediately begin to dephase due to application of imaging gradients. Immediately before application of the second RF pulse note the relative rotation direction of the leading and trailing spins. The second RF pulse essentially flips the spin system like a pancake, but physically, each spin is in the same location and experiences the same gradients. Therefore, following the second RF pulse spins continue to rotate relative to each other, but in the opposite direction. By this means the spins continue to come together and eventually refocus, resulting in an echo peak. The timing of the echo peak ($2\,T_W$) occurs after an equal time has elapsed between the first and second RF pulses ($T_W$). Following the echo peak the spins continue to dephase, resulting in a trail off of the echo signal.

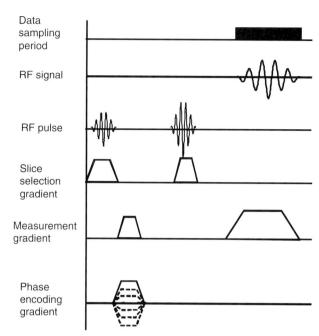

**FIGURE 3-10** Spin echo imaging sequence is illustrated, showing the sampled signal, the first applied radio frequency (RF) pulse being the initial slice selection RF pulse (transmitted to the body) and the second pulse being the refocusing pulse, these are applied in conjunction with the slice selection gradients, the primary read-out or measurement gradient applied on either side of the refocusing RF pulse, the phase encoding gradient is represented by the dashed lines indicating that this gradient is applied at varying amplitudes, and each applied during a separate application of the basic sequence, with each gradient step corresponding to the acquisition of one line of k-space.

## High Performance Gradients

In common with the GRE sequence, gradient slew rate has a direct effect on spin echo images, but the spin echo sequence may allow some further room for image optimization. One property that influences image quality is the BW of signal reception, which is directly influenced by the availability of high performance gradients. The BW per pixel essentially determines the thermal noise that contributes to each pixel and is governed by the formula:

$$BW\ per\ pixel = 1/sample\ time$$

Consider the case of low performance gradients, where the sample time (ST) is set at 10 ms. Under these circumstances the BW per pixel is 100 Hz. Now, consider the situation if high performance gradients are available, and the ST is set at 2 ms. This dictates that the BW per pixel is 500 Hz. The BW per pixel contributes to the BW of the acquisition (which is more commonly quoted in scanner systems) and is given by the formula:

$$Total\ BW = BW\ per\ pixel \times No.\ of\ pixels$$

Therefore, for 256 points per line, the total BW would be:

Low performance gradients; BW = 25 kHz

High performance gradients; BW = 128 kHz

Therefore, we note that high performance gradients allow generation of images with higher noise contributions, because they permit higher BWs to be used. After selecting the repetition times (TRs) and TEs for a spin echo sequence, it may be possible to select a lower BW than that defaulted by the scanner. Sometimes, using all the gradient power available to the scanner may be counter-productive, and the spin echo sequence allows this to be set for higher quality.

# STIMULATED ECHO

There are three echo types, as follows:

- Gradient echo
- Spin echo
- Stimulated echo

In the progression established thus far, GRE requires one RF pulse, spin echo requires two RF pulses, and so it is not surprising that stimulated echo requires three RF pulses. Referring to Fig. 3-11, which outlines the state of the spin system at each stage of the stimulated echo sequence: following the initial RF pulse (90 degrees), the spin system dephases; at the time of application of the second RF pulse (90 degrees), only the component of spins orthogonal to the RF pulse are affected, and this component is sent back along the z-axis; in the delay between the second and third RF pulses, the spins along the z-axis do not dephase in the presence of any gradients, because only spins in the transverse plane are affected by gradients; the third RF pulse brings the spins down from the z-axis into the transverse plane in such a manner that they refocus under the same gradient conditions that pertained following the first RF pulse; following this, the spins refocus and form the stimulated echo.

## Stimulated Echo Features

Even when applied with the optimal RF pulses for each of the three pulses (90 degrees), only half of the signal is available for imaging use, because the action of the second RF on completely dephased spins only affects the spin component orthogonal to the RF field direction. Therefore, the sequence is only 50% efficient. While image contrast is dependent on T1 and T2 characteristics, T2 weighting is not as prominent as in a comparable spin echo sequence: this is because during the period when spins are aligned back along the z-axis, no T2 dephasing takes place. In the basic form just described, largely due to the loss of signal, stimulated echo imaging is rarely used in commercial imaging sequences.

## High Efficiency Stimulated Echo

An important lesson to take away from the basic stimulated echo sequence is that spins can be realigned along the z-axis by application of RF pulses, and therefore realignment along the z-axis can occur much faster than relying on T1 relaxation to realign spins. However, we also saw in the stimulated echo sequence that alignment of spins along $B_0$ was only 50% efficient, which may negate the benefits of this rapid spin realignment. However, by paying close attention to spin conditions pertaining at the time of the second RF it is possible to align all spins along $B_0$. Under conditions that the spins are dephased at the time of the second RF pulse, consider the spins split into two orthogonal components, and note that the RF pulse affects only one component. In this case, the spins are dephased due to the influence of imaging gradients applied following the initial RF pulse. Under conditions where all gradients are applied in the form of a gradient echo, it is possible

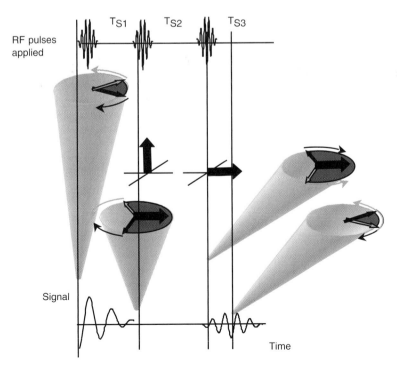

**FIGURE 3-11** The stimulated echo spin conditions are illustrated. The positions of the three radio frequency (RF) pulses are indicated on the top line. Following the first RF pulse, the signal is generated and decays during the initial period $T_{S1}$. Following the second RF pulse, no signal is seen during the second period $T_{S2}$. Following the third RF pulse, a stimulated echo is seen during the period $T_{S3}$. Following the first RF pulse, spins in the transverse plane are dephased. At the time of the second RF pulse only the component of spins orthogonal to the RF pulse (indicated by the large solid arrow) are sent back along the longitudinal ("Z") axis. The spins that remain in the transverse plane dephase further and do not contribute to the signal. During the period $T_{S2}$ spins continue to relax due to the T1 process. At the time of the third RF pulse the spins along the longitudinal axis are brought down into the transverse plane and continue their rephasing process to form the signal echo. In effect the second and third RF pulses can be regarded as a split refocusing pulse as is used in the spin echo sequence.

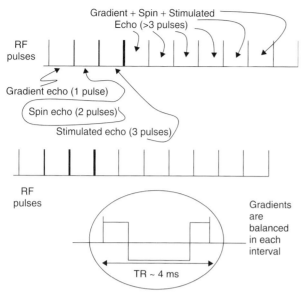

**FIGURE 3-12** The conditions for steady state free precession (SSFP) are illustrated. The SSFP sequence requires that all RF pulses are applied at equal intervals and are of equal amplitude. From the first pulse a single gradient echo is formed (with suitable gradients applied); from the second radio frequency (RF) pulse a gradient echo and a spin echo are formed; from the third RF pulse a gradient echo, spin echo, and stimulated echo are formed. For all subsequent RF pulses, the three types of echo are formed each time. By arranging for the pulses to be spaced equally, all three echoes will occur at exactly the same time in each interval. By this means the signal is boosted by addition of all three echoes. The lower panel indicates the form of the gradient echo applied during each RF interval. In this case, the gradient is balanced, i.e. it is symmetric, and there are equal positive and negative areas, making the net gradient by the end of each sequence balance to zero.

to arrange for the spins to rephased at the time of the second RF pulse. Under these conditions the second pulse will act on all the spins, thereby making the sequence 100% efficient. Therefore, by ensuring that all gradients refocus the spins between the first and second RF pulses, and arranging for the phase of the RF pulse to be appropriately aligned, the stimulated echo sequence becomes more attractive for use.

## High Efficiency Imaging

As stated earlier, there are only three echo types (gradient, spin, and stimulated). If the three echoes could be combined, then the signal to noise ratio (SNR) of any imaging sequence based on the sum of three echoes could be substantially increased compared to any one echo used singly. What are the conditions required to combine them? As demonstrated for the enhanced stimulated echo system, echoes can be

combined by carefully controlling the phase of spin system. However, due to the T2 and T2* processes, control of the spin phase can only be accomplished with precision if short TRs and TEs are used. A sequence that incorporates all three echo types is the SSFP sequence (see Fig. 3-12). In the SSFP sequence, because all three echoes have to be exactly superimposed, it is essential that a uniform TR be used for each RF pulse: from the first pulse a gradient echo is formed; the second RF pulse also generates a gradient echo and in conjunction with the first RF pulse generates a spin echo at the exact same time; the third RF pulse generates a gradient echo, a spin echo, and a stimulated echo, each occurring at exactly the same time. All pulses thereafter will continue to generate this triplet of echoes, each superimposed, and producing a high SNR image.

## Steady State Free Precession

The conditions for maintaining the train of superimposed echoes are as follows:

- TR must be < T2*.

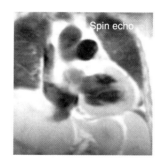
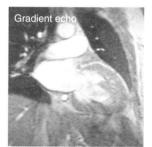
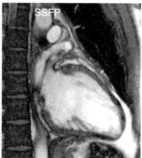
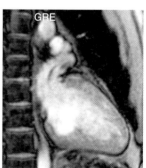

**FIGURE 3-13** Comparison of three basic imaging sequences: spin echo, gradient echo, and steady state free precession. The spin echo sequence is a black-blood sequence, and is used for morphologic imaging; gradient echo is a bright-blood approach, where the bright signal is due to flow refreshment; and steady state free precession (SSFP) is a bright-blood approach where signal is due to spin properties which are independent of blood flow. Note the almost uniform contrast of blood and myocardium in the SSFP image compared to the gradient echo image, where variations in blood flow lead to variations in blood–myocardial contrast.

- RF pulses must be applied at a uniform rate.
- Gradients in each TR interval must be exactly balanced (i.e., the net effect of each gradient must be canceled before application of each RF pulse).

The optimal RF pulse angle to maintain each echo at a uniform level is a compromise between the conditions for each of the three echo types. For cardiac imaging at 1.5 T, the optimum angle is approximately 45 degrees when the TR is approximately 4 ms. Under conditions that a uniform signal is generated for each echo, the system is said to be in the "steady-state". The imaging sequence based on this train of echoes is termed SSFP. Common acronyms for SSFP are as follows:

- FIESTA (fast imaging employing steady-state acquisition)
- Balanced FFE (balanced [gradient] fast field echo)
- True FISP (true fast imaging with steady precession)

Although in a spin echo sequence, moving blood is generally lost (black blood) and in gradient echo, moving blood is generally bright (bright blood) but dependent on flow conditions, in SSFP imaging blood signal is effectively independent of motion and is predominantly dependent on the T1 and T2 properties of spins. The advantage of this is that blood–myocardial contrast is effectively constant and is not dependent on local flow properties.

## SUMMARY

Gradient echo requires one RF pulse per k-space line and is sometimes called a bright blood sequence. Spin echo requires two RF pulses per k-space line, and is sometimes termed a black-blood sequence. Stimulated echo requires three RF pulses per k-space line and is rarely used as a primary imaging sequence. SSFP requires uniform application of RF pulses at short TRs with balanced gradients, such that all three echoes simultaneously contribute to each k-space line. SSFP produces images that are essentially flow independent and with high SNR (see Fig. 3-13).

# PART II

# Clinical Application

# CHAPTER 4

# Cardiovascular Magnetic Resonance Imaging Positioning

June Yamrozik

## INTRODUCTION

The heart is an oblique structure in the body. Specific positioning techniques are needed to image this dynamic organ. This chapter will focus on the imaging planes of the heart. Step-by-step imaging techniques will be provided to perform these positions. The cardiac anatomic structures will also be shown on the resultant cardiac images. This will enable the novice technologist to become familiar with cardiac terminology, anatomy, and the cardiac planes of the heart.

## IMAGING PLANES OF THE BODY

It is imperative to have a full understanding of the imaging planes for magnetic resonance imaging (MRI) positioning. The body is divided into three planes and a detailed description of each plane is as follows (see Fig. 4-1):

- The Z plane, also known as transverse or axial plane, cuts the body from top to bottom or superior to inferior.
- The Y plane, also known as the coronal plane cuts the body from front to back or anterior to posterior.
- The X plane, also known as the sagittal plane cuts the body from right to left.

## CARDIAC IMAGING PLANES

### Two-Chamber or Vertical Long Axis (VLA) View

To acquire a two-chamber image (VLA), center parallel to the long axis of the left ventricle and left atrium from an axial or transverse breath-hold image (see Fig. 4-2A). To ensure accurate positioning always center from a breath-hold image. The resultant image will demonstrate the LV, left atrium, left atrial appendage, and mitral valve (MV) (see Fig. 4-2B).

### Aliased Two-Chamber View

The field of view (FOV) that was selected was too small for this body habitus and fold over or wrap has marred this image (see Fig. 4-3).

### Four-Chamber or Horizontal Long Axis (HLA) View

To acquire a four-chamber image (HLA), center parallel to the long axis of the two- chamber image (VLA) (see Fig. 4-4A).

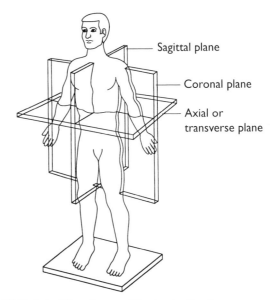

Sagittal plane

Coronal plane

Axial or transverse plane

**FIGURE 4-1** The planes of the body: **Z** = **transverse or axial**, divides the body superior to inferior or top to bottom, **Y** = **coronal**, divides the body anterior to posterior or front to back, **X** = **sagittal**, divides the body from right to left.

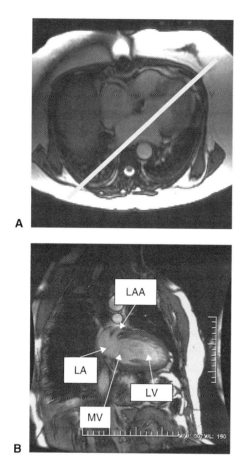

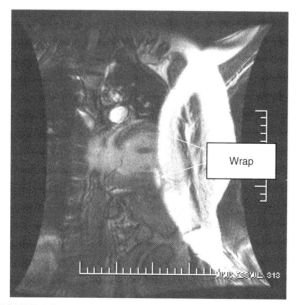

FIGURE 4-2 **(A)** Center parallel to the long axis of the left ventricle and left atrium from a transverse or axial breath hold image. **(B)** A properly positioned 2 chamber (VLA) image will demonstrate the left ventricle (LV), left atrium (LA), left atrial appendage (LAA) and mitral valve (MV).

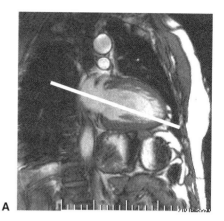

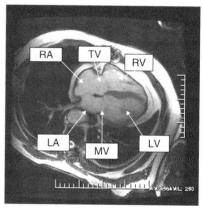

FIGURE 4-4 **(A)** Center parallel to the long axis of the left ventricle and left atrium from the 2 chamber (VLA) image. Do not center directly in the middle of the left ventricle but a little lower to avoid the aortic valve. **(B)** A properly positioned 4 chamber (HLA) will demonstrate the left ventricle (LV), right ventricle (RV), left atrium (LA), right atrium (RA), mitral valve (MV) and tricuspid valve (TV).

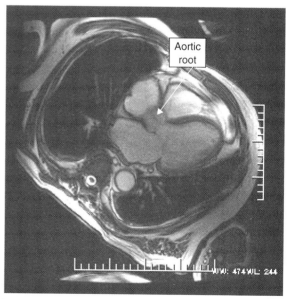

FIGURE 4-3 Wrap or aliasing producing a nondiagnostic two-chamber (VLA) image. This is produced by selecting an incorrect field of view (FOV).

FIGURE 4-5 This image was centered a bit too superior resulting in having the aortic root in the image. It is wise to take more than one image to save time.

The resultant image will demonstrate the right and left ventricle, the right and left atrium, mitral and tricuspid valve (see Fig. 4-4B).

## Malpositioned Four-Chamber View

This image was positioned too superior on the two-chamber view. It is wise to set up two to three slices to get an accurate output image. The resultant image has the aortic root making it a five-chamber image (see Fig. 4-5).

## Short Axis View

To acquire a short axis (SA) view, center perpendicular to the septum on the four-chamber view (HLA) (see Fig. 4-6A). The resultant image will demonstrate the left and right ventricle in a nice circular shape (see Fig. 4-6B).

## Short Axis with Motion Artifact

This image demonstrates impaired image quality because the patient had difficulty holding their breath (see Fig. 4-7).

## Additional Positioning to Acquire the Two- and Four-Chamber Images

There are additional ways to acquire the aforementioned images. A good mid-SA image that demonstrates the papillary muscles can be used to position the two- and four-chamber view. To acquire a four-chamber or HLA view, center in between the papillary muscles and at the base of the RV (see Fig. 4-8A). The resultant image known as the four-chamber or HLA view will demonstrate the right and left atrium, the RV and LV, and MV and tricuspid valve (see Fig. 4-8B).

The same SA image can be used to demonstrate the two-chamber view. Center perpendicular to the LV (see Fig. 4-9A) and the resultant image will demonstrate the LV, left atrium, left atrial appendage, and MV (see Fig. 4-9B).

It is wise to know both of these positioning methods, because sometimes for whatever reason (patient anatomy) one position might work better than the other. Therefore, make sure you know both ways of acquiring these images so it will not be difficult to deviate from your routine when one position is not working.

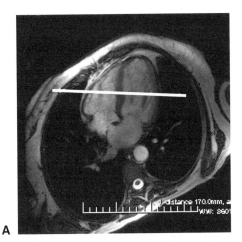

A

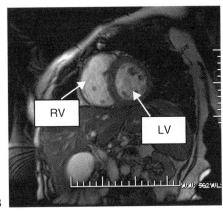

B

**FIGURE 4-6** **(A)** Center perpendicular to the septum from the 4 chamber (HLA) image and parallel to the mitral annulus. **(B)** A properly positioned short axis image will demonstrate the left ventricle (LV) and the right ventricle (RV) in a nice round circular shape.

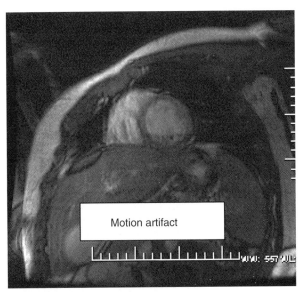

**FIGURE 4-7** This patient had difficulty holding their breath causing motion on this image. To remedy this problem different parameters can be set on the machine. For instance, decrease field of view (FOV), or decrease matrix, or decrease number of excitations or try parallel imaging.

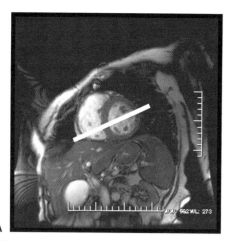 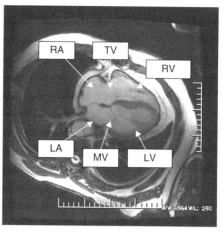

**FIGURE 4-8** **(A)** Center in between the papillary muscles and at the base of the right ventricle (RV) from the short axis (SA) image to acquire a 4 chamber (HLA) image. **(B)** A properly positioned 4 chamber (HLA) will demonstrate the left ventricle (LV), right ventricle (RV), left atrium (LA), right atrium (RA) ,mitral valve (MV) and tricuspid valve (TV).

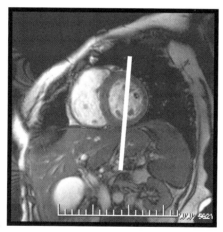 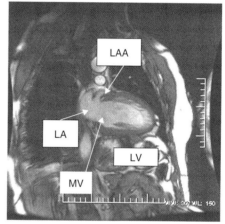

**FIGURE 4-9** **(A)** Center perpendicular to the mid left ventricle from the SA view. **(B)** A properly positioned 2 chamber (VLA) image will demonstrate the left ventricle (LV), left atrium (LA), left atrial appendage (LAA) and mitral valve (MV).

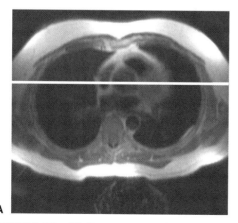 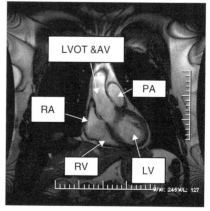

**FIGURE 4-10** **(A)** Center perpendicular to the aorta on a breath hold transverse or axial image. **(B)** The resultant image will show the left ventricle (LV), aortic valve (AV) and outflow tract. The pulmonary artery (PA), right atrium (RA), right ventricle (RV) will also be seen on this view.

## Left Ventricular Outflow Tract (or Coronal Image)

Center perpendicular to the aorta on a breath-hold transverse or axial image (see Fig. 4-10A).

The resultant image will demonstrate the LV, aortic valve (AV), and outflow tract (see Fig. 4-10B).

## Flow Artifact

Sometimes turbulent flow in the aorta will cause a flow artifact on left ventricular outflow tract (LVOT) image (see Fig. 4-11). This problem can be resolved by adjusting the frequency peak on the machine to water. Due to different patient body types sometimes the frequency peak will adjust to fat. If this does not eliminate the problem perhaps substitute to a standard gradient echo sequence. Normally, steady state free precession (SSFP) imaging is desired; however, gradient echo imaging is a good substitute when all else fails.

## Para Axial Aorta

Center parallel to the AV using the LVOT (coronal) image (see Fig. 4-12A). The resultant image will demonstrate the cusps of the AV (see Fig. 4-12B).

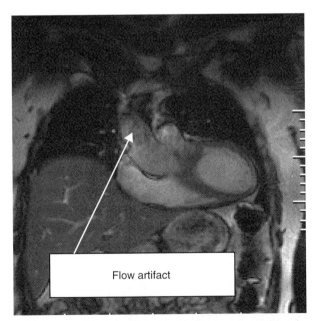

**FIGURE 4-11**   Flow artifact can hinder image quality. Sometimes, the frequency peak is adjusted to fat instead of water causing this artifact. Adjust the frequency peak to try to solve this problem. Sometimes standard gradient echo imaging needs to be substituted if the prior does not remedy the problem.

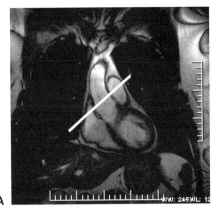

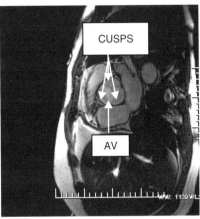

**FIGURE 4-12**   **(A)** Utilize the coronal (LVOT) image and center parallel to the aortic valve (AV). **(B)** The resultant image demonstrates the AV and cusps of the valve.

## Three-Chamber View

Center parallel to the long axis of the LV and aorta as shown on the LVOT (coronal view) (see Fig. 4-13A). This image can also be acquired using a basal SA image that has the AV captured on the image. Center parallel to the aortic root as demonstrated on a SA image (see Fig. 4-13B). Both positions will demonstrate the AV, MV, LV, and a portion of the RV (see Fig. 4-14). Become familiar with both of these positioning techniques because sometimes one might work better than the other.

## Malpositioned Three-Chamber View

The MV and AV are missed in this position (see Fig. 4-15). During set up, it is wise to take two to three images to ensure accurate positioning.

## Parasagittal Aorta

This image is acquired by centering parallel to the ascending and descending aorta from a breath-hold transverse or axial image (see Fig. 4-16A). The resultant

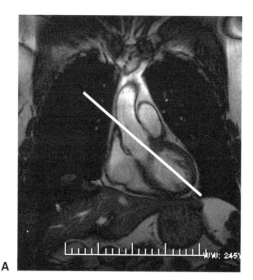 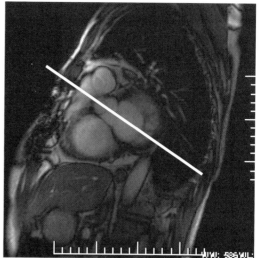

**FIGURE 4-13**   **(A)** Center parallel to the long axis of the left ventricle (LV) and aorta as shown in the left ventricular outflow tract (LVOT) coronal view. **(B)** Center parallel to the aortic root as shown on the basal short axis (SA) image.

image will demonstrate the aorta in a candy-cane view (see Fig. 4-16B).

## Off-Centered Parasagittal

This image was not centered quite parallel to the ascending and descending aorta. The entire aorta is not demonstrated in this plane (see Fig. 4-17).

## Right Ventricular Outflow Tract

This image is acquired by centering perpendicular to the pulmonic valve (PV) from a breath-hold transverse or axial image (see Fig. 4-18A). The resultant image will demonstrate the pulmonary artery (PA), PV and RV (see Fig. 4-18B).

## Right Ventricular Outflow Tract Flow Artifact

Sometimes turbulent flow in the pulmonary will cause a flow artifact on the right ventricular outflow tract

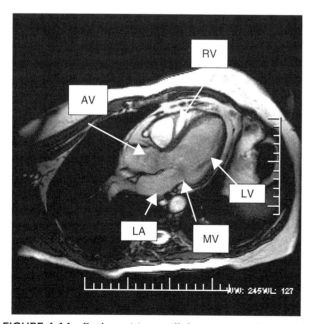

**FIGURE 4-14**   Both positions will demonstrate the aortic valve (AV), mitral valve (MV), left ventricle (LV) and a portion of the right ventricle (RV).

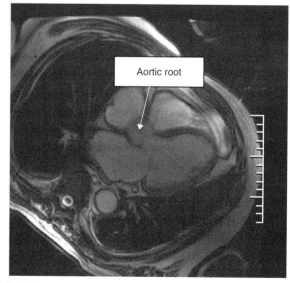

**FIGURE 4-15**   The mitral valve (MV) and aortic valve (AV) are not visualized well on this image. During setup, it is wise to take more than one image.

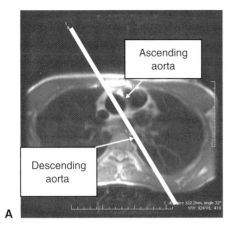

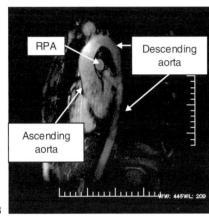

FIGURE 4-16    **(A)** Center parallel to the ascending and descending aorta from a breath-hold transverse (axial) image. **(B)** The resultant image shows the ascending and descending aorta in a candy cane shaped image. The right pulmonary artery is also seen (RPA).

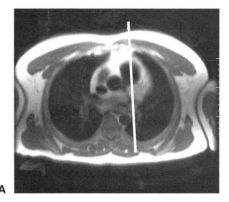

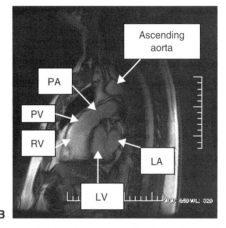

FIGURE 4-18    **(A)** Center perpendicular to the pulmonic valve on a transverse (axial) breath hold image. **(B)** This image is done to show the pulmonary artery (PA), pulmonic valve (PV) and right ventricle (RV). The ascending aorta, left ventricle (LV) and left atrium (LA) can also be seen.

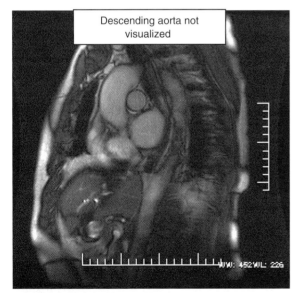

FIGURE 4-17    This image does not show the entire aorta. It is wise to take more than one image parallel to the ascending and descending aorta in order to demonstrate it in the parasagittal plane.

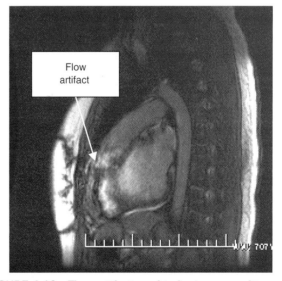

FIGURE 4-19    Flow artifact can hinder image quality. Sometimes, the frequency peak is adjusted to fat instead of water causing this artifact. Adjust the frequency peak to try to solve this problem. Sometimes standard gradient echo imaging needs to be substituted if the prior does not remedy the problem.

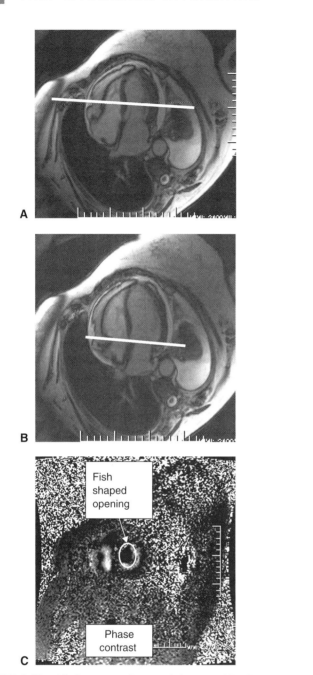

**FIGURE 4-20** **(A)** Center at the tip of the mitral leaflets for patients with diastolic dysfunction. **(B)** Center at the mitral annulus or slightly more basal for patients with mitral regurgitation. **(C)** The resultant image will show the mitral valve (MV) in a fish shaped appearance.

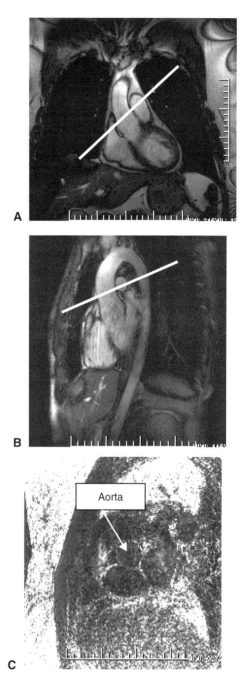

**FIGURE 4-21** **(A)** Center parallel to the pulmonary artery and the ascending aorta from a coronal (LVOT) image. **(B)** Center parallel to the pulmonary artery and the ascending aorta from a parasagittal image. **(C)** The ascending aorta is shown in a circular shape.

(RVOT) image (see Fig. 4-19). This problem can be resolved by adjusting the frequency peak on the machine to water. Due to different patient body types sometimes the frequency peak will adjust to fat. If this does not eliminate the problem perhaps substitute to a standard gradient echo sequence. Normally, SSFP imaging is desired; however, gradient echo imaging is a good substitute when all else fails.

## Mitral Valve Phase Contrast–Magnetic Resonance

This image is acquired by centering perpendicular to the MV leaflets on a four-chamber or HLA view. A patient with the diagnosis of diastolic dysfunction is centered at the tip of the leaflets when the valve is opened

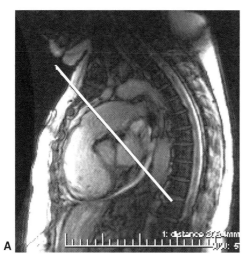 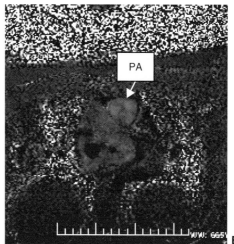

FIGURE 4-22 **(A)** Center parallel to the pulmonic valve (PV) on a right ventricular outflow tract (RVOT) image. **(B)** The pulmonary artery (PA) will be demonstrated in round shape.

(see Fig. 4-20A). For mitral regurgitation center when the valve is closed usually at the mitral annulus (see Fig. 4-20B).

The resultant image will demonstrate the MV and will resemble an open fish mouth appearance (see Fig. 4-20C).

## Aortic Phase Contrast–Magnetic Resonance

This image is acquired by centering parallel to the ascending aorta on either an LVOT (coronal) (see Fig. 4-21A) or parasagittal image of the aorta (see Fig. 4-21B). The resultant image shows the aorta in a circular shape (see Fig. 4-21C).

## Pulmonary Phase Contrast–Magnetic Resonance

This image is acquired by centering parallel to the PV on an RVOT view (see Fig. 4-22A). Make sure that the position is above the valve. The resultant image will demonstrate the PA in a circular shape (see Fig. 4-22B).

## SUMMARY

The novice cardiac MRI technologist needs to know and understand the imaging planes and specific cardiac planes. A complete understanding of the positioning explained in the preceding text will help one master the techniques of cardiac imaging. It is essential to become familiar with the terminology by incorporating it in your everyday language while imaging the heart. In the beginning, it may be difficult because an MRI technologist is familiar with axial (transverse), coronal, sagittal, and para (coronal or sagittal) imaging planes of

the entire body. Cardiac imaging focuses on the planes of the heart. Therefore, when an SA image of the heart is imaged the plane of the heart is in SA whereas the plane of the body is in sagittal or parasagittal. When one can differentiate between the two, cardiac imaging will be mastered.

## QUIZ

### How much have we learned about cardiac positioning?

1. The below view is acquired by centering parallel to the two-chamber view.
   a. LVOT
   b. RVOT
   c. Four-chamber view or (HLA)
   d. Coronal

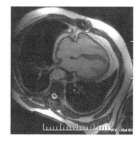

2. The below image:
   a. Is called a parasagittal image.
   b. Can be called candy-cane view.
   c. Is accomplished by centering parallel to the ascending and descending aorta in an axial view.
   d. Is both a and c
   e. Is all of the above

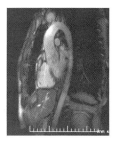

3.  This image can also be called a VLA view.
    a.  True
    b.  False

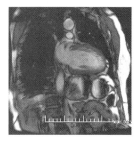

4.  This view is called:
    a.  RVOT image
    b.  Coronal image
    c.  Transverse image
    d.  None of the above

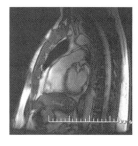

5.  What view will this position demonstrate?
    a.  Two-chamber
    b.  Four-chamber
    c.  Short axis
    d.  LVOT

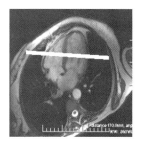

6.  The left atrial appendage is best seen on what view?
    a.  Two-chamber or (VLA)
    b.  Coronal
    c.  RVOT
    d.  Five-chamber

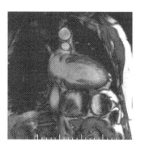

7.  This view is called:
    a.  LVOT
    b.  Coronal
    c.  Four-chamber
    d.  Both a and b

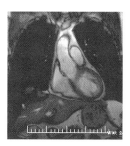

8.  This image can also be called an HLA view.
    a.  True
    b.  False

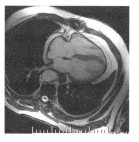

9.  The three-chamber image best demonstrates which of the following structures?
    a.  AV, MV and LV, and some RV
    b.  PA and PV
    c.  Ascending and descending aorta
    d.  Tricuspid valve, MV, left and right atrium

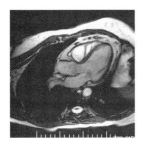

10. The four-chamber (HLA) image best demonstrates which of the following structures?
    a. Tricuspid valve, MV, left and right atrium
    b. AV, MV LV, and some RV
    c. RV, PA, and PV
    d. LV and RV, left and right atrium, tricuspid and MVs

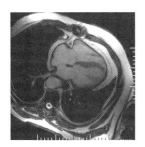

## Quiz Answers

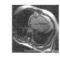 1. c

 2. e

 3. a

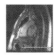 4. a

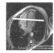 5. c

 6. a

 7. d

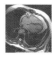 8. a

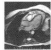 9. a

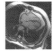 10. d

# CHAPTER 5

# Cardiovascular Magnetic Resonance Imaging Protocols

June Yamrozik

This chapter discusses imaging protocols. Different protocols vary from institution to institution; so let this serve as a guideline to assist cardiac imaging. The cardiac magnetic resonance imaging (MRI) technologist will learn the proper sequences and positions for specific examinations.

## OVERVIEW

### Positioning

#### Two-Chamber or Vertical Long Axis View

To acquire a two-chamber view (vertical long axis [VLA]), center parallel to the long axis of the left ventricle (LV) on an axial or transverse breath-hold (BH) image (see Fig. 5-1A). To ensure accurate positioning always center from a BH image. The resultant image will demonstrate the LV, left atrium, left atrial appendage (LAA), and mitral valve (MV) (see Fig. 5-1B).

#### Four-Chamber or Horizontal Long Axis View

To acquire a four-chamber view (horizontal long axis [HLA]), center parallel to the long axis of the two-chamber view (VLA) (see Fig. 5-2A). A mid short axis (SA) slice that shows the papillary muscles can also be used (see Fig. 5-2B). The resultant image will demonstrate the right and left atrium, right ventricle (RV) and LV and MV and tricuspid valve (see Fig. 5-2C).

#### Three-Chamber View

Center parallel to the long axis of the LV and aorta as shown on the left ventricular outflow track (LVOT[coronal view]) (see Fig. 5-3A). This image can also be acquired using a basal SA image that has the aortic valve (AV) captured on the image. Center parallel to the aortic root as demonstrated on an SA image (see

Fig. 5-3B). Both positions will demonstrate the AV, MV, LV, and a portion of the RV (see Fig. 5-3C). Become familiar with both of these positioning techniques because sometimes one might work better than the other.

## CARDIOVASCULAR MAGNETIC RESONANCE PROTOCOLS

Two to three of the images shown earlier are performed on all of our cardiac protocols. These views enable the physician to get a sufficient display of heart function. These sequences are considered routine at our facility.

Double inversion recovery–spin echo (DIR-SE) (black blood) non–breath-hold (NBH) transverse (axial) from the pulmonary artery (PA) to the base of the heart for morphology and diameter of vessels are also routine at our imaging modality. With no further ado, let us proceed to cardiovascular magnetic resonance (CMR) protocols.

## CARDIOVASCULAR MAGNETIC RESONANCE IMAGING PROTOCOLS

### Arch Cardiovascular Magnetic Resonance Imaging Protocol

A patient suffering from the following indications is most likely to be scheduled for an arch MRI/magnetic resonance angiography (MRA):

1. Dissection
2. Coarctation
3. Aneurysm
4. Marfan disease

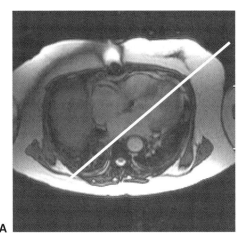
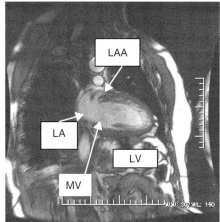

**A**                                                                                 **B**

FIGURE 5-1   **A:** Center parallel to the long axis of the left ventricle and left atrium from a transverse or axial breath-hold image. **B:** A properly positioned two-chamber (vertical long axis [VLA]) image will demonstrate the left ventricle (LV), left atrium (LA) left atrial appendage (LAA) and mitral valve (MV).

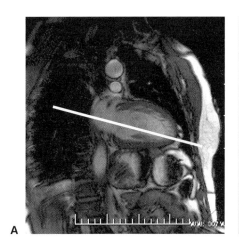
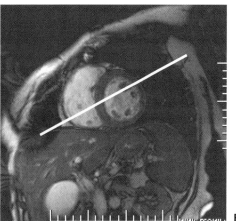

**A**                                                                                 **B**

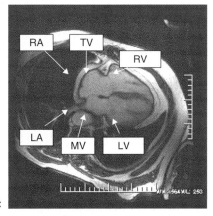

**C**

FIGURE 5-2   **A:** Center parallel to the long axis of the left ventricle and left atrium from the two-chamber (vertical long axis [VLA]) image. Do not center directly in the middle of the left ventricle but a little lower to avoid the aortic root. **B:** Center in between the papillary muscles and at the base of the right ventricle from the short axis (SA) image to acquire a four-chamber ([HLA]) image. **C:** A properly positioned four-chamber (HLA) will demonstrate the left ventricle (LV), right ventricle (RV), left atrium (LA), right atrium (RA), mitral valve (MV) and tricuspid valve (TV).

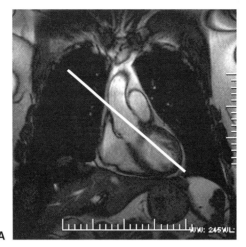
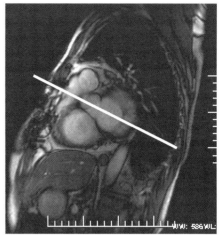
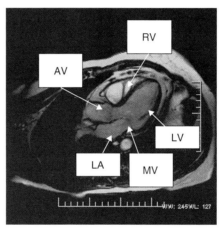

**FIGURE 5-3** **A:** To acquire a three-chamber image, center parallel to the long axis of the left ventricle (LV) and aorta as shown in the (left ventricular outflow track [LVOT]) coronal view. **B:** Another way to acquire a three-chamber is to center parallel to the aortic root as shown on the basal short axis (SA) image. **C:** Both positions will demonstrate the aortic valve (AV), mitral valve (MV), LV and a portion of the right ventricle (RV).

## Protocol Set Up

A three-plane (Z transverse, Y coronal, X sagittal) BH localizer scout is performed to ensure that the patient is properly positioned on the cardiac coil. The scout images should look as shown in Fig. 5-4A–C. A BH transverse (axial) scout image is then used to set up for the two-chamber images. Please look at Fig. 5-5A, B.

## Sequences Performed

1. Two-, three- and four-chamber imaging steady state free precession (SSFP/cine)
   a. White blood imaging
   b. Demonstrates heart function
   c. Always center from a BH image (see Fig. 5-6A–C)
2. DIR-SE transverse (axial) NBH imaging
   a. Start at the level of the apices of the lung and terminate at the renal arteries

   b. DIR-SE
   c. Black blood (see Fig. 5-7A, B)
3. Parasagittal imaging (SSFP/cine)
   a. Center parallel to the ascending and descending aorta from a transverse (axial) BH image (see Fig. 5-8A)
   b. Aortic arch seen in a candy-cane view (see Fig. 5-8B)
   c. White blood sequence
   d. This image is done to look for the following:
      • Coarctation
      • Dissection
4. LVOT also known as *coronal imaging (SSFP/cine)*
   a. Center perpendicular to the aorta from a BH transverse (axial) image (see Fig. 5-9A, B)
   b. This image is done to look for the following:
      • Aortic dilatation
      • Aortic regurgitation

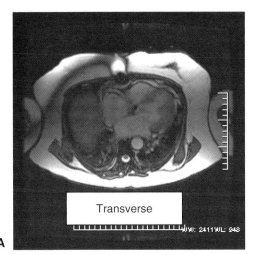

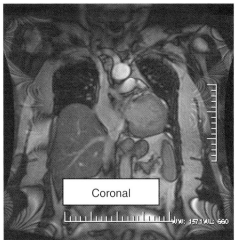

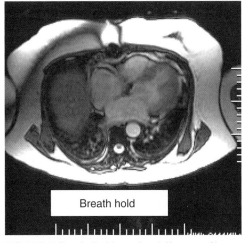

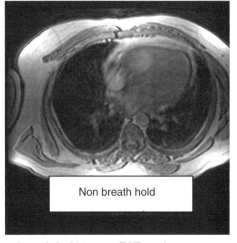

**FIGURE 5-4    A–C:** The signal intensity is in the heart area representing proper positioning of the patient and coil placement. Each image is a breath-hold which will produce consistent output images.

**FIGURE 5-5    A, B:** Note the difference between a breath-hold image (BHI) and a non–breath-hold image (NBHI). The heart is sharp and clear on the BHI whereas the heart is difficult to visualize on an NBHI. If one were to position a BHI from a NBHI the output image would not be a consistent representation of the resultant image due to heart motion.

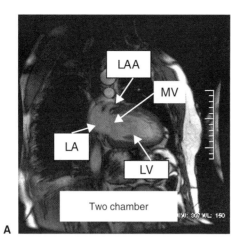

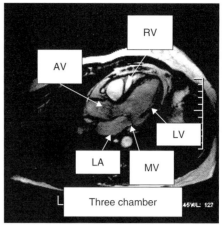

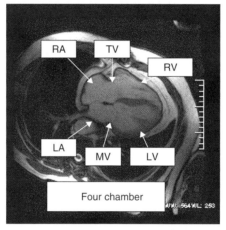

FIGURE 5-6  **A–C:** Routine imaging at our facility; two-, three- and four-chamber images. The two-chamber (vertical long axis [VLA]) image will demonstrate the left ventricle (LV), left atrium (LA) left atrial appendage (LAA) and mitral valve (MV). The four-chamber (horizontal long axis [HLA]) will demonstrate the left ventricle (LV), right ventricle (RV), left atrium (LA), right atrium (RA), mitral valve (MV) and tricuspid valve (TV). The three-chamber image will demonstrate the aortic valve (AV), mitral valve (MV), LV, and a portion of the RV.

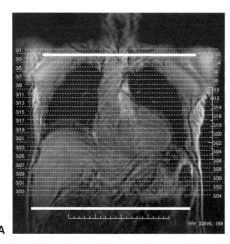

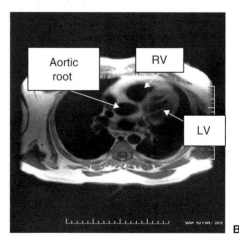

FIGURE 5-7  **A:** Position set for non–breath-hold image (NBHI). Double inversion recovery-spin echo (DIR-SE) imaging from the apices of heart to renal arteries. **B:** Black blood image in the transverse position. This image shows morphology of the heart. RV, right ventricle; LV, left ventricle.

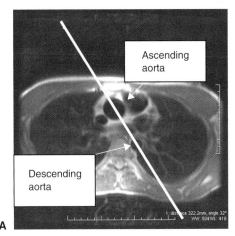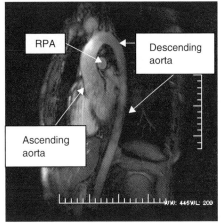

**FIGURE 5-8** **A:** Center parallel to the ascending and descending aorta from an axial (transverse) breath-hold (BH) image. **B:** Aortic arch demonstrated in a candy-cane view. Ascending and descending aorta is visualized in one view. RPA, right pulmonary artery.

- Aortic aneurysm
- Aortic stenosis (see Fig. 5-10A, B).
5. Para-axial AV (SSFP/cine)
   a. Center parallel to the AV from a coronal (LVOT) image as seen in Fig. 5-11A, B
   b. BH DIR paraxial is optional
   c. It is imperative to perform aortic valve imaging if Marfan's or coarctation is suspected
      - Bicuspid AV is critical to assess for these two diagnoses
      - Examples of AV (see Fig. 5-12A, B)
6. Precontrast parasagittal arch imaging (3D time of flight [TOF]) gradient echo (GE)
   a. Perform a prerun parasagittal 3D volume centered parallel to the ascending and descending aorta from an axial (transverse) image

   b. Coronal 3D volume may also be used depending on physician preference
   c. 10- to–20-second BH scan duration
   d. This is done to ensure that the proper field of view (FOV) is used to accommodate the structure of the heart (see Fig. 5-13A, B).
   e. Timing test run (GE)
      - Various methods can be performed, as follows:
         - Bolus tracking
         - Smart prep
         - Real time
         - Fluoroscopy
      - Basic timing to a parasagittal image will be discussed
         - This method has been found to be most accurate at our institution

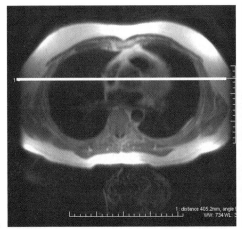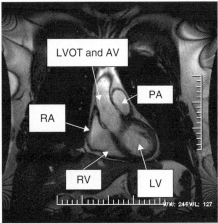

**FIGURE 5-9** **A:** Center perpendicular to the aorta from an axial (transverse) image. **B:** The left ventricular outflow track (LVOT) (coronal) will demonstrate the left ventricle (LV), aortic valve (AV) and outflow tract. RA, right atrium; PA, pulmonary artery; RV, right ventricle.

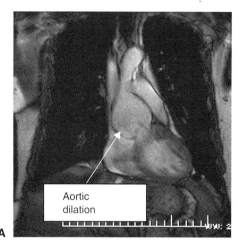
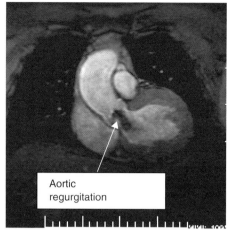

Aortic
dilation

A

Aortic
regurgitation

B

**FIGURE 5-10** **A:** Left ventricular outflow track (LVOT) (coronal) image demonstrating aortic dilation of the ascending aorta. **B:** LVOT (coronal) image demonstrating aortic regurgitation. Notice the black jet representing flow going back into the LV.

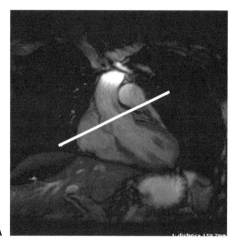
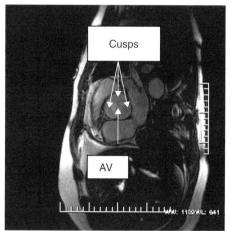

A

Cusps

AV

B

**FIGURE 5-11** **A:** Center parallel to the aortic valve from a breath-hold (BH) coronal (left ventricular outflow track [LVOT]) image. **B:** The cusps of the valve are demonstrated. This is a normal tricuspid aortic valve (AV) demonstrating three cusps.

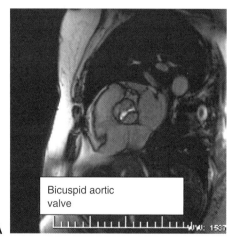
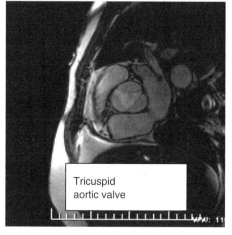

Bicuspid aortic
valve

A

Tricuspid
aortic valve

B

**FIGURE 5-12** **A:** Abnormal aortic valve. Notice the slit in the valve which demonstrates two leaflets. This is known as a *bicuspid aortic valve.* **B:** This is an image demonstrating a normal tricuspid aortic valve with three leaflets.

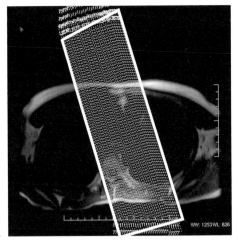 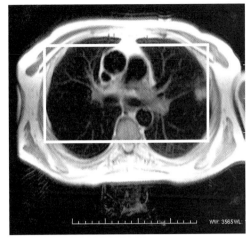

**FIGURE 5-13  A:** This is a pre–3D volume centered parallel to the ascending and descending aorta. Always do a prescan to ensure proper centering and field of view. Haste makes waste and when contrast administration is used always do a prescan image.
**B:** Coronal pre–3D volume centered perpendicular to the ascending and descending aorta.

f.  Timing run (GE)
   - Center parallel to the ascending and descending aorta from a transverse (axial) image (this need not be BH)
   - Take 60 scans at 1-second intervals
   - This makes setting the injector with ease
   - Set the injector: flow rate : 2 mL per second, contrast 2 to 3 mL and saline with the same flow rate
     - A 3 mL per second flow rate is sometimes used when a patient is suffering from slow flow

   - Hand injecting is not recommended because it can be inaccurate
   - Inject

g.  Resultant images
   - Review the images and select the image that shows contrast in the ascending aorta for the appropriate scan delay (see Fig. 5-14A, B)
     - Always add 2 seconds to the scan delay because it is better to error with too much contrast than not enough

h.  Calculating dosage

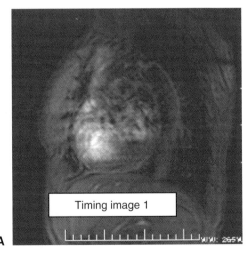 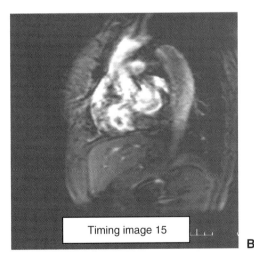

**FIGURE 5-14  A:** The start of the timing sequence. The first image is free of contrast.
**B:** Scroll through the timing images and find an image that has contrast in the ascending aorta as the one illustrated above. Contrast is also seen in the descending aorta. The image number is 15. Contrast is visualized well on this image. This will be the appropriate scan delay plus add 2 seconds because it is better to error with too much contrast than not enough. Scan delay would be 17 seconds.

- From reviewing the timing images, the scan delay value is determined by how much dosage is required to adequately image the aorta
- 0.1 mmol per kg of a paramagnetic compound (gadolinium) is used at this institution and is called *a single dosage*
  i. Formula for calculating dosage
  - Weight in kg $\times \frac{0.1}{1\text{ kg}} \times \frac{1\text{ mL}}{0.5\text{ mmol}}$
  - Example:
    - 70 kg $\times$ 0.1 $\times$ 2 = 14 mL (Single dosage)
    - 70 kg $\times$ 0.05 $\times$ 2 = 7 mL (Half dosage)
    - 704 kg $\times$ 0.2 $\times$ 2 = 28 mL (Double dosage)
  - There are several brands of paramagnetic compounds to select from and the formula given earlier appears to be the universal dosage chart but it is always wise to check the manufacturer's insert
7. Postcontrast parasagittal 3D TOF GE
   a. Perform the 3D volume run with the appropriate scan delay
   - Always add 2 seconds to the scan delay because it is better to error with too much contrast than not enough
     - 10- to 20-second scan delay is a normal delay
     - 30- to 50-second scan delay is used for slow flow
     - Set the injector with the appropriate flow rate of 2 to 3 mL per second
     - Set the saline factor the same flow rate and a dosage of 20 mL
     - Timing is everything
   b. Calculate dosage
   - 0.1 mmol per kg (single dosage)
   - For example, if the patient weighs 80 kg what is the dosage?
     - 80 kg $\times$ 0.1 $\times$ 2 = 16 mL
     - Set the injector with the appropriate dosage and scan delay
     - Resultant image (see Fig. 5-15)
   c. Aortic arch abnormalities (see Fig. 5-16A, B)

## Viability Cardiovascular Magnetic Resonance Imaging Protocol

A patient having the following indications is most likely to be scheduled for cardiac viability protocol.

1. Question of myocardial infarction
2. Acute or chronic myocardial infarction

## Sequences Performed

1. Routine three-plane scout as illustrated in Fig. 5-4A–C
2. Two-, three- and four-chamber imaging (SSFP/cine)
   a. White blood imaging

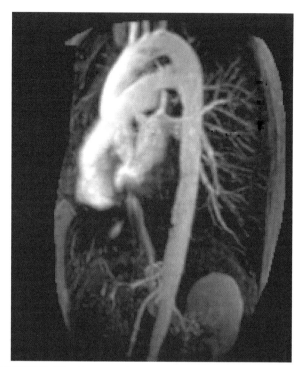

**FIGURE 5-15** Contrast 3D magnetic resonance angiography (MRA) with very nice enhancement of the aorta plus visualization of renal arteries.

   b. Demonstrates heart function
   c. Always center from a BH image (see Fig. 5-6A–C)
3. DIR-SE transverse (axial) NBH imaging
   a. Start at the top of the PA and terminate at the base of the heart
   b. DIR-SE
   c. Black blood
4. SA images from the base of heart to apex
   a. Center perpendicular to septum and parallel to mitral annulus
   b. 8-mm zero gap at this institution
   c. Image from base of heart to apex (see Fig. 5-17)
   d. The function of the heart is then analyzed to obtain an exact ejection fraction
   - Measurement analysis will be discussed in the next chapter
5. Precontrast imaging (perfusion and delayed hyper enhancement) (GE) fast gradient echo with inversion recovery (FGE-IR) prepared pulse
   a. Always take precontrast images before injection for positioning purposes
   b. Utilize the four-chamber image and take two SA scout precontrast sequences before injection
   - First pass perfusion (GE)
     - 5 to 7 SA slices and 20 to 30 phases per image
   - Delayed hyperenhancement (FGE-IR)
     - 400 inversion time (TI) to null the myocardium.

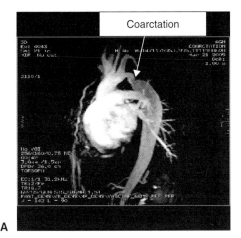
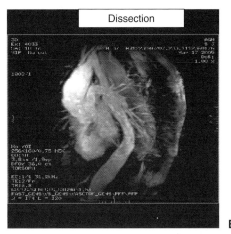

**A**                                                                 **B**

**FIGURE 5-16**    **A:** Contrast 3D magnetic resonance angiography (MRA) demonstrating coarctation of the aorta. **B:** A large type B dissection is demonstrated on the 3D contrast MRA image.

- Center mid-heart
- Center perpendicular to the septum on the four-chamber image (see Fig. 5-18A–C)
- Once images are checked and meet the appropriate specifications, contrast imaging should follow

6. Perfusion contrast imaging (GE) FGE-IR prepared pulse
   a. Dosage is 0.05 mmol per kg (half dosage)
      - Example: If Pat is 80 kg what is the dosage?
         - 80 kg × 0.05 × 2 = 8 mL

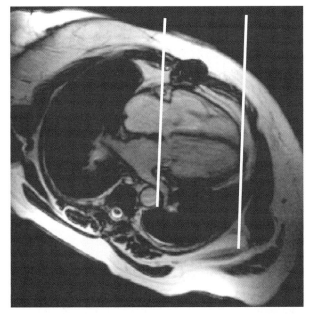

**FIGURE 5-17**    Center from base of heart to and including apex by 8 mm with zero gap. Make sure position is parallel to mitral annulus and perpendicular to the septum.

- It has been studied that a lower perfusion dosage more accurately demonstrates the hypointensity of the myocardium
- Set the injector with the appropriate factors
   - Flow rate is set at 5 mL per second at our institution
   - Gadolinium dosage as calculated (8 mL)
   - Dosage of 20 mL saline is always used to follow the contrast and utilize the same flow rate for saline
   - Inject, wait 2 seconds, or set scan delay to two and scan
   - 5 to 7 SA first pass perfusion slices and 20 to 30 phases per image are acquired
   - Resultant images (see Fig. 5-19A, B)

7. Delayed hyperenhancement imaging (DHE) FGE-IR prepared pulse
   a. An additional 0.15 mmol per kg is administered after the first pass perfusion injection for the hyper enhancement images
      - Double dosage (0.05 + 0.15) = 0.2
      - As previously discussed in the above example, if a 0.05 dosage is 8 mL, what is the remaining 0.15 dosage?
         - 80 kg × 0.15 × 2 = 24 mL
      - It has been studied that a 0.2 mmol per kg dosage of gadolinium demonstrates the hyperintensity of the myocardium more accurately
   - DHE images are acquired 10 and 20 minutes postcontrast.
      - The DHE images must be centered identically to the first pass perfusion sequence This is critical for diagnosis
      - The TI normally varies between 160 and 250
         - A black nulled myocardium is of vital importance

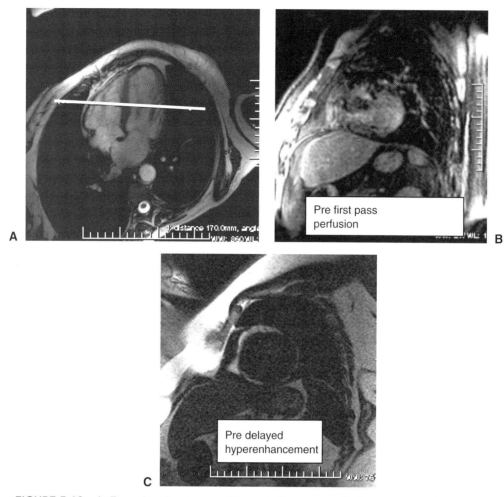

**FIGURE 5-18** **A:** Four-chamber image with centering perpendicular to septum for scout imaging. **B:** Pre perfusion set to make sure field of view (FOV) and coverage is accurate for enhancement imaging. **C:** Pre delayed hyperenhancement with nulled myocardium.

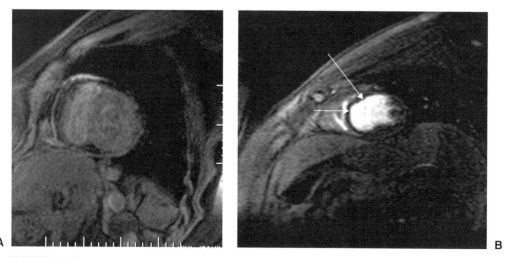

**FIGURE 5-19** **A:** First image of post perfusion set. **B:** Middle image of postperfusion set demonstrating some hypointensity at the area of the septum.

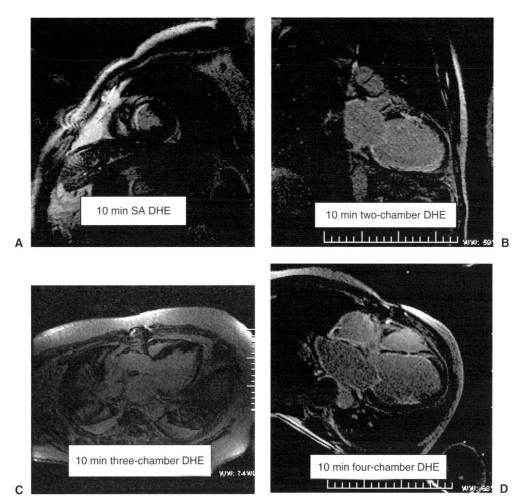

**FIGURE 5-20** **A–D:** Delayed hyperenhancement (DHE) images that are nulled well. These areas of hyperintensity signify damage to the myocardium. The short axis (SA) image shows hyperintensity in the anterior septal region; hyperintensity is also noted in the anterior, inferior and apical region of the heart in the two-chamber view. The four-chamber shows hyperenhancement in the septal and lateral regions of the heart. The three-chamber shows minimal hyperenhancement in the posterior aspect of the heart.

- Take several SA images at different TIs between the 10- minute time interval in order to properly null the myocardium
- Many manufacturers are incorporating sequences to automatically detect the appropriate TI
- Two-, three- and four-chamber 10-minute DHE images are also required (see Fig. 5-20A–D)
- Repeat the 10-minute delayed hyperenhancement set at 20 minutes' postcontrast
- SA DHE
- Two-, three-, and four-chamber DHE
- Center identical to the 10 minute post set
- In between sets take single images at different TIs to maintain proper TI

8. Tag imaging (GE) when necessary
   a. Sometimes tag images are acquired to look at cardiac wall motion
   b. Center identical to the SA images (see Fig. 5-21)

## Atrial or Ventricular Septal Defect Cardiovascular Magnetic Resonance Imaging Protocol

A person suffering from an atrial septal defect (ASD) or a ventricular septal defect (VSD) has a hole in the heart. This hole is located in between the atria and septum or ventricles and septum. The following indications warrant a cardiovascular magnetic resonance imaging (CMRI):

1. Increased pulmonary pressures
2. Pulmonary hypertension

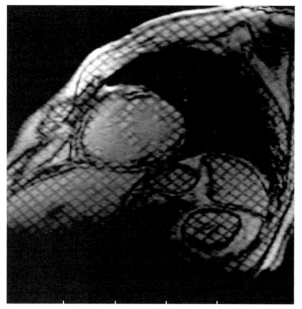

**FIGURE 5-21**   Short axis (SA) tag image showing cardiac wall motion.

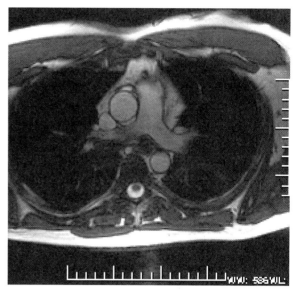

**FIGURE 5-22**   Steady state free precession (SSFP) transverse breath-hold (BH) image starting at the pulmonary artery.

3. Heart murmur
4. Increased palpitations
5. Shortness of breath
6. Leg swelling

## Sequences Performed

1. Routine three-plane scout as illustrated in Fig. 5-4A–C.
2. Two- and three-chamber imaging (SSFP/cine)
   a. White blood imaging
   b. Demonstrates heart function
   c. Always center from a BH image
3. Four-chamber imaging (SSFP/cine)
   a. Take four to five images to try to capture the ASD or VSD
   b. White blood imaging
4. DIR-SE transverse (axial) NBH imaging
   a. Start at the top of the PA and terminate at the base of heart
   b. DIR-SE
   c. Black blood
5. SSFP/cine transverse (axial) BH imaging
   a. Image the entire heart from PA to diaphragm
      • 8-mm zero gap at this institution
      • Staring image (see Fig. 5-22)
   b. SA imaging from atria to base of heart can be substituted (see Fig. 5-23)
      • Whichever way is selected, the RV and LV will be measured to check ejection fraction and stroke volume
      • Measuring will be discussed in the measurement analysis chapter

6. Right ventricular outflow tract (RVOT) SSFP/cine imaging
   a. Center perpendicular to the pulmonic valve (PV) from a transverse (axial) BH image (see Fig. 5-24A, B)
7. Phase contrast magnetic resonance (PCMR) of the aorta and PA
   a. These sequences are done to see the volume of flow coming in from the PA and out of the aorta.

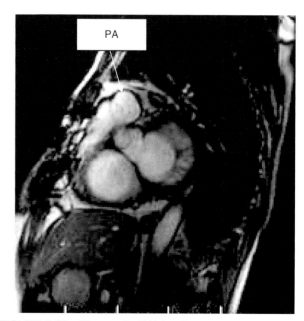

**FIGURE 5-23**   Short axis (SA) basilar imaging staring at pulmonary artery. PA, pulmonary artery.

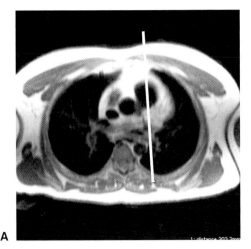
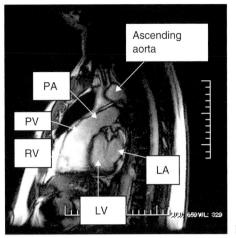

FIGURE 5-24  **A:** Center perpendicular to the pulmonic valve (PV) from a breath-hold (BH) transverse image. **B:** Resultant image will demonstrate the pulmonary artery (PA), PV, and right ventricle (RV). This is also known as the *right ventricular outflow tract image.* LA, left atrium; LV, left ventricle.

A flow ratio quantification is than calculated and will be discussed in the measurement analysis chapter.

b. Center parallel and one inch above the PV from a RVOT image for the PA PCMR
   • Velocity encoding (VENC) is normally 150 to 200 cm per second
   • Slice or through-plane direction
   • (see Fig. 5-25A, B)
c. Center parallel to the PA and aorta from a parasagittal image or a coronal (LVOT) image
   • VENC is normally 150 to 200 cm per second
   • Slice or through-plane direction (see Fig. 5-26A–C)

8. PCMR of the ASD or VSD
   a. Utilize the four-chamber view that demonstrates the ASD or VSD
   b. Do PCMR at that level
      • A low VENC between 30–50 is utilized for better visualization of the jet. All or inplane direction (see Fig. 5-27A, B)
9. Examples of ASD and VSD images (see Fig. 5-28A, B)

## Pulmonary Stenosis CMRI Protocol

A person suffering from the following indications might suggest pulmonary stenosis

1. Shortness of breath
2. Rheumatic fever in the past

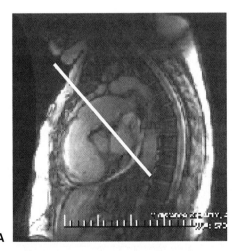
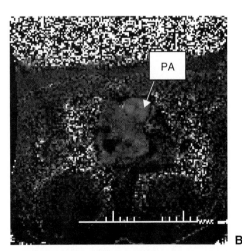

FIGURE 5-25  **A:** Positioning for pulmonary artery (PA) phase contrast magnetic resonance. Center parallel and 1 in. above the pulmonic valve. **B:** Phase contrast image showing the PA.

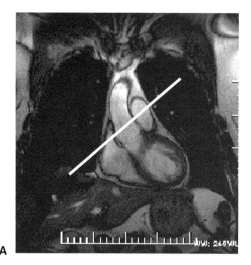
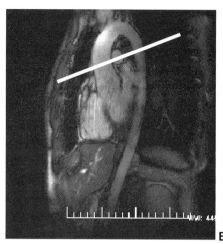
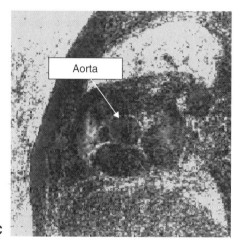

**FIGURE 5-26**    **A–C:** Positioning for an aortic phase contrast magnetic resonance (PCMR). **A:** Center parallel to the pulmonary artery (PA) and aortic valve (AV) from a coronal (left ventricular outflow track [LVOT]) image. **B:** Center parallel to the PA and ascending aorta from a parasagittal image. **C:** The resultant image shows the PA in a nice circular shape.

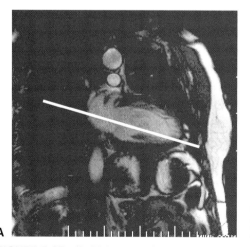
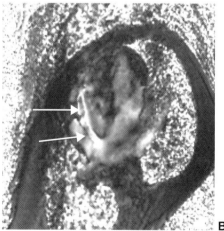

**FIGURE 5-27**    **A:** Make sure the positioning is identical to the four-chamber image that shows the atrial septal defect (ASD). Utilize the two-chamber image to set up for the accurate position. **B:** The resultant image demonstrating the ASD. Notice the white jet in between the atria.

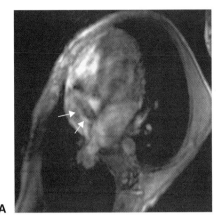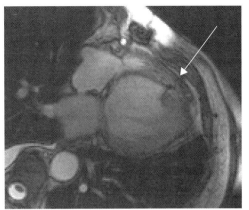

**FIGURE 5-28    A:** Atrial septal defect (ASD) in between the atria. Note the black jet. **B:** A small ventricular septal defect (VSD) in between the ventricles. Note the black jet.

3. Endocarditis in the past
4. Fatigue
5. Chest pain

## Sequences Performed

1. Routine three-plane scout as illustrated in (see Fig. 5-4A–C)
2. Two-, three- and four-chamber imaging (SSFP/cine)
   a. White blood imaging
   b. Demonstrates heart function
   c. Always center from a BH image (see Fig. 5-6A–C)
3. DIR-SE transverse (axial) NBH imaging
   a. Start at the top of the PA and terminate at the base of the heart.
   b. DIR-SE
   c. Black blood

4. RVOT SSFP/cine imaging
   a. Center perpendicular to the PV from a transverse (axial) BH image (see Fig. 5-24A, B)
5. SA para axial SSFP/cine of PV
   a. Center parallel and on the PV for an SA image (see Fig. 5-29A, B)
6. PCMR of the PA
   a. Center parallel and 1 in. above the PV from a RVOT image for the PA PCMR
      • VENC is normally 150 to 200 cm per second.
      • Slice or thru plane direction (see Fig. 5-25A, B)

## Arrhythmogenic Right Ventricular Dysplasia Cardiovascular Magnetic Resonance Imaging Protocol

A person suffering from the following indications is most likely to be scheduled for an arrhythmogenic right

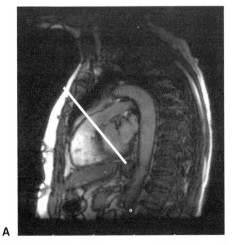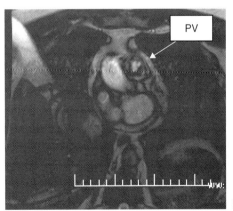

**FIGURE 5-29    A:** Center parallel to the pulmonic valve and on the valve. **B:** Short axis (SA) image of the pulmonary artery (PA) demonstrating the leaflets of the pulmonic valve (PV).

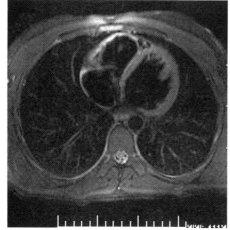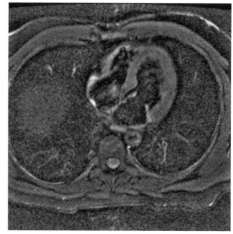

**A**                                                         **B**

**FIGURE 5-30** **A:** Triple inversion recovery suppressing fat along the right ventricle. There appears to be some bright signal around the right ventricle. **B:** Image intensification is used to suppress this signal to make sure it is not fat.

ventricular dysplasia (ARVD) cardiovascular magnetic resonance (CVMR):

1. Heart palpitations
2. Arrhythmias
3. Episodes of ventricular tachycardia

## Sequences Performed

1. Routine three-plane scout as illustrated in Fig. 5-4A–C
2. Two-, three- and four-chamber imaging (SSFP/cine)
   a. White blood imaging
   b. Demonstrates heart function
   c. Always center from a BH image (see Fig. 5-6A–C)
3. DIR-SE transverse (axial) NBH imaging
   a. Start at the top of the PA and terminate at the base of the heart
   b. DIR-SE
   c. Black blood
4. SSFP/Cine transverse (axial) BH imaging
   a. Image the entire heart from PA to the diaphragm
      • 8-mm zero gap at this institution
      • Staring image (see Fig. 5-22)
5. Triple inversion recovery, fast spin echo inversion recovery (FSE-IR), short inversion time inversion recovery (STIR) imaging
   a. Center identical to the SSFP/cine imaging
   b. This sequence suppresses the fat to get a clear look at the RV
   c. Image intensification factor is sometimes used to suppress slow blood flow in the RV. Slow blood flow and fat appear bright on the MRI image and

both these factors need to be suppressed for an accurate diagnosis (see Fig. 5-30A, B).
6. RVOT SSFP/cine imaging
   a. Center perpendicular to the PV from a transverse (axial) BH image (see Fig. 5-24A, B)
7. SA SSFP/cine image
   a. One single slice is obtained to look at function
   b. Centering is from a four-chamber image and at the tip of the MV (see Fig. 5-31A, B)

## Positive ARVD

1. If ARVD is present enhanced imaging is required
2. DHE most likely in the plane with the area of interest

## Right Ventricular Abnormalities

See Figs. 5-32A, B; 5-33A, B

## Pericarditis Cardiovascular Magnetic Resonance Imaging Protocol

A person suffering from the following indications would most likely be scheduled for a CMRI to evaluate the pericardium

1. Retrosternal chest pain
2. Sharp stabbing pain
3. Pain while breathing

## Sequences Performed

1. Routine three-plane scout as illustrated in Fig. 5-4A–C.

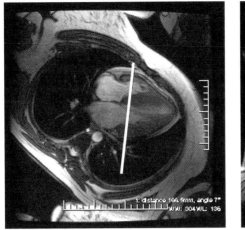
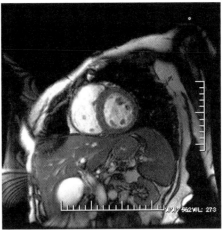

**A**    **B**

**FIGURE 5-31    A:** Center on the tip of the mitral valve. **B:** This will show function of the heart in a short axis (SA) image.

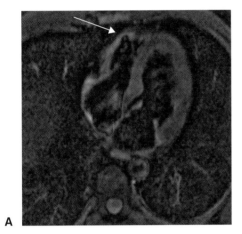
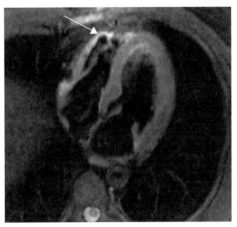

**A**    **B**

**FIGURE 5-32**    Right ventricular abnormalities. **A, B:** There is a thinned mid right ventricle (RV) with aneurysm. A small outpocketing upon contraction. Image **A:** an axial triple inversion recovery (TIR) with image intensification and in **B** an axial TIR image is used to demonstrate this abnormality.

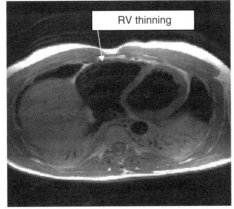
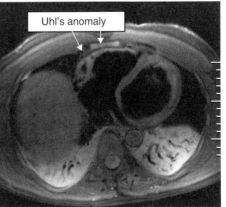

**A**    **B**

**FIGURE 5-33    A, B:** Axial double inversion recovery (DIR) image demonstrates right ventricle (RV) thinning and in **B** using axial triple inversion recovery (TIR) the thinning is also seen. This patient is suffering from UHL's anomaly.

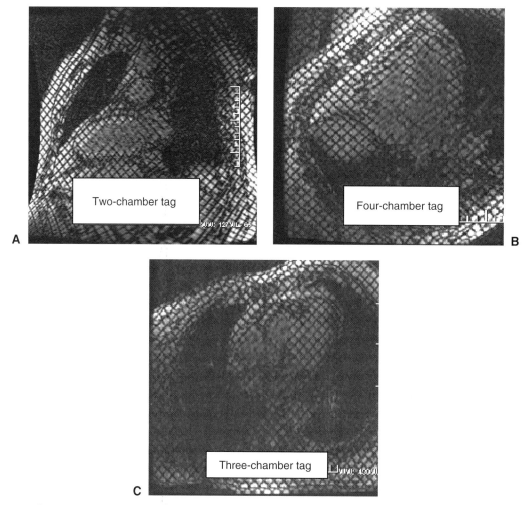

**FIGURE 5-34** **A–C:** Two-, three- and four-chamber tag imaging done to see the how well the pericardium is moving with the heart. This sequence will show constriction and adherence of the pericardium.

2. Two-, three-, and four-chamber imaging (SSFP/cine)
   a. White blood imaging
   b. Demonstrates heart function
   c. Always center from a BH image (see Fig. 5-6A–C)
3. Two-, three-, and four-chamber imaging (GE tag imaging)
   a. Demonstrates how well the pericardium is moving around the heart (see Fig. 5-34A–C)
4. DIR-SE transverse (axial) NBH imaging
   a. Start at the top of the PA and terminate at the base of the heart
   b. DIR-SE
   c. Black blood
5. SSFP/cine and GE tagging SA imaging
   a. Three SA images
      • Do base, mid and apex imaging (see Fig. 5-35A–C; see Fig. 5-36A–C)
      • Utilize both sequences and make sure centering is identical

   b. Transverse SSFP/cine and/or DIR-SE fat saturation or triple inversion recovery (TIR) might also be required

## Pericardial Abnormalities

See Fig. 5-37

## Cardiac or Viability Cardiovascular Magnetic Resonance Imaging Protocol

1. A patient in question with the following condition will most likely undergo a cardiac MRI
   a. Myocarditis
   b. Sarcoidosis
   c. Amyloidosis
2. The following protocol is identical to the viability protocol already explained in the beginning of this chapter. Please review. The only difference is that

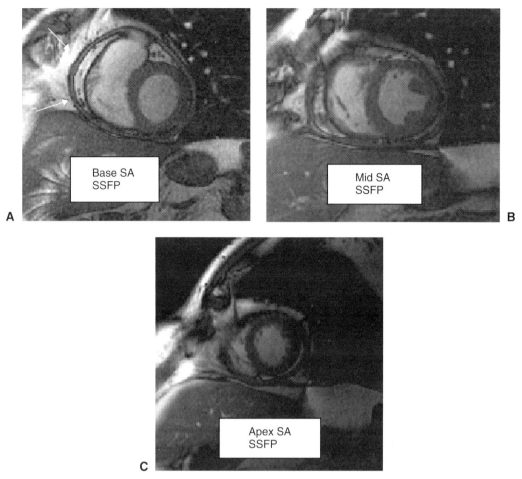

**FIGURE 5-35** **A–C:** Three short axis (SA) steady state free precession (SSFP) images taken at base, mid and apex of the heart. Notice the pericardial thickening in *A*.

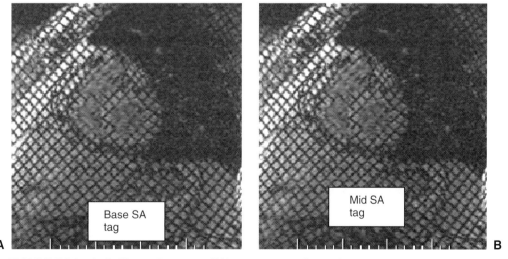

**FIGURE 5-36** **A–C:** Three short axis (SA) tag images taken at base, mid, and apex of the heart. This demonstrates pericardial movement and if any adherence pattern or constriction is present.

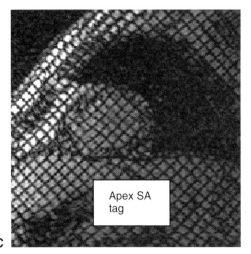

**FIGURE 5-36** (*Continued*)

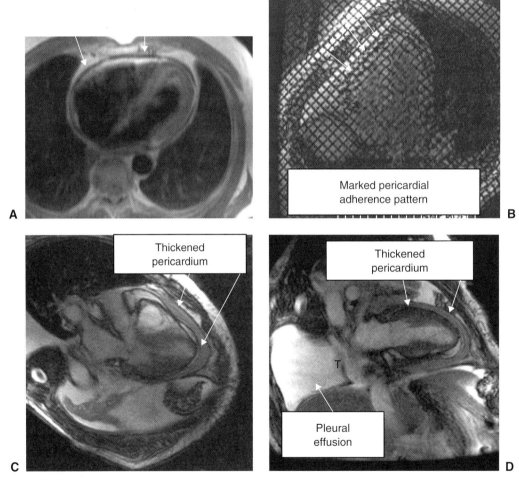

**FIGURE 5-37** **A:** Double inversion recovery (DIR) or black blood sequence demonstrating a thickened pericardium. **B:** A four-chamber tagged gradient echo (GE) image showing an adherence pattern in the right ventricular region. **C:** A three-chamber steady state free precession (SSFP) image showing a large pericardial thickening. **D:** A two-chamber SSFP image also showing pericardial thickening and pleural effusion of the lung.

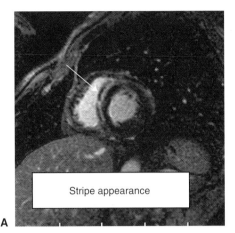
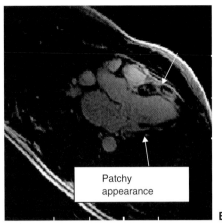

**FIGURE 5-38**    Two images diagnosing myocarditis of the myocardium. In **A:** short axis (SA) delayed hyper enhancement (DHE) image shows a striped enhancement in the septal region of the heart. **B:** The four-chamber DHE image shows a patchy enhancement on the walls of the myocardium. This was biopsied after magnetic resonance imaging (MRI) and was confirmed as giant cell myocarditis.

DHE images are taken 2 minutes' postcontrast instead of 10 minutes.

3. Continual improvements in cardiac MRI are making it easier to diagnose the aforementioned conditions. Until recently, sarcoidosis of the heart could only be diagnosed through biopsy. Also, myocarditis is being imaged well with the use of CMRI. The following images (see Figs. 5-38A, B; 5-39A, B) demonstrate this point very well.

## Thalassemia Cardiovascular Magnetic Resonance Imaging

Thalassemia is a condition whereby the hemoglobin of the blood does not break down properly and can cause increased amounts of iron deposition in the myocardium. A GE sequence, varying the echo time (TE) by every 2 milliseconds, is utilized in determining this condition. At our institution, we use a fast-spoiled gradient-echo imaging (FSPGR) sequence with a flip angle of 20, repetition time (TR) = 26.6, TE = 3.2 − 21.2 increasing by 2 milliseconds for a total of 10 images, matrix $256 \times 128$ and bandwidth 8.06. A series of SA images, centered at the same location, varying the TE are acquired. After the images are acquired, a region of interest (ROI) is placed on the septum, at the region of the right ventricular insertion point (see Fig. 5-40A) and the iron content of the heart is measured related to T2*. The series of images obtained at the range of TE values provides enough information to extract the

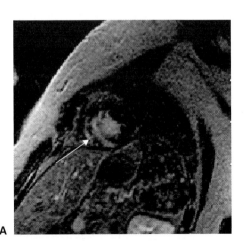
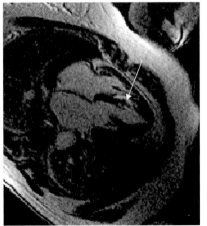

**FIGURE 5-39**    Two images diagnosing sarcoidosis of the heart. **A:** The short axis (SA) delayed hyperenhancement (DHE) image **A** shows hyperenhancement in the septal wall. **B:** The four-chamber image shows hyperenhancement in the anterior wall.

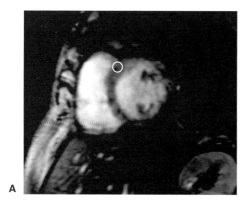

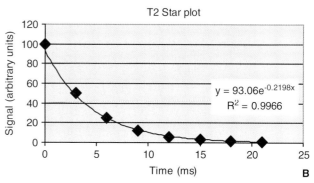

**FIGURE 5-40** **A:** Short axis (fast-spoiled gradient-echo imaging [FSPGR]) demonstrating region of interest (ROI) in quantitating T2* for early detection of iron overload in the myocardium. **B:** The formula describing how signal attenuates due to T2* is: Signal = Constant × e (−Te/T2*).

T2* value. The calculation of T2* can be conduced in the spreadsheet program, Excel. Enter one column of the TE values (in milliseconds) and enter a corresponding column of signal values measured in the myocardium. Use the plot graph feature, selecting the X-Y option, to generate the graph shown in Fig. 5-40B. Select the trend line fitting routine, choosing the exponential fit with the equation and R2 value printed on the graph. The program will plot a fitted line. The R2 value indicates how good the data fit is, with a value close to 1 indicating a good fit. The formula printed on the graph shows that the constant in the equation is 93 and that the T2* has a value of 1/0.2198 millisecond, or 4.5 milliseconds. This technique has proved to be beneficial in predicting iron overload in the heart. A normal cardiac measurement is 52 ± 16 milliseconds.

An abnormal cardiac measurement <20 milliseconds signifies substantial myocardial iron uptake.

## SUMMARY

The novice CMRI technologist is now familiar with positioning and the proper sequences needed to diagnose an abnormality of the heart. The aforementioned protocols are guidelines to get the technologist acquainted with imaging routines. There will be many more protocols that the technologist will learn in the future. I recommend writing a protocol book, and having it at your disposal while imaging patients. This will make imaging go very smoothly in the beginning.

# CHAPTER 6

# Measurement Analysis

June Yamrozik

Many manufacturers have software packages available to analyze the mechanics of the heart. This chapter will show the cardiac magnetic resonance imaging (MRI) technologist how to measure the right ventricle (RV) and left ventricle (LV). The terms *end diastole volume* (EDV), *end systole volume* (ESV), *stroke volume* (SV), *ejection fraction* (EF) will be defined and easily understood. Phase contrast magnetic resonance (PCMR) will be illustrated and provide the technologist with an understanding of how to calculate this data and the type of flow that is being analyzed. A brief description of wall motion and delayed hyperenhancement imaging will be discussed.

## MEASUREMENT ANALYSIS OF THE RIGHT AND LEFT VENTRICLE

Cardiac MRI is one modality that gives accurate measurements of cardiac function. People with cardiomyopathy, congestive heart failure, myocardial infarction, pulmonary hypertension, and arrhythmogenic right ventricular dysphasia (ARVD) will have a cardiac function study done at our institution. Also, cardiac function MRI is sometimes ordered as a comparison to other studies because of its precise results, especially in circumstances for pacemaker placement where an accurate EF is necessary.

## SHORT AXIS PLANE POSITIONING OF THE RIGHT AND LEFT VENTRICLE

### Measuring Short Axis Images of Left Ventricle in Diastole and Systole

A stack of SA images from the base of heart to the apex with an 8-mm slice thickness and zero gap is performed at our institution. This is positioned from a

four-chamber image and is centered parallel to the mitral annulus and perpendicular to the septum as shown in Fig. 6-1. The sequence that is utilized is steady state free precession (SSFP).

After the images are processed, they are analyzed to access heart function. The images are measured from the base of heart to the apex. The starting point is at the mitral valve level of the LV. It is important to exclude the left atrium. The epicardial and endocardial borders of the heart are measured in diastole. Diastole is when the heart is at maximum dilation. It is normally the first phase of the SSFP cine sequence (see Fig. 6-2). The heart also needs to be measured in systole. Systole is when the volume of the heart cavity is squeezed to peak contraction. To locate systole, start with the first image of the heart which is normally diastole and sort

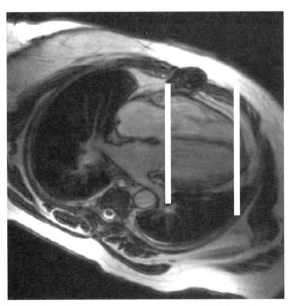

**FIGURE 6-1** Positioning for short axis (SA) function imaging. Center perpendicular to the septum and parallel to the mitral annulus from a four-chamber image.

**FIGURE 6-2** Illustration of a short axis heart in diastole. The outer outline represents the epicardial border and the inner outline represents the systolic border of the left ventricle. Notice that the atrium is excluded from the most basilar slice and is not measured. The epicardial border is measured in the most apical slice and the endocardial blood cavity is not seen and therefore not measured.

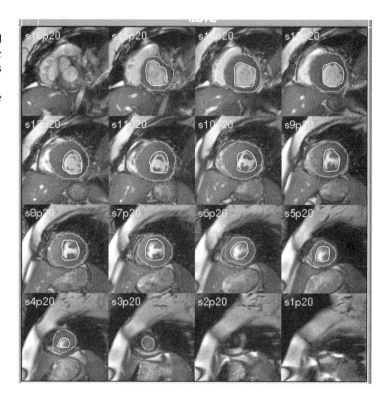

through the images one by one, to watch the heart contract. When the heart is at its maximum contraction the following image will dilate. Measure the endocardial borders of the heart in systole from base to apex (see Fig. 6-3).

## Measuring Right Ventricle from Short Axis Image in Diastole and Systole

Diastole and systole will be the same phases of the heart that were measured on the LV. The RV is difficult to

**FIGURE 6-3** Illustration of a short axis heart in systole. The outlined areas represent the endocardial borders.

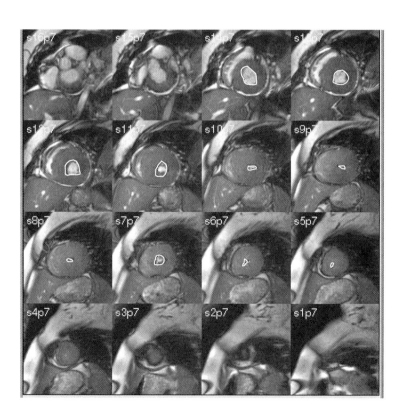

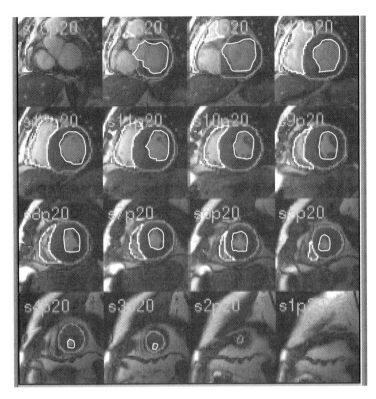

**FIGURE 6-4**  Illustration of a short axis heart in diastole. In addition to the left ventricle (LV) epicardial and endocardial borders, the right ventricle (RV) endocardial border is now outlined. Notice the RV in the most basilar slice; it is arising from the pulmonary artery.

locate on the base image. The right ventricular outflow tract (RVOT) is what to look for on the basilar image. The beginning of the RV will be seen coming off the pulmonary artery (PA) region. Measure the endocardial borders of the RV in diastole. Make sure that the right atrium is excluded (see Fig. 6-4). Measure the endocardial borders of the RV in systole (see Fig. 6-5).

## TRANSVERSE PLANE POSITIONING OF THE RIGHT AND LEFT VENTRICLE

### Measuring Right Ventricle and Left Ventricle in Transverse Plane

Transverse (axial) SSFP images are obtained from the PA to the apex of the heart with an 8-mm slice thickness

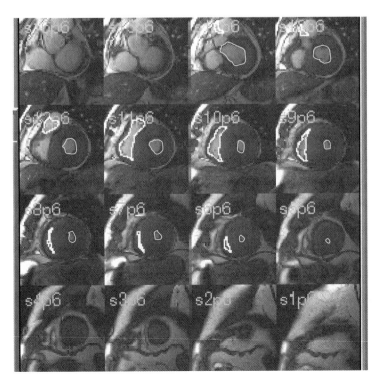

**FIGURE 6-5**  Illustration of short axis heart in systole. The endocardial borders of the right ventricle (RV) and left ventricle (LV) are outlined.

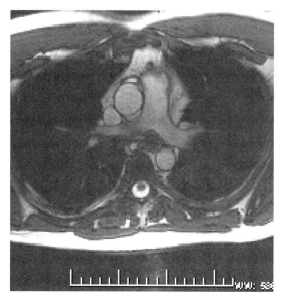

**FIGURE 6-6** Transverse image of the heart staring at the level of the pulmonary artery.

the RV and LV (see Fig. 6-8). The epicardial borders of the RV are not measured routinely at our institution because the myocardium around the RV is much thinner in comparison to the LV. The epicardial borders of the RV are measured on patients with pulmonary hypertension and right-sided heart failure to quantify RV mass.

## Data Analysis of the Right and Left Ventricle

When the measurements are completed the particular software package will calculate the EF, mass, EDV, ESV, and SV. The EF shows how well the heart is pumping during each heart beat. A normal EF is within the range of 55% to 70%. The mass shows the size of the myocardial muscle. EDV demonstrates the amount of blood left in the cavity during dilatation of the heart. ESV demonstrates the amount of blood left in the cavity during contraction of the heart. The SV is determined by taking the amount of blood during dilatation or relaxation of the heart (EDV) and subtracting the amount of blood left in the cavity during contraction (ESV).

*Example:*
120 mL (EDV) − 70 mL (ESV) = 50 mL (SV)

The EF can be calculated by taking the SV and dividing it by the EDV and multiplying by 100.

*Example:*
50 mL (SV)/120 mL (EDV) × 100 = 41.6% (EF)

and zero gap. The starting image is demonstrated in Fig. 6-6. Once again diastole and systolic measurements are performed. Look for the beginning of the RV coming from the PA. Start measuring the LV at the left ventricular outflow tract (LVOT) region. Measure the epicardial and endocardial borders of the LV in diastole. Measure the endocardial borders of the RV in diastole as shown in Fig. 6-7. In systole, measure the endocardial borders of

**FIGURE 6-7** Transverse images of the heart in diastole. The epicardial and endocardial borders of the LV are measured in diastole. The endocardial border of the right ventricle (RV) is measured in diastole.

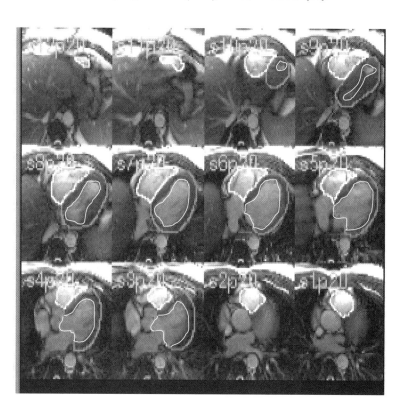

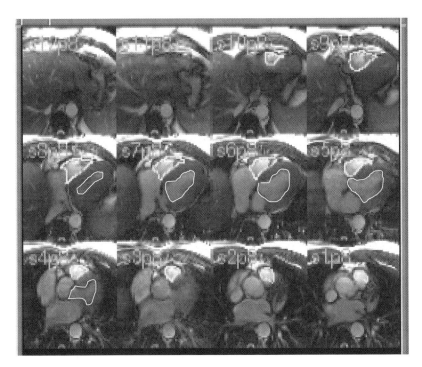

FIGURE 6-8 Transverse images of the heart in systole. The endocardial borders of the right ventricle (RV) and left ventricle (LV) are highlighted.

## PHASE CONTRAST MAGNETIC RESONANCE IMAGING

### Circulation of Blood Flow to the Heart

Let us review the circulation of blood flow to the heart. Deoxygenated blood from the body flows to the right atrium and is pushed through the tricuspid valve. It enters the RV and travels through the pulmonic valve to push blood to the lungs and then to the pulmonary arteries. Oxygenated blood will come in through the pulmonary veins and empty into the left atrium. It will travel through the mitral valve and into the LV and then through the aortic valve to the rest of the body.

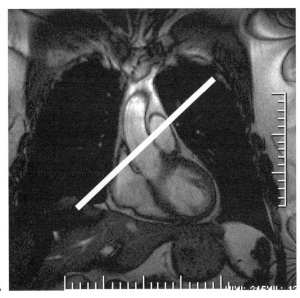
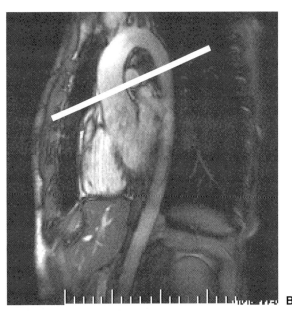

A
B

FIGURE 6-9 **A:** A coronal (left ventricular outflow tract [LVOT]) of the heart. Center parallel and to the tip of the aortic leaflet for the phase contrast magnetic resonance (PCMR) aortic image. **B:** A parasagittal image of the aorta. Center parallel to the pulmonary artery and aorta for the PCMR aortic image.

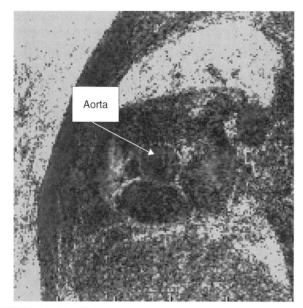

**FIGURE 6-10** Phase contrast magnetic resonance (PCMR) image of the aorta.

PCMR is a means to measure and quantify blood flow. It provides the physician with an estimation of left ventricle flow, stenotic flow, and the ratio of flow in right and left ventricle due to congenital abnormalities. Whenever a scan is ordered to assess aortic, mitral, tricuspid, and pulmonary regurgitation or stenosis, a

PCMR is normally performed. Regurgitation is a condition that occurs when the valves of the heart are not closing properly and is causing backward flow to the heart. Stenosis occurs when the valves of the heart are not opening properly causing blocked forward flow to the heart. Also, in congenital heart disease with conditions such as atrial septal defect (ASD), ventricular septal defect (VSD), and patent ductus arteriosus (PDA) where blood flow deviates from the norm, a PCMR is performed. An ASD occurs when blood flow is communicating between the right and left atrium. A VSD is when blood flow is communicating between both ventricles. A PDA is communication between the aortic and PA.

## Aortic Regurgitation Phase Contrast Magnetic Resonance

Center parallel to the aortic valve from a coronal (LVOT) image. A parasagittal image can also be utilized and center parallel to the aortic valve and PA (see Fig. 6-9A and B). Center one inch above the valve and the velocity encoding factor (VENC) depending on the regurgitation should be in between (250 to 550 cm/second). The higher the regurgitation the higher the VENC. The phase contrast image will look as shown in Fig. 6-10. A morphologic image and a phase contrast image will be acquired (see Fig. 6-11A and B). Normally

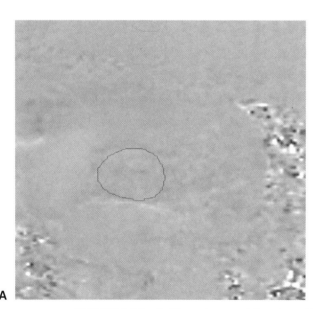

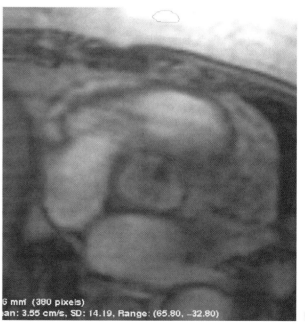

6 mm² (380 pixels)
an: 3.55 cm/s, SD: 14.19, Range: (65.80, -32.80)

A    B

**FIGURE 6-11** **A:** Phase image of the aorta. Normally 40 to 60 phases are acquired and measured as shown by the contour around the aorta. **B:** Morphologic image of the aorta. This image is acquired simultaneously with the phase contrast magnetic resonance (PCMR) sequence. The aorta is best visualized on this view and is the set that is contoured. The contours will also be displayed on the phase set.

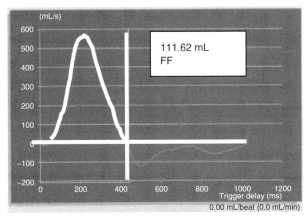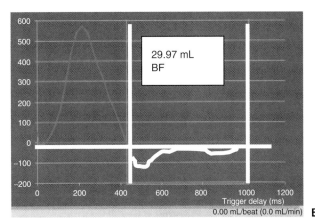

**FIGURE 6-12    A:** The chart illustrating forward flow of the aorta. The white slope illustrates flow from diastole to systole and the number is recorded. For example: 111.62 mL. **B:** The chart illustrating backward flow of the aorta. The flow between the white lines represents the regurgitant flow. Notice it is below the line on the chart. This flow is recorded. To calculate the regurgitant flow, take the amount of regurgitant flow and divide it by the forward flow. For example: 29.97 mL/111.62 mL = 26.8%. FF, forward flow; BF, backward flow.

40 to 60 phases of the aorta are obtained. The data is analyzed by contouring the aorta at each phase. After contouring the aorta, a flow curve is illustrated. Forward flow is the amount of blood flowing out of the aorta and to the rest of the body (see Fig. 6-12A). Backward flow is the amount of blood going back into the LV (see Fig. 6-12B). With this information the amount of regurgitant flow can be calculated. The amount of regurgitation is calculated by taking the backward flow and dividing it by the forward flow and multiplying by 100. As the chart demonstrates, the backward flow is 29.97 mL and the forward flow is 111.62 mL.

*Example:*
29.97 mL/111.62 mL $\times 100 = 26.8\%$

Mild regurgitation is defined as <30%, moderate = 30% to 49%, severe is ≥50%. This patient is suffering from mild regurgitation.

## Aortic Stenosis Phase Contrast Magnetic Resonance

The positioning remains the same as in the previous example; however, we are now quantifying the data to

| Image | Velocity |
|---|---|
| 1 | 200 |
| 2 | 256 |
| 3 | 180 |
| 4 | 200 |
| 5 | 350 |
| 6 | 310 |
| 7 | 360 |
| 8 | 380 |
| 9 | 270 |
| 10 | 260 |
| 11 | 180 |
| 12 | 100 |
| 13 | 70 |

**FIGURE 6-14**   When the peak velocity is selected, the velocity will correlate with the selected image. In this instance image 8 is peak systole. The peak velocity is 380 cm per second or 3.8 mm Hg. From this information, the peak gradient is determined by using the Bernoulli formula:

$$4 \times (\mathbf{PV})^2$$
$$\mathbf{PV} = \mathbf{3.8\,mm\,Hg}$$
$$4 \times (\mathbf{3.8\,mm\,Hg})^2 = \mathbf{57.76\,mm\,Hg}$$

**FIGURE 6-13**   The chart illustrating the systolic peak velocity of the aorta. This is when the heart is in peak contraction.

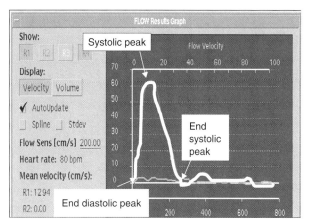

**FIGURE 6-15**   The mean velocity on the aortic flow needs to be calculated. The chart demonstrates the beginning of end diastolic flow and end systolic flow of the heart.

| Image | Velocity |
|---|---|
| 1 | 200 |
| 2 | 256 |
| 3 | 180 |
| 4 | 200 |
| 5 | 350 |
| 6 | 310 |
| 7 | 360 |
| 8 | 380 |
| 9 | 270 |
| 10 | 260 |
| 11 | 180 |
| 12 | 100 |
| 13 | 70 |

**FIGURE 6-16**   All these velocities need to be added and averaged to get the mean flow. In this example, 13 velocities are added and divided by 13. The mean velocity is 2.39 mm Hg. The mean gradient can be determined by using the Bernoulli formula. The mean gradient is 22.84 mm Hg.

look at the velocity of blood flow going out of the aorta. Stenosis is when the valve is not opening properly and is causing blocked forward flow. After contouring the aorta, a report shows the velocities of the heart from end diastole to end systole. First, the systolic peak velocity (PV) is determined (see Fig. 6-13). This is when the heart is in peak contraction. The systolic PV correlates to image 8 of the aortic contours (see Fig. 6-14). The PV is 380 cm per second or 3.8 m per second. Next we calculate the **peak** gradient using the Bernoulli formula. The formula is as follows:

$$\text{Peak gradient} = 4 \times (\text{PV})^2$$
$$\text{PV} = 3.8 \text{ m per second}$$
$$\text{Peak gradient} = 4 \times (3.8)^2 = 57.76 \text{ mm Hg}$$

The peak gradient is 57.76 mm Hg. We then calculate the mean velocity flow. This is done by averaging the numbers from end diastole to end systole (see Fig. 6-15). Image 1 represents end diastole and image 13 represents end systole (see Fig. 6-16). Add all the velocities together and divide by the total number of velocities. In this example, divide by 13. After the data has been calculated, the resultant number is 3116/13 = 239.69 cm per second or 2.39 m per second. Now it is time to calculate the **mean** gradient using the Bernoulli formula:

$$\text{Mean gradient} = 4 \times (\text{PV})^2$$
$$\text{PV} = 2.39 \text{ m per second}$$
$$\text{Mean gradient} = 4 \times (2.39)^2 = 22.84 \text{ mm Hg}$$

Mild stenosis is defined as 0 to 25 mm Hg, moderate 25 to 40 mm Hg, and severe >40 mm Hg. In the aforementioned example, this patient is suffering from mild stenosis.

## Atrial Septal Defect Phase Contrast Magnetic Resonance

This is when blood flow is traversing between the right and left atrium (see Fig. 6-17). A PCMR of the pulmonary and aortic artery needs to be quantified to assess this defect. This will quantify the ratio of blood flow coming in through the PA and exiting through the aorta. The positioning of the aorta remains the same as in the previous two examples (see Fig. 6-18A and B). A PCMR of the PA also needs to be performed. The positioning is as follows: center parallel to the pulmonic valve from a RVOT (coronal) image and center 1 in above the valve (see Fig. 6-19). A morphologic and phase contrast image

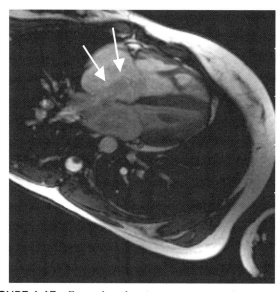

**FIGURE 6-17**   Four-chamber image representing an atrial septal defect (ASD). The white arrows show blood flow between the right and left atrium.

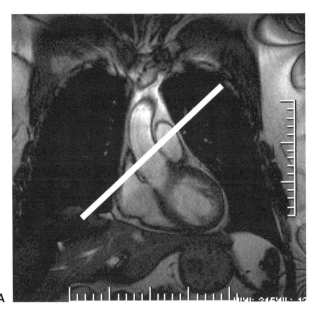

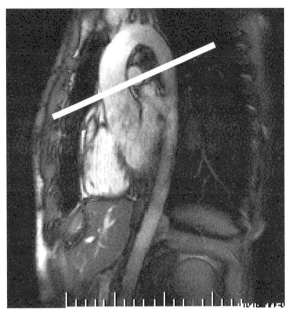

**FIGURE 6-18**   **A:** A coronal (left ventricular outflow tract [LVOT]) of the heart. Center parallel and to the tip of the aortic leaflet for the PCMR aortic image. **B:** A parasagittal image of the aorta. Center parallel to the pulmonary artery and aorta for the phase contrast magnetic resonance (PCMR) aortic image.

will be generated (see Fig. 6-20). Contour both the aorta and PA images which are normally 40 to 60 phases. After the contouring is completed, a flow curve from the data is produced. It is at this time that we can calculate the ratio of blood flow between the right and left ventricle

**FIGURE 6-19**   Center parallel to the pulmonic valve from a right ventricular outflow tract ([RVOT]) image and center 1 in above the valve.

(see Fig. 6-21A and B). To quantify the defect, take the PA flow and divide it by the aortic flow.

$$85.91 \text{ mL}/52.70 \text{ mL} = \text{QP} : \text{QS} = 1.63 : 1$$

The information calculated will determine the ratio of pulmonary arterial flow to systemic flow, which is referred to as the QP:QS ratio. The QP:QS ratio in this example is 1.63:1. In this instance, there is more blood flow in the right side of the heart indicating a left-to-right shunt. This patient is suffering from a moderate ASD. The following is a list of QP:QS ratios.

1 = Normal
1 to 1.5 = Mild
1.5 to 2 = Moderate
2+ = Severe

## TISSUE TAGGING WALL MOTION ANALYSIS

Tissue tagging is a means to measure the motion of the myocardial wall. Radio frequency grid lines are placed over the heart to evaluate the strain of the myocardium. Using 1D and 3D tag analysis, myocardial wall motion can be analyzed (see Fig. 6-22). An entire stack of SA tagged images starting from the base of heart of 8-mm slice thickness and zero gap are acquired. Images are analyzed from base of heart excluding aortic root to the apex of heart where myocardium is still visible. The

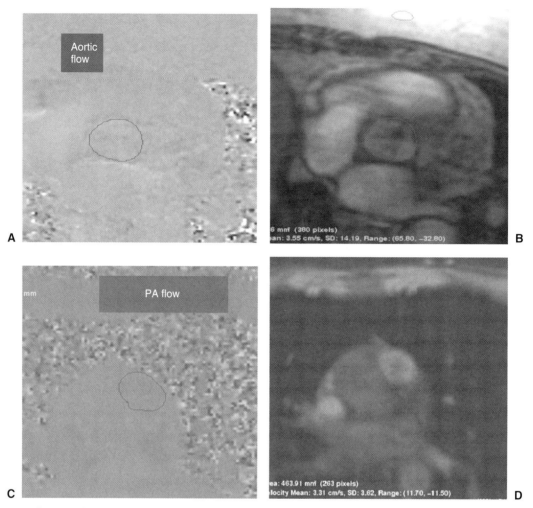

**FIGURE 6-20** **A–D:** Phase and morphologic images of the aorta and pulmonary artery. The aorta and pulmonary artery are contoured.

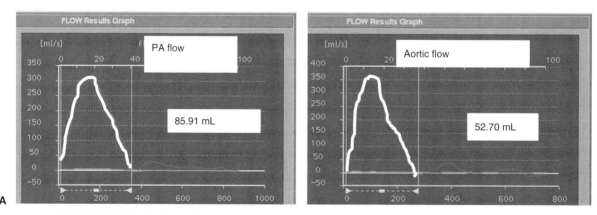

**FIGURE 6-21** **A:** Chart illustrating pulmonary artery flow or can be stated as forward flow of the pulmonary artery. The flow is calculated as 85.91 mL. **B:** Chart illustrating aortic flow or can be stated as forward flow of the aorta. The flow is calculated as 52.70 mL. The defect is calculated by taking the pulmonary artery (PA) flow and dividing it by the aortic flow. In this example, 85.91 mL/52.70 mL, the ratio of pulmonary arterial flow to systemic flow can be calculated. It is referred to as the QP:QS ratio, which is 1:63 to 1. This patient has a left-to-right shunt with a moderate atrial septal defect (ASD).

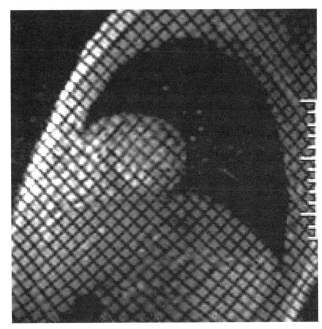

**FIGURE 6-22**  Short axis tag imaging of the heart. The grid lines are placed over the heart to illustrate the wall motion of the heart.

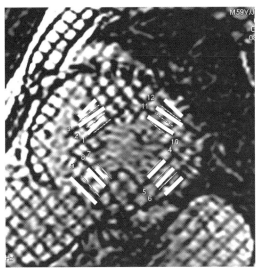

**FIGURE 6-24**  One-dimensional (1D) data analysis measuring the epi-, mid-, and endocardial borders of the LV acquired in a short axis view. The septal, anterior, inferior, and lateral segments of the heart are measured. This is a very tedious and time-consuming process.

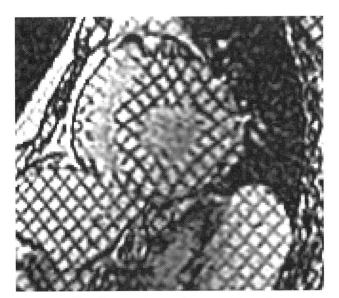

**FIGURE 6-23**  Short axis tagged image of heart in systole. The deformation and the strain of the grid tag lines are best defined in systole.

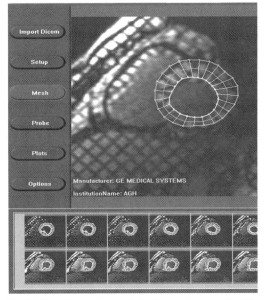

**FIGURE 6-25**  3D analysis of the heart in systole. The epicardial and endocardial borders of the LV are measured in systole. The software program measures all the phases of the LV to analyze the myocardial strain.

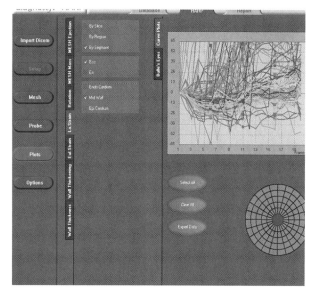

**FIGURE 6-26** The results are illustrated on the chart and analyzed to determine the strain.

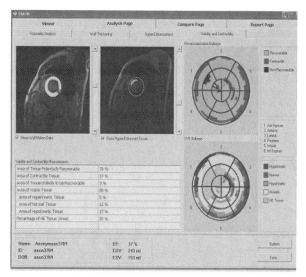

**FIGURE 6-28** In the uppermost left image, the large area highlighted is demonstrating kinetic tissue of the myocardium and the small area highlighted is normal tissue. The next image demonstrates an infarct.

data is analyzed in systole, when the heart is in peak contraction and when the deformations of the grid lines are best demonstrated (see Fig. 6-23). Until recently, without any software programs at our disposal this information was measured using 1D analysis.

Each segment of the LV in systole (septal, anterior, lateral, and inferior) is measured in endo-, mid-, and epicardial borders (see Fig. 6-24). This is a time-consuming process but once the data is gathered, the motion and strain of the LV is determined. A 3D analysis of the heart is a much easier and faster method. HARP (harmonic phase) is a software program that we have been utilizing at our research center. The measuring is less tedious as well as less time consuming. The

epicardial and endocardial border of the LV is measured in systole (see Fig. 6-25). The results are displayed and reviewed to determine the strain of the myocardium (see Fig. 6-26).

## DELAYED HYPERENHANCEMENT ANALYSIS

This software program can measure the percentage of infracted myocardial tissue (see Fig. 6-27). Wall motion abnormalities can also be deciphered utilizing this software (see Fig. 6-28). New software programs are

**FIGURE 6-27** Delayed hyperenhancement region highlighting an infarct.

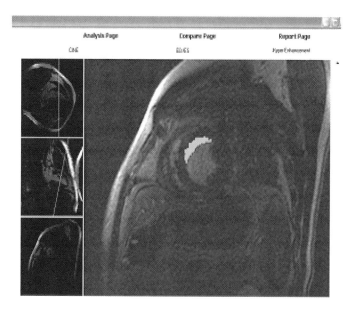

being developed to help understand the dynamics of cardiac MRI imaging.

## SUMMARY

The cardiac MRI technologist is now familiar with a basic understanding of how to measure a heart for cardiac function. The terms *end diastolic volume* (EDV), *end systolic volume* (ESV), *stroke volume* (SV), and *ejection fraction* (EF) will become a part of the technologist's everyday jargon. The application and usage of phase contrast magnetic resonance (PCMR) should be understood. Also, there are several programs available to concentrate on the mechanics of cardiac function.

# CHAPTER 7

# Cardiovascular Anatomy

Robert W. W. Biederman

Innumerable textbooks have been solely devoted to dissertations on cardiac anatomy over the centuries. Most of these have focused on practical, autopsy-based anatomy with few depicting image-based, non-autopsy or pragmatic clinical anatomy. The natural question that one may ask is, "What is the difference? Why does it matter?" The answer is that the difference becomes clinically relevant when the anatomic features that are visible on images approach or exceed those observable to the naked eye at autopsy or in the surgical suite. Is it possible that the evaluation of closed-chest cardiovascular anatomic features could actually be seen with better clarity and precision than when the postmortem body is explored or view directly on the operating table? Investigations by us and others suggest that the answer to that question is, "Yes". Specifically, many features of the heart are visible in the beating, contracting state that are paradoxically masked when the heart stops. When the heart finally stops beating, upon natural death or arrested for surgical purposes, rather then stopping at an arbitrary point in the cardiac cycle, the heart ceases beating when calcium cycling terminates, resulting in massive calcium overload and frank tetanus, and obligatorily ending the cardiac cycle in *systole*. Therefore, the heart stops in the contractile state, in fact in a *massive* state of hypercontraction with resultant emptying of most of the ventricular volume such that, when combined with the extreme vasodilatory state, due to absent venous return, the heart is at a markedly unnaturally small and shrunken state. This results in rigorous retraction of the otherwise subtle but important anatomic features, such as the valvular/papillary muscle relationship, trabeculae carnae, as well as deflation of the venous and arterial system, with subsequent distortion of the relative relationships of the normal cardiac structures to each other.

The cardinal notion here then is that cardiovascular magnetic resonance (CMR), with its high spatial resolution and modest temporal resolution, permits imaging in the *normal*, unadulterated state, permitting a more realistic and "natural state" assessment, often portraying features of the left ventricle (LV) not recognized by the pathologist or the surgeon. In this chapter, details of the cardiac and related cardiovascular anatomy will be delineated; their relations in the normal state will be illustrated and presented in standard CMR imaging planes.

In general, imaging in our hands starts with a series of multislice transverse axial acquisitions, obtained in either the double inversion recovery sequence or a steady state free precession (SSFP) sequence. In the following figures, CMR images will be demonstrated in the SSFP sequence, with the moving anatomy viewable in the accompanying digital video disc (DVD). The motion during the natural cardiac cycle often helps to define the interrelationships based on an anatomicophysiologic basis. Figures 7-1 to 7-5 display the multislice axial transverse acquisitions from the great vessels through to the diaphragm; Figs. 7-6, 7-7 show coronal anatomy; Figs. 7-8, 7-9 show parasagittal views; Figs. 7-10, 7-11 show short axis views. Figures 7-12, 7-13, and 7-14 are two-chamber, three-chamber, and four-chamber views, respectively, with Fig. 7-15 showing the paraxial aortic valve (AV) view. Here, descriptions and discussions of integral anatomic segments of the heart and vascular and there interrelations are presented, generally without specific reference to any particular view. Table 7-1 gives an explanation of abbreviations used in text and figures.

## CARDIAC ANATOMY

The heart is considered to have three segments: the atria, ventricles, and the great vessels. The atria and ventricles are each partitioned into two compartments, the left and right sides, with two atrioventricular valves that connect the respective ventricle to the atria and the semilunar valves that connect the great vessels to the ventricles.

The heart is a central mediastinal organ that lies generally in the left chest and aligned with the long axis

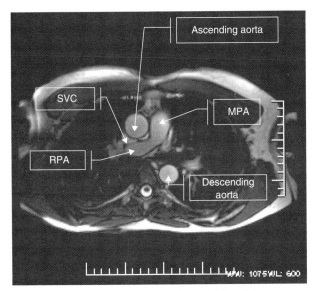

**FIGURE 7-1**  Transverse image (see Table 7-1 for abbreviations).

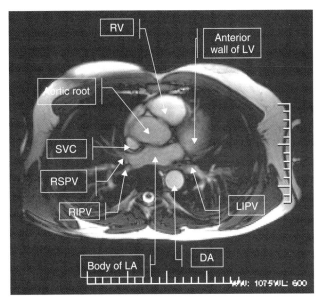

**FIGURE 7-3**  Transverse image (see Table 7-1 for abbreviations).

traveling from the posterior right shoulder to the left nipple, as related to the sagittal plane of the body. This is the standard position, defined as normal or levocardia. Infrequently, the heart is in the opposite chest, with a mirror image denoted as dextrocardia. An even rarer finding is that of mesoposition, where the heart occupies the midline position.

## SIDEDEDNESS

In healthy individuals, the cardiovascular, gastrointestinal, and respiratory organs are asymmetric such that

sidedness occurs. The cardiovascular side is defined by the position of the morphologic right atrium. This is determined specifically by the size and shape of the right atrial appendage. Importantly, it is not decided by position of the LV, ventricular apices, relationship of the great arteries, or more importantly, by the particular side that the gastrointestinal or respiratory system occupies. Similarly, definitions of sidedness for the pulmonary and gastrointestinal system can be defined by the relationship of the lungs to the liver/inferior vena cava system. Sidedness has many variants: situs solitus is normal as described in the preceding text,

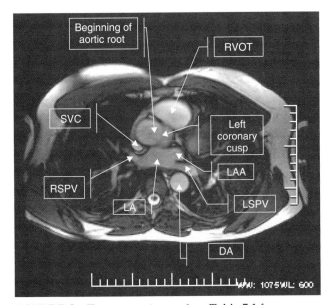

**FIGURE 7-2**  Transverse image (see Table 7-1 for abbreviations).

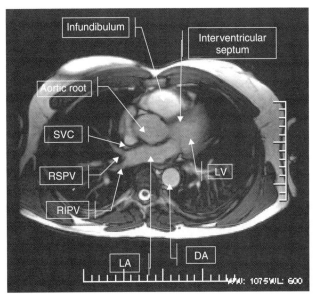

**FIGURE 7-4**  Transverse image (see Table 7-1 for abbreviations).

**FIGURE 7-5** Transverse image (see Table 7-1 for abbreviations).

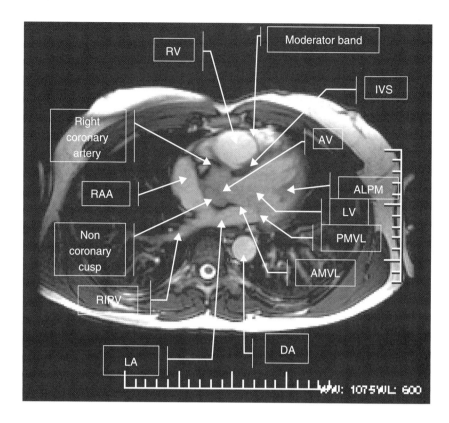

whereas situs inversus is the mirror image of the entire mediastinal respiratory and gastrointestinal system. Situs isomeric defines a more symmetric pattern with situs indeterminate and situs ambiguous defining less clear relationships of the three systems to each other. Finally, right isomerism is when there is bilateral right-sided symmetry and left isomerism is when there is bilateral left-sided symmetry. In the former, there is a bilateral morphologic right atria (two) while the spleen is absent, known as *asplenia syndrome*.

## ATRIA

An understanding of the morphologic features of the right and left atria in healthy individuals is critical. While seemingly mundane, a well-founded anatomic understanding in healthy individuals is essential to allow insight into pathologic states, especially in congenital heart disease. The right atrium has small–to–absent pectinate muscles and, as a large tricorn appendage, receives the superior and inferior vena cava, as well as the coronary sinus. An important feature, helping to define the right atrium, is a subtle projection from the inside of the right atrium called the *crista terminalis*. The projection of this feature as viewed from the pericardial side is the *sulcus terminalis*. The morphologic left atrium is smaller than the right, has slightly thicker walls, and has a windsocklike appendage with larger pectinate muscles. There is no *crista terminalis*

and the body of the left atrium receives the four pulmonary veins. The left atrium has a septum primum, whereas the right atrium has the septum secundum, which forms the interatrial septum. Not seen by current imaging techniques, are the foramina venarium minima, which are small venous openings returning venous flow directly from the cardiac muscle. The right atrium is superior and rightward to the heart. The entrance to the right atrium can be traced from three pathways: superior vena cava (SVC) (superior), inferior vena cava (inferior), and the coronary sinus (located inferior and posterior and below the floor of the left atrium). A fourth entrance is through the tricuspid valve. Entrance into the left atria, however, is through the four pulmonary veins, which are normally located as two right (upper and lower) and two left (upper and lower). The position and number of pulmonary veins can vary considerably from four, and the appearance on images is quite variable. In patients referred for pulmonary vein isolation, we and others have described as many as seven veins and as few as two. Frequently, the pulmonary veins do not lie in a superior–inferior direction, but enter the body of the atrium in one plane, making it difficult for an electrophysiologist to locate the anatomic variants. A considerable amount of variability is sometimes not recognized, and therefore not reported. Especially, when more than four pulmonary veins are identified, one can imagine the difficulty encountered when the electrophysiologist isolates the first four pulmonary veins and,

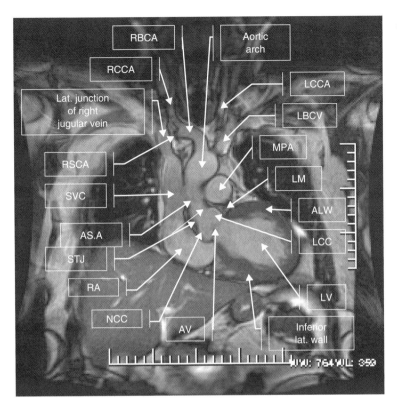

**FIGURE 7-6** Coronal image (see Table 7-1 for abbreviations).

unknown to him, there are several more. CMR has a unique ability to define these anatomic variants and relate them in space using SSFP or three-dimensional magnetic resonance angiography (MRA) reconstruction techniques.

## VENTRICLES

### Right Ventricle

The right ventricle (RV) receives the deoxygenated blood of the superior and inferior vena cava, as well as deoxygenated coronary blood flow from the coronary sinus and the small Thebesian veins, which drain from the right ventricular myocardium directly into the right ventricular chamber. Anterior to the RV is the pericardium and sternum, whereas inferiorly is the diaphragm, to the left and posteriorly is the ventricular septum. The RV is essentially crescent shaped and consists of three parts: the inflow, outflow, and body. The outflow portion known as the *infundibulum* is a tubular-shaped channel that leads to the pulmonary valve. A thick muscular ridge called the supraventricular crest separates the pulmonary and tricuspid orifices. Trabeculae carnae are rounded and irregular projections that arise from the body of the RV and are embryologically remnants from the mesocardium, whose purpose is somewhat ambiguous. Some authors believe that they may be helpful in redirecting flow in an efficient manner from the inflow to the RV body and into the outflow infundibulum. Others believe, including us, that they aid in a more efficient contractile and ejection patterns to exclude blood. The pattern of myocardial fiber orientation is less mechanically effectively organized in the RV compared to the LV. The ultimate trabeculae carnae are the papillary muscles, which are attached to chordae tendonae, which parachute out towards the tricuspid valve. The RV, as compared to the LV, is recognized by its morphology, with a moderator band, which houses the right bundle branch electrical conduction system for the right ventricular free wall. In many hearts a septal–parietal band is present, which houses the origination of the papillary muscles, as opposed to arising off the floor of the right ventricular apex. The RV is well seen on transverse axial slices, whereas sagittal view depicts the inlet and outlet portions in relation to the infundibulum and pulmonic valve exceptionally well, and the traditional four-chamber view, which demonstrates the right ventricular free wall and body, and papillary muscle structure which is orthogonal to the plane of the tricuspid valve. For three-dimensional volumetric analysis, the short axis slices depict the RV in the most anatomically and favorable manner for contouring. At the inlet or outlet segments, as the tricuspid valve is approached, the RV appears as a blunted crescent, becoming thinner as the apex is approached. The normal thickness for the RV free wall is highly variable, being thickest at the base and tapering

**FIGURE 7-7** Coronal image (see Table 7-1 for abbreviations).

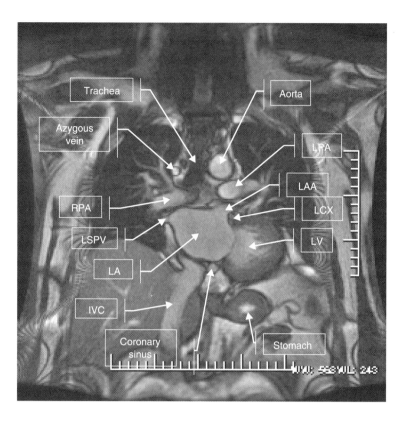

gradually and irregularly (due to the trabecular pattern). In general, the RV should not be thicker than 3.5 mm.

## Left Ventricle

The LV is the main pumping chamber for the body. It is a larger and thicker-walled chamber than the RV and possesses the geometric configuration that approximates to a prolate ellipse of rotation. It forms the major portion of the left surface of the heart. The mitral valve is behind and to the left of the aortic semilunar valve. Interestingly, despite the LV being at least 50% larger than the RV, the mitral valve is 50% smaller in surface area than the tricuspid valve. Presumably, teleologically, this is due to the more efficient diastolic filling from the left, as opposed to the right atrioventricular valve into the respective ventricular chamber. The LV has a small outflow tract, as opposed to the aforementioned muscular right ventricular outflow tract. The LV contains a fibrous aortic vestibule leading into the semilunar AV. The mitral annulus is in continuity with the fibroannular skeleton through a fibrous connection known as the *central fibrous body* that can occasionally be seen on a modified parasagittal view, where the infundibulum is well seen in connection with the main pulmonary artery trunk and sinus of Valsalva. As with the supraventricularis crest, the inflow and outflow of the LV is separated by a thin subaortic curtain,

which forms a rather acute angle between them. This central fibrous body is thin and mobile, and this flexibility is presumably to allow alterations in the shape of the mitral annulus during cardiac contraction, permitting optimization and regulation of valve motion with subsequently more efficient blood flow. There are two large papillary muscles—the inferior-medial, which arises from the more diaphragmatic sternal-costal surface, and a posterior-lateral, which is derived from the more lateral wall. As intimated in the opening paragraph, CMR depicts these muscles, not as arising from the floor of the LV apex as a solid muscle, but as fingerlike roots that gradually coalesce to form the solid papillary muscle that we classically know from autopsy and surgery. We have termed this lacylike projection the *cypress root* formation. Only during native contraction in a relaxed state are the cypress root formations visible, and then only with high-fidelity imaging such as CMR, and in some cases computed tomography (CT). It should be noted that, often, papillary muscles have bifed or even trifed heads. More importantly, the chorda tendonae that are derived from the muscle, typically spread not only to the ipsilateral mitral leaflet, but send important and prominent chordae tendonae to the contralateral leaflet. Rarely, there is just one papillary muscle supplying both mitral leaflets, and this is termed a *parachute mitral valve.*

As in the RV, the LV is defined by (a) an inlet portion containing the mitral apparatus, (b) the trabecular zone,

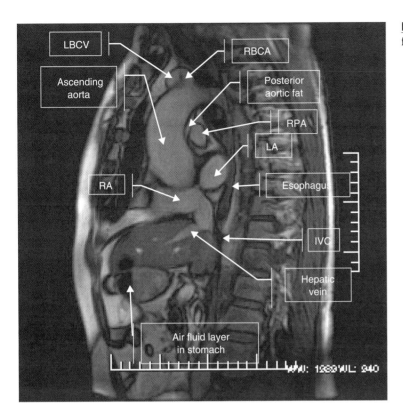

**FIGURE 7-8** Parasagittal image (see Table 7-1 for abbreviations).

which is the body of the LV, and (c) the outflow as described earlier. It should be noted that the morphologic LV has a much finer trabecular pattern than the RV. It does not have a moderator band, in that the left ventricular electrical communication is through the ventricular septum, which is the bundle of His and Purkinge fibrous system, forming the left bundle branch system. Again, as opposed to the RV, the right bundle branch is visualized as a moderator band, whereas the left bundle system is buried within the ventricular septum and invisible by standard CMR techniques.

Assessment of the LV, as in the RV can be obtained in multiple common projections. Transverse-axials give the relationship to the remainder of the cardiac and cardiovascular structures, while the two- and four-chamber views depict the left relationship to the atria and adjacent RV and septum, respectively. This classical two-chamber view shows the LV as a V-shaped structure, orthogonal to the mitral valve apparatus, with the left atrial appendage seen anterior to the left upper pulmonary vein. Specifically in this projection, the fibrous connection of the posterior wall of the left atrial appendage, serving as the anterior wall of the left upper pulmonary vein, is well appreciated and is sometimes called the *Q-tip sign* as popularized in transesophageal echocardiography. As for the RV, short axis projections are used to assess function in conjunction with endocardial and epicardial contouring. A standard three-chamber view,

analogous to the parasternal long axis in transthoracic echocardiography, depicts the anterior septum and the posterior wall, and elegantly depicts the anterior mitral leaflet (A2) and posterior mitral scallop (P2).

The AV is similar to the pulmonary valve and consists of three semicircular collagen scallops. Similar to the pulmonic valve, there is an aortic sinus; however, it is named the *sinus of Valsalva*. It should be noted that the pulmonic valve possesses a sinotubular junction and has an unnamed sinus. This is important because the LV classically possesses a prominent sinotubular junction above the AV, which is well recognized, while a similar anatomic structure above the pulmonic valve can be occasionally misinterpreted as the supravalvar pulmonic stenosis. The AV cusps are symmetrically and equilaterally placed at 120 degrees from each other, helping to classify the presence of a bicuspid AV by the absence of this symmetric geometric relation. Although a pseudoraphe may be present, and appears to be a nearly normal trileaflet, failure to detect the 120-degree structures helps to clarify pathologic from the normal AV. The AV has three cusps: noncoronary cusp; left cusp, which houses the left main artery; and the anterior or right coronary artery cusp. The right coronary artery typically comes off higher than the left coronary artery from the respective sinuses. During diastole, the closed AV maintains structural integrity, such that it supports a column of relatively stationary blood at high pressure. As left ventricular–developed pressure climbs

**TABLE 7-1**

List of Abbreviations Used in Text and Figures

| Abbreviation | Explanation |
|---|---|
| ALPM | Anterior lateral papillary muscle |
| ALW | Anterior lateral wall of left ventricle |
| AMPM | Anterior medial papillary muscle |
| AMVL | Anterior mitral valve leaflet |
| ASA | Ascending Aorta |
| ASW | Anterior septal wall |
| AV | Aortic valve |
| DA | Descending aorta |
| ILW | Inferior lateral wall of left ventricle |
| IVC | Inferior vena cava |
| IVS | Interventricular septum |
| LA | Left atrium |
| LAA | Left atrial appendage |
| LAD | Left anterior descending |
| LBCA | Left brachiocephalic artery |
| LBCV | Left brachiocephalic vein |
| LCCA | Left common carotid artery |
| LCC | Left coronary cusp |
| LCX | Left circumflex |
| LIPV | Left inferior pulmonary vein |
| LM | Left main coronary |
| LPA | Left pulmonary artery |
| LSPV | Left superior pulmonary vein |
| LSCA | Left subclavian artery |
| LV | Left ventricle |
| LVOT | Left ventricular outflow tract |
| MPA | Main pulmonary artery |
| MV | Mitral valve |
| NCC | Noncoronary cusp |
| PV | Pulmonic valve |
| PLPM | Posterior lateral papillary muscle |
| PMPM | Posterior medial papillary muscle |
| PMVL | Posterior mitral valve leaflet |
| PW | Posterior wall |
| RA | Right atrium |
| RAA | Right atrial appendage |
| RBCA | Right brachiocephalic artery |
| RCA | Right coronary artery |
| RCC | Right coronary cusp |
| RCCA | Right common carotid artery |
| RIPV | Right inferior pulmonary vein |
| RPA | Right pulmonary artery |
| RSCA | Right subclavian artery |
| RSPV | Right superior pulmonary vein |
| RVOT | Right ventricular outflow tract |
| RV | Right ventricle |
| SMA | Superior mesenteric artery |
| STJ | Sinotubular junction |
| SVC | Superior vena cava |
| TV | Tricuspid valve |

during systole, the AV opens. Because there is differential collagen deposition, leading to varying elasticity, the sinus wall closest to the aortic root is virtually inelastic, whereas the most superior portion is more compliant and can increase in radius by upwards of 20%. Therefore, the AV commissures as they move apart, allows the aortic orifice to become triangular and the cusps assume a straight line between the three commissures. Importantly, during systole the leaflets open into, but do not touch, the sinuses. This natural protection serves as a gentle "cove" to shield high-pressure systolic blood flow during high systolic pressure, but shepherd diastolic coronary blood flow under relatively low pressures. It should be noted that CMR has helped to clarify the perception that *all* coronary blood flow occurs during diastole. Phase velocity mapping has demonstrated that predominantly, flow (80%) occurs during diastole for the LV, but flow is near symmetric for the RV, with 50% occurring during diastole and 50% during systole. Understanding hemodynamics of the right ventricular filling properties, having relatively low pressure during systole, as opposed to the higher LV transmyocardial pressures, helps to reconcile this observation.

## ATRIOVENTRICULAR SEPTUM

The atrioventricular septum is a muscular structure that divides the left and right atria as described earlier. A left septum is formed embryologically from the septum primum, while the right is formed embryologically from the septum secundum. Between the two is a small opening that forms, on occasion caudally, which is a patent foramen ovale, seen in upwards of 25% of the normal population. The inferior edge of this is known as the *limbus* of fossa ovalis. Portions of the septum interdigitate with the smooth-walled sinus venarium (venosus) as opposed to the more trabeculated, older portion of the right atrium. The limbus of this fossa ovalis is a muscular ridge, embryologically derived from septum secundum, which may be seen as a depression in the fossa ovalis. As the right atrioventricular valve is slightly apically displaced relative to the left interventricular valve, an underappreciated common inner atrial ventricular septum is formed. In this structure there is potential for a small defect (<0.8 cm) allowing blood to travel from the LV directly to the right atrium. This author has never seen this defect, but it has been described as a "mythical" Garbodie defect. SSFP images are ideal for defining the atrial septum, and are far preferred over double inversion recovery sequences, which due to through-plane motion and partial volume defects, might cause dropout of this structure and erroneous labeling of an atrial septal defect.

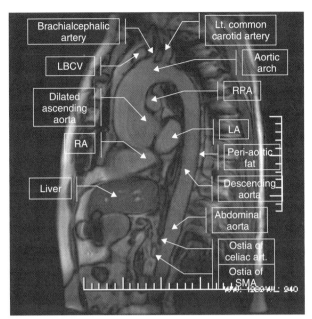

**FIGURE 7-9**    Parasagittal image (see Table 7-1 for abbreviations).

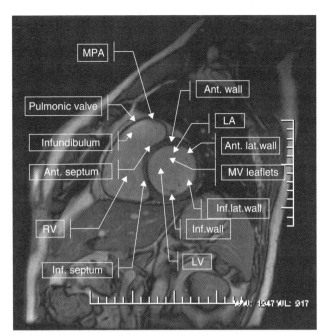

**FIGURE 7-10**    Short axis image (see Table 7-1 for abbreviations).

## INTERVENTRICULAR SEPTUM

The interventricular septum is defined as having the anterior muscular wall formed by Raffe fibers from the RV and discrete left ventricular fibers, forming a common muscle. Occasionally, the distinction between the right and left derived fibers can be seen by CMR as a discrete line known as the *linea alba*, as defined by echocardiography. The interventricular septum has three parts: (a) a perimembranous segment, which forms a thin fibrous junction at the anterior and right cusp of the AV; (b) a thick muscular segment; and (c) a small apical segment. Importantly, the most superior perimembranous septum is partly continuous with the fibrous infrastructure and fibrous-annular skeleton of the anterior and right aortic cusps. Defects in the most superior right portion of the septum cause a relatively rare atrial septal defect called a supracristal defect and cause structural loss of integrity of that portion of the septum or root structure, resulting in asymmetric aortic regurgitation, typically from the noncoronary cusp as that portion of the septum travels rightward and posterior. This is usually an indication for aortic root or valve repair independent of the degree of aortic regurgitation.

## PERICARDIUM

The pericardium encircles and closes the heart and the superior portions of the great vessels. It travels posteriorly to encircle the first several centimeters of the pulmonary veins, leading to a small posterior space behind the body of the left atrium. The fibers of the pericardium then pass to the central tendon into a small portion of the falciform ligament of the diaphragm. Pericardial fibers anchor the heart to the thoracic cavity and retain the heart in its proper location within the chest. Anteriorly, the heart generally does not approach the sternum, but is separated by the left lungs, especially inferiorly. The pericardium travels further in the cephalad direction to drape over the SVC right, and then inferiorly, toward the inferior vena cava whereas the latter is only minimally covered by the pericardial fibers. The pericardium is classically divided into the visceral and parietal pericardium, with the former being several cells thick, and is indistinguishable with the epicardial endothelial layer on CMR. The parietal pericardium is the fibrous sac that envelops the heart. Generally, <5 mL of serous fluid is present, and in most cases, this is detectable by CMR, especially using high-resolution SSFP imaging. It should be noted that variable amounts of epicardial fat are present along the epicardial layer and essentially obliterate and/or make negligible, the visceral pericardium. Additionally, substantial amounts of pericardial fat are also present. Both myocardium and fat, as well as pericardium and fat can be distinguished through the use of SSFP and double inversion or triple inversion recovery sequences. The pattern of epicardial fat is important. Generally, the largest amount of fat is at the base of the ventricles and chiefly occupies the right ventricular free basal wall. Specifically, the coronaries in the AV groove travel in a bed of fat, as does the left anterior descending artery, which travels in a small depression along the interventricular

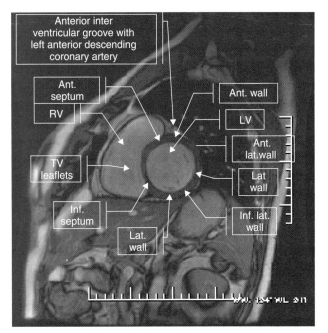

**FIGURE 7-11** Short axis image (see Table 7-1 for abbreviations).

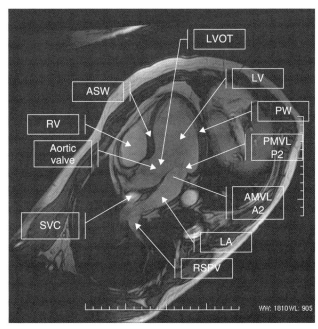

**FIGURE 7-13** Three-chamber image (see Table 7-1 for abbreviations).

septum known as the *intraventricular sulcus*. A posterior ventricular sulcus, less well described, houses the posterior descending artery branch from the right coronary artery, and also travels in a smaller bed of fat. Generally, fat dissipates as the apex is approached, becoming more prominent again at the apex proper. The basal lateral posterior wall is often devoid of fat.

This pattern appears not to be coincidental in that, teleologically, one can presume that the anterior right ventricular fat bed protects the heart against friction from the anterior structures such as the sternum, whereas the lateral and posterior wall, less subject to frictional forces from immovable structures, needs no such protection.

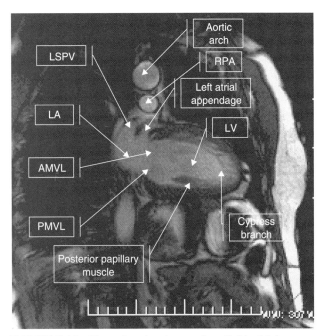

**FIGURE 7-12** Two-chamber image (see Table 7-1 for abbreviations).

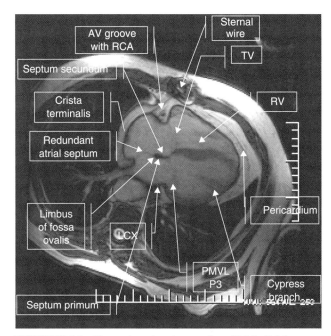

**FIGURE 7-14** Four-chamber image (see Table 7-1 for abbreviations).

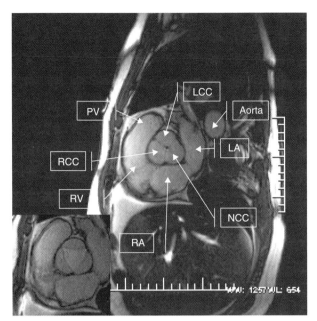

**FIGURE 7-15** Para-axial aortic valve with valve closed, and valve open in inset (see Table 7-1 for abbreviations).

## THE GREAT VESSELS

The pulmonary artery arises posteriorly to the aorta in healthy individuals and travels superiorly and posteriorly. The aorta originates from the LV in healthy individuals and courses superiorly and then slightly anteriorly towards the right, forming the proximal portion of the ascending aorta. The aortic arch is defined not by the most transverse segment of the aorta, but by the abrupt takeoff of the right brachiocephalic artery, which then divides to form the right common carotid artery and the right subclavian artery. Next, slightly rightward, and slightly posterior, is the left common carotid artery, followed in a similar manner by the right subclavian artery. In 1% to 3% of the population a bovine aorta is present, defined as a common origin of the right brachiocephalic and left common carotid arteries, such that only two great vessels are visualized. This information is important for the cardiothoracic surgeon and the interventional radiologists. The descending thoracic aorta travels to the left of the spine in the posterior mediastinum, passing behind the left atrium and continues down into the abdomen, giving rise to the celiac, superior mesenteric, and inferior mesenteric arteries. The right and left renal arteries, as well as normal accessory arteries, supply the respective kidneys. The main pulmonary artery originates from the distal portion of the infundibulum and pulmonic valve. It travels superiorly and posteriorly dividing into the right and left pulmonary branches. The left pulmonary originates from the trunk as a continuous vessel, and travels posteriorly to the left, and superior to the left main bronchus. However, the right pulmonary arises from the main pulmonary artery. The right pulmonary artery comes off in a more angulated fashion to travel behind the aortic arch, anterior to the right main bronchus initially, and then travels beneath the right main bronchus in a more distal pattern. The pulmonary arteries can be well defined in multislice transverse axials, as well as right parasagittal views. The right parasagittal projection is an excellent imaging view to visualize and distinguish between the left pulmonary artery and the aorta for a patent ductus arteriosum.

## TRACHEOBRONCHIAL TREE

The trachea travels down from the thorax, posterior to the head and carotid arteries and divides into the right and left bronchi at the level of the aortic arch. The two main stem bronchi travel caudally towards the carina, traveling to give rise to the branches adjacent to the pulmonary arteries. The left main bronchus travels underneath the left main pulmonary artery before it divides into upper and lower lobes. This bronchus to the left upper lobe is known as a *hyparterial bronchus*. The right main stem bronchus gives rise to the upper lobe of the right lung before it is crossed by the pulmonary artery to supply the middle and lower branches. This main branch is called the eparterial bronchus. The bronchus–pulmonary artery relationships are important in defining considerable pathologic features, which characteristically need identification in pediatric congenital heart disease.

## CONCLUSION

The capability of CMR to visualize large portions of the cardiac anatomy and place them in context with even larger segments of the cardiovascular system is one of the chief advantages that CMR provides to the clinician. The large field of view and ability to acquire images in virtually any conceivable plane makes CMR an unparalleled modality to define both normal and complex pathologic states. Classically defined using black-blood sequences, we opted to display the anatomy using the higher resolution and newer SSFP sequence, which we believe showcases the ability of CMR to illustrate important anatomic features previously not widely appreciated. When combined with the ability of CMR to portray anatomy and function, an unparalleled and often breathtaking window into the most important muscle in the body is unveiled, granting unprecedented anatomic and physiologic insights that eclipse even the surgeons and pathologists' view.

# CHAPTER 8

# Left and Right Ventricular Structure and Function

Robert W. W. Biederman

Perhaps no better utilization for cardiovascular magnetic resonance (CMR) can be seen in its application to evaluate the structure and function of the left ventricle (LV). Long established as the "gold standard" for accurate quantification of ejection fraction, CMR has remained the reference standard for nearly the last two decades. The high resolution offered by CMR, initially in the form of fast gradient-recalled echoes (GREs) and, for most of the early 2000s, steady state free precession (SSFP)-based sequences, have permitted an unparalleled ability to accurately delineate myocardium and blood pools. This capability allows accurate differentiation between blood and myocardium, generating highly reproducible and clinically relevant measurements of wall thickness and chamber volume (see Figs. 8-1 to 8-8).

Why is LV/right ventricle (RV) functional assessment by CMR the "gold standard"?

1. High resolution (matrices ranging from $128^2$ to $512^2$)
2. High endocardial and epicardial intrinsic contrast
3. Absence of foreshortening, due to exact placement of anatomy by prescription
4. Near absence of any user-dependence limitation
5. Reproducibility and accuracy to within 5 mL of volume
6. Not dependent on any geometric assumptions
7. Ability to perform three-dimensional (3D) imaging for exact measurements quickly (no absolute need for 2D anymore)
8. Volume-time measurements
9. Regional LV quantification; visually and/or quantitatively
10. Moderate to high temporal resolution

The assessment of left and right ventricular function is performed by measuring changes in volume between diastole and systole. While many techniques have the capability to perform this, the reliability, reproducibility, and accuracy of CMR have placed it at the forefront as

the "gold standard" for over two decades in that reliance on 2D techniques are not necessary. 3D CMR techniques carrry with them the critically important advantage of being not only user independent and geometrically not reliant on mathematical formulas to derive quantitative measurements but also to be applicable in a variety of pathologies. Deformed ventricles from a variety of pathologic conditions, including ischemic heart disease, no longer "fit" into the classical prolate ellipsoid, and as such, deviate from the underlying assumptions of a natural ellipse of rotation. Contiguous short-axis slices therefore, when contoured and assembled in order, provide the capability to measure the most unusual and distorted LVs and RVs. For conditions in which reliable measurements of volume, despite distortion, are required, for instance, in cases of LV aneurysms being considered for LV reduction surgery (Dor procedure) or for measurement of ejection fraction in the dilated and irregular ventricle for the placement of an automatic internal cardiac defibrillator (AICD), an accurate mechanism to quantitate LV function is important for the patient, physician and for socioeconomic considerations, avoiding needless placement of expensive technologies or inadvertent withholding of life-saving interventions.

As interventions become more and more advanced, they will, no doubt, be restricted to the population by inclusion and exclusion criteria in large part determined by ejection fraction. Therefore, a technique that has the lowest standard deviation and variance should be considered to be the ideal test to assess these patients. CMR, as stated in the preceding text, has long held that distinction.

Similarly, but to an even greater degree, the evaluation of the RV is classically difficult because of its inability to conform easily to any standard geometric formulae. Therefore, techniques that are reliant on 2D evaluations will always be inferior to those that use 3D. This becomes extraordinarily cumbersome and

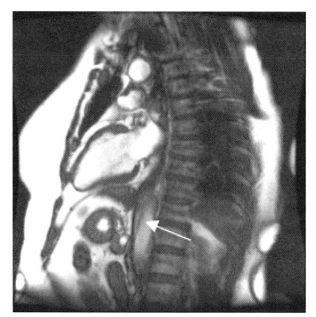

**FIGURE 8-1**   Steady state free precession (SSFP) image demonstrating the two-chamber (long-axis) plane. The two-chamber view is acquired from the axial plane and provides the most comprehensive information of LV structure and function because it specifically delineates the territory subtended by the left anterior descending (LAD), that is, the anterior and apical walls. The inferior wall territory is also demonstrated. Mitral valve anatomy and pathology can be well appreciated in this plane when seen in motion. Note the subtle descending aortic dissection (*arrow*) also seen in the "normal" patient. Left ventricular anatomic determination is made possible due to the unconstrained ability to obtain images in any plane, necessary independent of the orientation of the LV to the axis of the body. This allows cardiovascular magnetic resonance (CMR) to depict anatomy in a true cardiac axis perspective independent of the distortion due to cardiac perturbations such as congenital heart disease or due to extra cardiac deformities such as *pectus excavatum*.

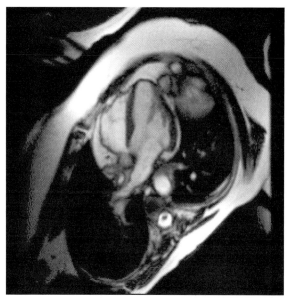

**FIGURE 8-2**   Acquired from a two-chamber view, this acquisition provides information about the inferior septum and lateral wall, and is the most definitive view for assessment of the right ventricle, including evaluation of tricuspid annular excursion (TAPSE). Additional information regarding the mitral and tricuspid valves, including morphology and pathology (regurgitation and stenosis can also be obtained).

frustrating, as we recognize so many manifestations of disease that effect the RV, often to an even greater extent than the LV. Assessment of diseases such as pulmonary arterial hypertension, arrhythmogenic right ventricular dysphasia (ARVD), right-sided valvular heart disease, most congenital heart disease, and other right ventricular cardiomyopathies is greatly aided by the use of CMR, that can be used to measure not only the thin-walled RV, providing mass estimations, but also provide volumetric information. As is true for the LV, Simpson rule is applied to stacks of contiguous slices contoured for either volume or mass, and is now routinely performed in most laboratories, using breath-hold images obtained using SSFP in <10 minutes, including contouring when using automatic or semiautomatic software (see Figs. 8-6 and 8-7).

Evaluation of left ventricular systolic function is performed in a variety of approaches as shown in Fig. 8-9, incorporating 2D and 3D SSFP sequences to define ejection performance, regional motion abnormalities, as well as allow quantification of left ventricular mass. In this example, a 67-year-old white man presents with a 2-week history of chest pain that culminated in syncope while at church. His examination demonstrated a harsh 5/6 systolic ejection murmur radiating up to the right carotid artery. He had a prominent and focal nondisplaced point of maximal intensity (PMI) with a palpable $S_4$, and as expected, an auscultatable $S_4$. He presents for CMR under the presumption that he had severe aortic stenosis. In the top panels the extensive left ventricular hypertrophy (LVH) is appreciated in the presurgical state whereas the lower panels depict the CMR images 6 months following aortic valve replacement. Note the decrease in LV size, extent of LVH, and the minimal paramagnetic effect from the artificial valve. Additionally, the right panels depict intramyocardial strain (radiofrequency [RF] tissue tagging) and visually, the improvement in mechanical deformation is easily and dramatically detectable, despite very severe prevalve replacement left ventricular ejection fraction (LVEF).

Analysis of ventricular function can be performed in several ways. We acquire standard 2D images of

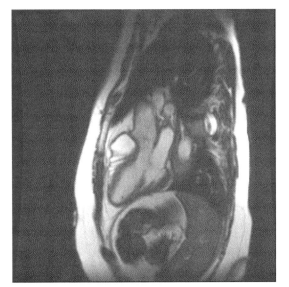

**FIGURE 8-3** Acquired from either a coronal or a short-axis slice, this view details the anterior septum, apex, and infralateral walls, and is the key view for certain 1D left ventricle (LV) measurements. Mitral and aortic valve pathology can be evaluated, as can the right ventricle (RV) outflow tract.

the two-, three-, and four-chamber views to allow systematic interrogation of segmental wall motion in a manner analogous to nuclear and echocardiographic techniques. This permits rapid overview using the American Society of Echocardiography–approved 17-segment model. CMR evaluation of the short axis in a

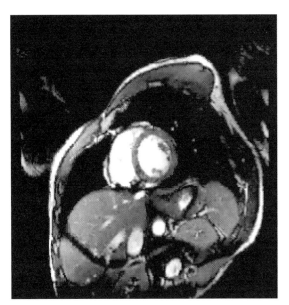

**FIGURE 8-4** Acquired from either the two- or four-chamber view, the short-axis acquisition provides the 2D or 3D acquisitions. Contiguous imaging from base to apex of stacks of left ventricle (LV) (and right ventricle [RV]) short-axis slices yields high quality, reproducible, and accurate volumetric and functional data.

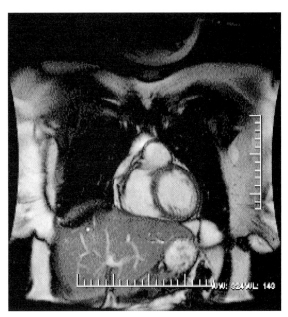

**FIGURE 8-5** Additional evaluation of both the left ventricle (LV) and right ventricle (RV) can be obtained in nonconventional views, afforded by the ability of CMR to image in any plane. This plane provides additional information about segmental wall motion, the mitral, aortic, and tricuspid valves. This plane often yields substantial anatomic detail about extracardiac anatomy.

contiguous manner permits semiquantitative evaluation and confirmation of the 2D visual analysis. We use a five-point scale for semiquantitative regional wall motion analysis:

0 = normal segmental function
1 = mild segmental hypokinesis
2 = moderate segmental hypokinesis
3 = severe segmental hypokinesis
4 = akinetic segment
5 = hyperkinetic segment

The summation of these regions divided by the number 17 gives a global semiquantitative measurement. The scores can be combined with ejection fraction, to provide a regional wall motion abnormality score, which often adds more specific and focal information than ejection fraction used alone. For example, in the setting of a large anterior wall myocardial infarction, with compensatory inferior wall hyperkinesis, the ejection fraction may be normal, borderline, or only mildly depressed, belying the otherwise important anterior wall hypokinesis. The apparent "normal" LVEF is better described by use of segmental analysis such as described in the preceding text. An important caveat is necessary: in the setting of the pathologic ventricle, often endocardial excursion is misinterpreted as segmental wall thickening (local shortening fraction). The ability of CMR to define visually and quantitatively the endocardial and epicardial borders

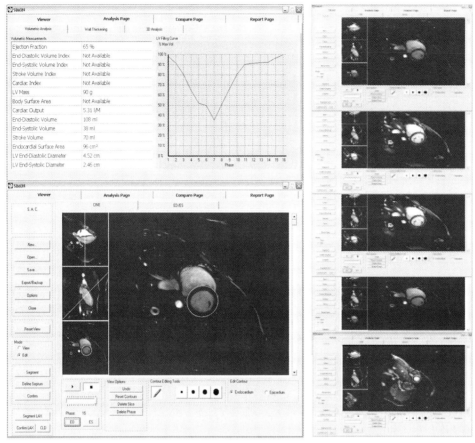

**FIGURE 8-6**   Representative semiautomated processing using prototype software (Chase Medical, Dallas, Texas) demonstrating the ability to quickly outline and measure endocardial and epicardial borders while tracking them through time to yield easily understandable and clinically relevant metrics (upper left panel). Note the time-volume curve in the same panel, which gives the rate of change of systolic and diastolic volumes.

allows for accurate determination of true systolic wall thickening versus localized adjacent wall tethering (see DVD). Especially, as the ischemic heart becomes more remodeled and scarred, the collagen formation in the chronic infarct is subjected to the forces of the adjacent myocardium, such that apparent movement toward the left ventricular centroid gives the illusion that there are close to normal mechanical contractile properties (tethering). Therefore, a careful recollection that "true" systolic function is only present when there is wall thickening, not simply displacement, is an important concept to keep in mind. Yet, when it comes to considerations for interventional possibilities, failure to recognize that myocardial contraction can be isometric not yielding active, displacement, leads to a disservice to the patient who could otherwise potentially benefit from reinstitution of blood flow to the area and subsequent return to more normal systolic thickening patterns.

Some investigators prefer to use the centerline method to interrogate LV function, in which serial slices are interrogated and wall thickening is scored, generally using 100 points, to determine segmental function. Briefly, endocardial and epicardial contours are drawn, and starting from a constant point on the ventricle, a series of 100 lines are placed perpendicular to the endocardial epicardial contours, uniting them. If performed in diastole and tracked throughout systole, local shortening fractions can be determined, and used to generate regional and global information about left ventricular segmental function.

Another method that has been used by us and originally described by Leon Axel MD, PhD is RF tissue tagging (see Fig. 8-9). This is perhaps the most common and complete method to define contractile properties within the myocardium. Although other invasive techniques such as sonomicrometry and tantalum markers provide local quantitation of intramyocardial mechanics, the very process of the measurement is invasive and locally destructive, not only to the patient, but to the specific measurements required. Obviously, this technique has limited capability in clinical practice, but a technique such as RF tissue tagging which possesses

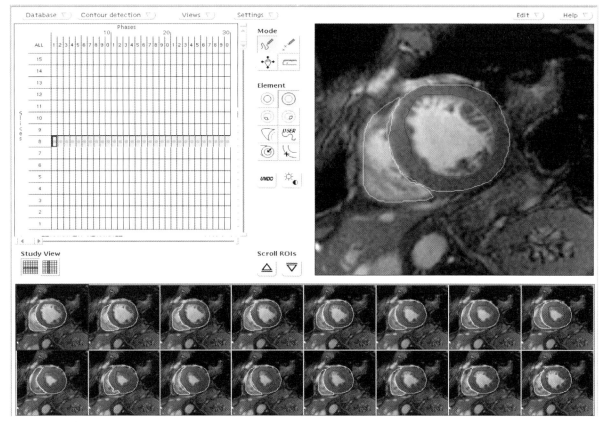

**FIGURE 8-7** Using endocardial and epicardial contours the entire left ventricle (LV) can be evaluated, yielding important clinical metrics such as left ventricular ejection fraction (LVEF), left ventricular end diastolic volume (LVEDV), left ventricular end systolic volume (LVESV), left ventricular stroke volume (LVSV), and LV mass. These can be indexed by normalization to body surface area. Also shown is the right ventricle (RV) endocardial contour, which generates similar metrics for the RV.

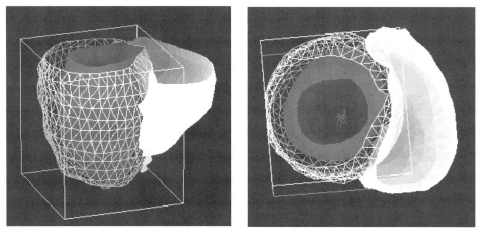

**FIGURE 8-8** 3D representation of a cine (best seen in the DVD) depicting left ventricle/right ventricle (LV/RV) interactions demonstrating the ability to comprehensively assess both LV and RV function. This snake algorithm is easily generated using contiguous epicardial and endocardial contours from most commercially available postprocessing software. Therefore, both standard clinical metrics, that have immediate clinical translation, as well as more complex interrogations, that shed greater insight into pathologic mechanisms, are possible. Manipulation in any plane or orientation is possible as shown in both figures and grants greater clarity for disease understanding, especially when depicted in cine mode.

Pre-AVR

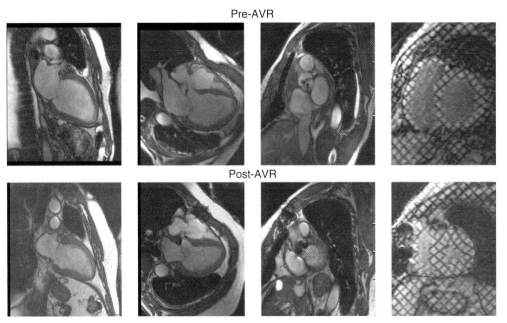

Post-AVR

**FIGURE 8-9**  A 67-year-old presents with severe aortic stenosis with an ejection fraction of 19% by the Simpson rule. The top panel demonstrates the decompensated nature of both the left the structure and function with severe quantitated left ventricular hypertrophy (LVH) and global systolic dysfunction. Not shown, phase velocity mapping demonstrated a peak and mean gradient of 72 and 40 mm Hg, respectively, indicating considerable myocardial reserve and an extreme example of afterload mismatch. After considerable discussions with the surgical team, the patient was felt to be a candidate for aortic valve replacement and the bottom panel demonstrates the structure and function of the patient 6 months following mechanical aortic valve replacement. From left to right views are the two-chamber, four-chamber, and short-axis at the base, near the mechanical valve. The right panels (upper and lower) are examples of the same region with radiofrequency tissue tagging applied. Note in the pre–aorta valve replacement (pre-AVR) intramyocardial strain pattern that there is minimal systolic stripe deformation, as evidence by little change in the square tiling pattern. However, 6 months after AVR, as seen in the lower right panels, there is, in addition to the sternal wire artifact, a dramatic improvement in intramyocardial systolic strain. This patient underwent only an AVR without concomitant coronary artery bypass surgery.

the noninvasive ability to track intramyocardial properties would have intrinsic appeal to the clinician and the clinician or investigator. The basic concept applied magnetization patterns to the myocardium to "tag" specific material points and to track their motion as the underlying myocardium deforms. The altered magnetization of the tagged region shows up as a dark line, and as the underlying tissue moves, the altered magnetized region necessarily moves as well, revealing the subtended tissue motion (see Fig. 8-10). The noninvasively applied tag lines persist as a property of the intrinsic T1 time, and the number of signal-read acquisitions performed per cardiac cycle. In general, the tagged myocardium retains a property of memory so that tags persist in the order of 400 to 800 milliseconds, allowing complete determination of systolic contraction, and depending on the persistence of the tags, diastolic

function can often be assessed. The exact physical deposition of the tagline is discussed in Chapter 28, but in general can be envisioned as a prepulse, analogous to inversion recovery or fat saturation pulses, that can be used in combination with a GRE sequence. Current techniques do not permit its use with SSFP pulse sequences, but would be ideal for even greater resolution. Qualitative visual assessment of the underlying tag motion throughout the cardiac cycle is, obviously, the easiest method of interrogation of local contractile properties. The true full potential of the tagged studies can be achieved only through more sophisticated quantitative analysis. Tracking material points throughout the cardiac cycle can be done manually for 1D and 2D methods, or can be performed in a semiautomated manner using prototype software. We use harmonic phase (HARP) (Palo Alto, CA) for clinical research evaluation

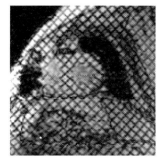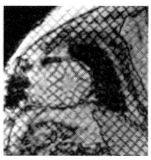

**FIGURE 8-10** Radiofrequency tissue tagging permits the tracking of intramyocardial mechanics throughout the cardiac cycle in a noninvasive way allowing for the estimation of contractile analysis defined as *strain*. In the left panel, an end-diastolic mid ventricular tagging example is shown with tags transiently imbedded within 10 to 15 milliseconds of the QRS spike detection. Note the near-perfect symmetric square tiling pattern. End-systole occurs 305 milliseconds later. Notice that as the underlying myocardium deforms, the noninvasively tagged myocardial stripes have followed the subtended myocardium, permitting measurement of segmental shorting properties (strain, %S). Analysis for 1D and 2D strain can be measured to yield circumferential and radial strain metrics. Acquiring multiple 2D contiguous slices permits the analysis of 3D strain, incorporating meridional (longitudinal) strain and can permit non-Cartesian coordinate analysis, yielding vector plots of directional mechanics. Clinically, this technique is often useful to ascertain the difference between endocardial excursion and adjacent to wall tethering in the acute and subacute infarct setting. More often, this is used in the assessment of the pericardium for constrictive pericarditis to differentiate between visceral and parietal pericardial adherence patterns and regional motion as related to the left and right ventricles.

of 1-, 2-, and 3D tissue tracking to define local deformation patterns in terms of circumferential, longitudinal, and radial strain metrics, defined as *local shortening fractions* (%S). Typically, only fiduciary material points are tracked when there is a saturated magnetized myocardial stripe; however, to define properties on the order of less than the tag stripe distance, interpolation schemes can be incorporated. Finally, any number of classical or innovative tag patterns can be placed. Commonly, orthogonal stripes are laid down but linear or radial tag stripes can also be performed to suit the specific nature of the investigation.

## CLINICAL ASSESSMENT

Ventricular evaluation is the primary use for CMR. In Fig. 8-11 a markedly dilated LV is present which, by most criteria, would be seen to have little evidence for revascularization as assessed by wall thinning criteria (left and middle panels). In right panel, the delayed hyperenhancement (DHE) sequence confirms the lack of reversibility, delineating a clear transmural infarct pattern, likely chronic (>1 year). Note that the anterior septum, however, demonstrates a thin subendocardial layer of infarct that is <25% scar, denoting a high likelihood of reversibility. More appropriately, although this tissue is deemed viable, the amount of myocardium represented as viable in the anterior septum is small and clinically insignificant and argues against revascularization. In this case, clinical decision making was formed mainly due to the high resolution afforded by CMR, allowing detection of a 1- to 2-mm thick rim of scar. This patient was referred for, and underwent, orthotopic cardiac transplantation. The surgical pathology confirmed the veracity of the CMR statements regarding the thin scar with mostly viable anterior septum. Note is also made in the DHE images that the RV or infundibulum was completely viable, assisting surgical considerations for intervention had the LV contained substantive viability.

An integrated approach to interrogating cardiomyopathies involves utilization of multiple sequences, each designed to delineate particular features of the LV, RV, their respective valves, presence of underlying myocardium perfusion, and the determination of the presence or absence of viability. The workhorse sequence of this workup is SSFP, which is used to assess ejection fraction and wall motion abnormalities. Used in either 2D or 3D mode, the prognostic information obtained is highly reproducible and accurate, allowing clinical decisions to be made with surety. In Fig. 8-12, the SSFP images provide volumetric information, and wall motion determinations. The images allow evaluation of the extent and magnitude of ventricular perturbations in 3D, aiding the diagnosis, and providing the capability to appropriately considered pharmacologic or interventional strategies. In this example, there is a prominent left bundle branch block, otherwise no regional abnormality, but moderate ventricular dilation, the extent of which is confirmed by a series of 3D, 8 mm contiguous acquisitions in the short axis. Perfusion information is incorporated to provide an estimate of the underlying coronary disease, if present. In this case, this 46-year-old white woman had a prodrome of 4 weeks of constitutional symptoms, fever, and malaise, culminating in weight gain, especially in her legs. Initially treated as an upper respiratory disease, she was admitted with congestive heart failure symptoms. The adenosine stress perfusion sequence (see Fig. 8-12, lower left panel) did not reveal a defect that corresponded to a coronary artery territory. Instead there were diffuse hypoperfusion abnormalities, mostly confined to the subendocardium and midwall.

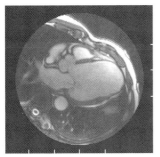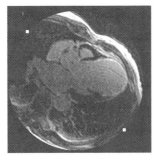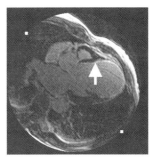

**FIGURE 8-11**   Severe left ventricular dilation, thinning, and left ventricular systolic dysfunction are present with a large amount of thinned and scarred myocardium by delayed hyperenhancement technique. Full thickness transmural scar is present, except for a small region (*arrow*) that reveals basal and mid anterior septal subendocardial infarction. The integration of left ventricular structure, viability, and function is a well-recognized capability of cardiovascular magnetic resonance (CMR).

The corresponding DHE images (see Fig. 8-12, lower right panel) do not demonstrate a subendocardial or transmural infarct pattern nor do they demonstrate a patchy, heterogeneous pattern. The data, as presented, is most consistent with a nonischemic cardiomyopathy. The patient underwent a coronary angiogram, which demonstrated normal coronaries, confirming the CMR diagnosis. The data, as acquired, argues for truncating her workup upon the completion of the CMR without the need for coronary angiography. A perfusion defect at adequate stress would depict substantive coronary artery disease (CAD). It should be noted that the concept of "balanced perfusion defects" does not exist in CMR such that high-grade three-vessel disease would be detectable by perfusion imaging. Adding the DHE sequence confirms the lack of a single large, or several smaller, subtler infarct patterns. Although the presence of some low-grade (but important) CAD could not be excluded, the immediate explanation of her presentation certainly can be ascertained noninvasively.

## DIASTOLIC FUNCTION

As described in the preceding text, for the assessment of systolic function CMR is the gold standard. We believe that CMR also possesses the ability to interrogate diastolic properties of the myocardium in a manner analogous to echocardiography. Using phase velocity mapping of mitral inflow, velocities can be tracked to generate both morphologic patterns, as well as quantitative velocities, similar to those performed in the echocardiography laboratory (see Fig. 8-13). Placing a short-axis slice parallel to the mitral valve plane (perpendicular to the long axis of the LV) and setting the velocity encoding at 30 cm per second and adjusting the phases to between 40 and 60 per slice allows for tracking of diastolic filling velocities over the cardiac cycle. When

interrogated for the entire diastolic filling time, one can easily determine whether there is a normal, impaired relaxation or restrictive filling pattern (see Fig. 8-13). A psuedonormal pattern can be determined if an impaired relaxation pattern is present, yet the relaxation time is <140 milliseconds. Diastolic function assessment adds, at most, an extra 2 minutes to the standard left

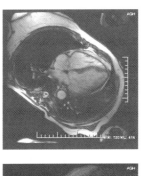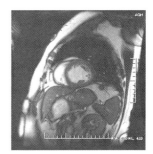
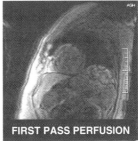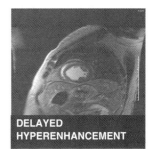

**FIRST PASS PERFUSION**    **DELAYED HYPERENHANCEMENT**

**FIGURE 8-12**   Integrating structure, function (top panel), perfusion (lower left panel), and viability (lower right panel) in this patient with cardiomyopathy, thought to be of nonischemic origin, reveals, in addition to a bundle branch block (best seen in DVD), no evidence of a perfusion defect or myocardial scar. This strongly suggests that in the absence of coronary artery disease; this is a nonischemic cardiomyopathy. No cardiac catheterization was performed, as CMR interrogation of the ostial, proximal, and mid coronary arterial tree revealed no evidence of disease (not shown).

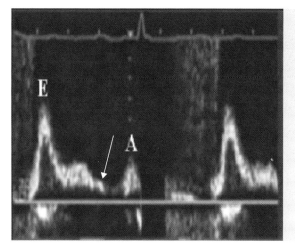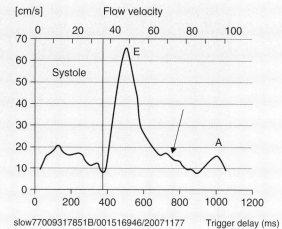

**FIGURE 8-13**   In the left panel, a representative cardiac cycle of mitral inflow velocities obtained by echocardiography is displayed, demonstrating a restrictive filling pattern; a poor prognostic finding. In the right panel, using phase velocity mapping in a near simultaneous acquisition (within 30 minutes), a virtually identical filling pattern is seen. Note the near exact reproducibility of subtle features in the morphologic pattern as depicted by the arrows. Diastolic function by CMR is not limited to an "icepick" view, as performed in the echocardiography suite, in that the entire blood flow domain can be interrogated and, as we have shown, contains important clinical information otherwise lost with a 1D approach.

ventricular function assessment but, more importantly, permits a more complete assessment of left ventricular structure and function. Indeed, the assessment of LV function is not complete without a diastolic assessment, as shown by our colleague, Dr. Vikas Rathi.

A more complete analysis can be performed by tracking diastolic myocardial velocities such as is done with tissue tracking in the echocardiography laboratory. In this case, aligning a phase velocity mapping slice parallel to the long axis of the LV to obtain myocardial velocities in various long axis projections can be easily obtained. In this case, the velocity-encoding factor (VENC) should be set to 10 cm per second. Great care must be exercised to cardiac-gate this sequence properly, as the velocity-encoded gradient is subject to considerable noise. However, quite reproducible tissue tracking signals can be obtained, and furthermore, can be assessed throughout the base, mid, and apical LV segments, not typically performed in classic echocardiography. It should be noted that there is no limitation to assess diastolic function solely in the LV, as the RV can be assessed in exactly the same manner. Finally, utilizing the previously mentioned RF tissue tagging, one can measure cardiac rotation and torsion. The latter has been shown by several investigators including us to be

highly reproducible and is related to the noninvasive measure of $\tau$ (tau). Systematic tracking of torsion can be used as a measure of underlying myocardial structural changes in response to surgical, pharmaceutical, or alternative therapeutic interventions. We believe that the unique ability of CMR to interrogate diastolic function across the entire blood flow range, in 3D, and incorporated torsion, will characterize CMR as the "go to" diastolic tool in the future, when accurate and reproducible lusitropic measurements are critical. As dedicated pharmaceutical agents, now in development, will modulate diastolic dysfunction through modification of the extra cellular matrix, calcium handling or resequestration mechanisms, become available, demonstrations of their efficacy for both LV mass regression and lusitropy will increase the need for the accurate and reproducible capabilities of CMR. These evaluations can be performed, and have been shown to be statistically significant, in small cohorts of patients due to the low measurement variance inherent in CMR. These aspects are expected to minimize cost and maximize speed of progression through the development and U.S. Food and Drug Administration (FDA) approval process, and this notion has not been lost on pharmaceutical research and development firms.

# CHAPTER 9

# Valvular Heart Disease

Robert W. W. Biederman

Cardiovascular magnetic resonance (CMR) is generally believed to be an excellent modality for nearly every cardiac or vascular application. However, if there is a perceived weakness related to non-coronary imaging of the cardiovascular system, the general perception in the non-CMR community is that valvular heart disease poses the greatest limitation for CMR. Consequently, echocardiography has assumed the major workload for clinical valvular assessments, and CMR has classically been relegated to a secondary modality upon the failure of echocardiography. As one might infer from the direction of this prose, this notion has clearly changed over the last 5 years, making many elements of CMR comparable, or, in some indications, superior to echocardiography. The main limitation that persists, with the greatest clinical impact, is the relatively limited ability for the CMR-based evaluation of endocarditis.

The severity of valvular heart disease can be assessed in a number of ways by CMR, providing another example of the diversity of the modality to perform a comprehensive cardiovascular examination, especially for valvular assessments. The steady state free precession (SSFP) and the phase velocity mapping (PVM) sequences offer the greatest ability to assess and quantitate the extent of disease. Less often, resorting to the older gradient-recalled echo (GRE) sequences with long echo times (TEs), offers more physiologic representation of the true severity of valvular lesions through loss of signal in jet flow due to the greater intervoxel dephasing phenomena.

By definition, the two lesions that dominate valvular evaluations are regurgitant and stenotic pathologies. Each is approached in a distinct manner, which will be illustrated here by means of case study examples.

In many CMR textbooks valve anatomy is not well described because it has traditionally not been well depicted by CMR. The image in Fig. 9-1 of the aortic valve and its cusp anatomy suggests that this:

notion is erroneous and outdated. Using this approach, planimetry of the aortic valve can be formally measured, not grossly estimated, as when employing various geometric formulae available to the echocardiographer or angiographer utilizing the continuity equation or the Gorlin formula. Theoretically and practically, this direct approach yields information closest to what might be obtained in the surgical suite. It would seem intuitive that the closer an imaging modality comes to demonstrating that which is visible to the eye the more accurate and robust the measurement generated would be. The following are a series of case studies and examples of valvular anatomy and lesions.

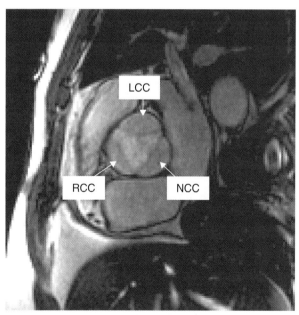

**FIGURE 9-1** Gradient-recalled echo (GRE) image demonstrating a cross-sectional and anatomic view of the normal trileaflet aortic valve. LCC, left coronary cusp; RCC, right coronary cusp; NCC, noncoronary cusp.

# CASE STUDIES

**Case Study 1.** SSFP imaging of all four valves in a healthy 38-year-old black man demonstrating the normal anatomic structure of each of the valves (see Fig. 9-2). Note also the incidental atrial septal aneurysm seen in middle panel, as well as tricuspid valve prolapse. In the right panels, the trileaflet aortic valve is shown in diastole and systole. Note the high resolution that can be obtained with standard imaging sequences.

**Case Study 2.** A 67-year-old man presents with syncope and several months of dyspnea on exertion (see Fig. 9-3). The examination demonstrated a harsh systolic ejection murmur radiating to the right upper sternal border, in addition to a diastolic murmur. Both lesions are depicted in the SSFP images (best seen in the DVD). Using PVM, the peak and mean gradients were 72 and 43 mm Hg, with the patient requiring aortic valve replacement (AVR). Using an SSFP sequence, visualization of the aortic valve and its associated intervoxel dephasing artifact gives substantial clinical information concerning the severity of the lesion. General severity can be gauged by the depth of radiation of the jet into the ascending aorta, with a more cranial excursion indicating worse severity (for constant scanner performance and variables). The extent of calcification can also be seen, as well as aortic root calcification, which is important for the cardiothoracic surgeon to plan a course of action. Additionally, the extent of the sinus of Valsalva, sinotubular junction, and ascending aortic dilation are easily appreciated.

**Case Study 3.** In aortic regurgitation (AR) (see Fig. 9-4 left and middle panels) the primary method for initially detecting disease severity is exactly the same as that used in echocardiography, in which the width of the jet relative to the left ventricular outflow tract (LVOT) dimension is related to severity of the regurgitant lesion. Specifically, mild corresponds to a jet less than one third, moderate to between one third and two thirds, and severe is greater than two thirds of the LVOT dimension in the three-chamber view. Although echocardiographically derived, this measurement in comparison with angiography, the CMR LVOT view reveals an eccentric jet of AR (left panel, arrow). The short-axis view shows two smaller jets of AR (middle panel, arrows) composing the one jet seen in the orthogonal view. CMR permits mathematical quantitation to be performed, providing the ability to track serial changes and/or assess response to management strategies.

**Case Study 4.** The Coanda effect is illustrated in the right panel (see Fig. 9-4), whereby a small jet of AR is seen radiating along the anterior mitral leaflet (arrow) but is underestimated by all semiquantitative techniques because of the energy dissipation that occurs as the jet travels along the leaflet. This is also an example of the imaging equivalent of the Austin Flint murmur.

**Case Study 5.** Evaluation of the mitral valve typically begins with an SSFP sequence in the short-axis view, depicting the anterior and posterior leaflets. Shown in Fig. 9-5 are images from a 56-year-old white woman demonstrating the individual anatomy of the mitral valve leaflets (single phase of an SSFP sequence taken from a short-axis acquisition). The individual scallops of the posterior leaflet are visible. This information is critical when considering mitral valve repair or replacement. Delineation of this information for the surgeon adds a clear extra dimension, as the leaflets are directly visualized and related to cardiac anatomy.

**Case Study 6.** A 43-year-old white man presents for routine evaluation with a dilated aortic root on transthoracic echocardiography and concern for bicuspid aorta, both confirmed by CMR (see Fig. 9-6). Note the underestimation of the ascending aortic dilation (right panel) but, just as importantly, the relative prolapse of the posterior cusp is well seen in this flagrant example of a bicuspid aortic valve (right panel). Believed to be a failure of neural crest cell migration, lack of proper migration of elastic fibers contributes to the above scenario, which also includes aortic coarctation (not present in this patient). In this case, the combination of SSFP (left and middle panels) and double-inversion recovery (DIR) (right panel) sequences answered the entire spectrum of clinical questions posed. PVM was performed to quantitate the degree of peak and mean gradient. 3D volumetrics complete the picture, with full delineation of mild left ventricular hypertrophy, suggesting the growing physiologic significance to this common congenital anomaly. Yearly follow-up and endocarditis prophylaxis were recommended with a high likelihood for requiring aortic valve surgery in the near future (<10 years).

Mitral regurgitation (ERO) (MR) has been shown to be associated with increased morbidity and mortality, even in asymptomatic patients. Yet, estimation of MR by echocardiography has been primarily limited to quantification of effective regurgitant orifice area derived from various geometric assumptions. CMR also permits indirect quantitation of MR. MR is the most ubiquitous valvular lesion for which a patient may present. Discussed in an earlier chapter, several aspects bear reiteration. First, MR is depicted as a dephasing intervoxel

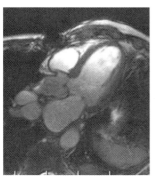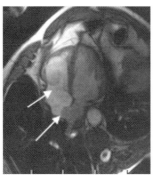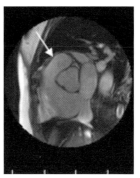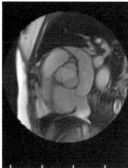

**FIGURE 9-2**   Steady state free precession (SSFP) images: far left panel is a standard three-chamber view demonstrating the mitral valve and aortic valve, middle left panel shows the redundant tricuspid valve leaflets and a moderate size atrial septal aneurysm, whereas the right panels shows a cross-section of both the aortic (systole far right, and diastole mid right) and pulmonic valve (arrow). Images relate to case study 1.

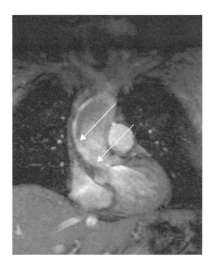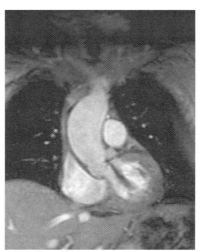

**FIGURE 9-3**   Combined valvular pathology due to calcified and restricted aortic leaflets in this gradient-recalled echo (GRE) sequence. In systole (left), the eccentric dephasing artifact of moderate aortic stenosis is present, whereas in diastole (right) the mild-moderate (1–2+) aortic regurgitation is present and represented as a pan-cyclic murmur on auscultation; this patient's initial presenting clinical finding. Images relate to case study 2.

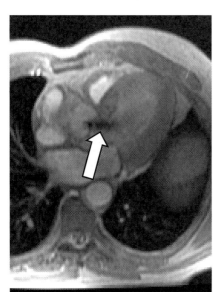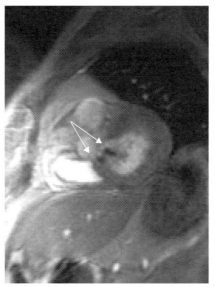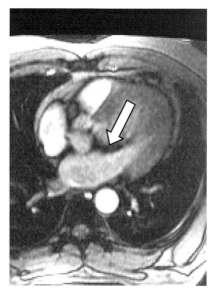

**FIGURE 9-4**   Gradient-recalled echo (GRE) images demonstrating combined aortic valvular heart disease. Left panel demonstrates aortic stenosis, with the right and middle panels showing aortic regurgitation. Images relate to case studies 3 and 4.

**FIGURE 9-5** Steady state free precession (SSFP) image of a short axis slice depicting the anterior and posterior mitral valve leaflets and scallops. Images relate to case study 5.

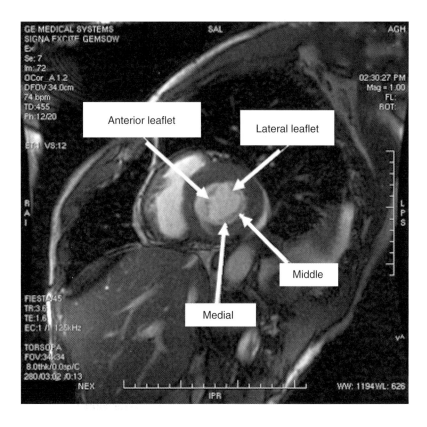

artifact and is used clinically to gauge semiquantitatively the extent of mitral valve leakage. Using PVM, the exact amount of regurgitation can be measured in a manner very distinct and very different from the many physiologic and geometric assumptions utilized by echocardiography. Measurement of all the blood volume that passes through a plane positioned parallel to the mitral valve annulus completely interrogates the extent (volume) of MR. Moreover, elements to define the underlying anatomic mechanistic perturbations can also be well defined by CMR. In Fig. 9-7, there are several metrics used surgically and clinically to better describe the etiology of MR, where, for two patients with essentially the same left ventricle (LV) metrics, there is a very discordant degree of MR. Examining the mitral valvular apparatuses demonstrates the explanation for the differences in MR (see Table 9-1). In patient A, as opposed to patient B, the mitral annulus, tenting angle, coaptation distance (valve closure point from mitral annulus), and tenting area (area of triangle formed by the junction of the mitral annulus and the valve closure point) are near normal.

Even in cases in which the regurgitant jet is eccentric or where the LVOT cannot be completely removed from the image plane as described earlier, other

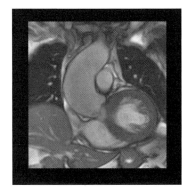 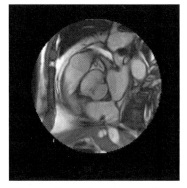 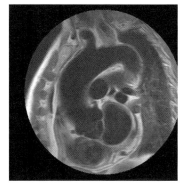

**FIGURE 9-6** Various views of the aortic root and ascending aorta: A bicuspid aortic valve and the sinuses of Valsalva (SSFP imaging; left and right panel) with their respective coronary arteries derived from the left and right and cusps (double inversion recovery [DIR] imaging on the right panel). Images relate to case study 6.

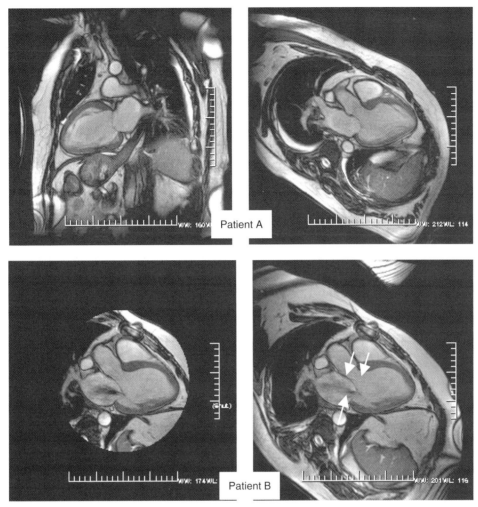

**FIGURE 9-7** Steady state free precession (SSFP) images of patients with nearly identical left ventricular structure and function, yet markedly different extent of mitral regurgitation. Table 9-1 demonstrates the precision and capability of cardiovascular magnetic resonance (CMR) to delineate the mechanism for this observation due to marked differences in mitral annular and structural changes. This is critically important for the cardiologist and cardiothoracic surgeon in determining the suitability for mitral valve repair.

CMR techniques, such as PVM or stroke volume (SV) analysis are available to mathematically determine the regurgitant volume or fraction. For instance, if one adds a single PVM plane at the level of the aortic root, when combined with standard 3D LV volumetrics, this method can accurately, rapidly, and easily quantitate MR by comparing the 3D volumetric imaging of the LV with an aortic PVM acquisition targeted to quantitate LV SV. This approach is applicable to patients without AR or intracardiac shunts. By subtraction of the PVM-derived SV ($SV_{PVM}$) from the volumetric-derived SV ($SV_{3D}$), in the absence of AR or shunt, the mitral regurgitant volume is found. Regurgitant fraction is defined as ($SV_{3D} - SV_{PVM}/SV_{3D}$)**.** This simple, reliable, and quick method can be easily incorporated into CMR studies, giving additional prognostic information, and may be an ideal tool for serial quantitative follow-up of regurgitant lesions.

The evaluation of AR follows an analogous methodology to MR where the PVM slice is placed parallel to the aortic root, at the level of, or just above, the sinotubular junction. Because all blood flow that is destined to regurgitate into the LV must, by definition, cross the midascending aorta, we standardize the acquisition plane as bisecting the right pulmonary artery. Similar to MR, direct quantitation of the AR volume and regurgitant fraction is possible (see Fig. 9-8). Regurgitant fraction is measured as the regurgitant volume divided by the forward SV. In the above example: 21 mL/86 mL = 24% regurgitant fraction (see Fig. 9-9). This is derived from a forward SV of 86 mL (area above the zero point) and regurgitant volume (area below the zero point).

## TABLE 9-1

Left Ventricle Volumetrics in Two Patients with Dramatically Different Degrees of Mitral Regurgitation

|  | Patient A | Patient B |
|---|---|---|
| Age | 66 | 66 |
| MR | Trace | 3–4+ |
| Gender | M | M |
| EF (%) | 21 | 22 |
| LV EDVI (mL/m$^2$) | 102 | 105 |
| LV ESVI (mL/m$^2$) | 21 | 23 |
| r/h | 0.81 | 0.82 |
| Mass/volume | 1.21 | 1.19 |
| Annulus (mm) | 33 × 32 | 40 × 38 |
| Tenting (degree) | 105 | 125 |
| Coapt (mm) | 9 | 15 |
| Tenting (mm$^2$) | 1.6 | 2.6 |

EF, ejection fraction; LVEDVI, left ventricular end diastolic volume index; LVESVI, left ventricular end-systolic volume index ; r/h, radius/wall thickness.

Using this technique, the addition of a 1- to 2-minute PVM (non–breath-hold, which we prefer for greater accuracy and patient comfort) or a 13- to 17-second (if breath-hold), quantitation of AR can be reported which compares more favorably with a "mild, moderate or severe grading." For uniformity, CMR regurgitant fraction is defined in Table 9-2.

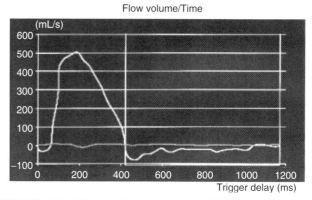

Flow volume/Time

**FIGURE 9-9**  Phase velocity mapping (PVM) demonstrates the presence of aortic regurgitation, and the display of quantitative flow, without reliance on semiquantitative techniques. Flow below the zero line is related to the regurgitant fraction.

Aortic regurgitant fraction >40% is an absolute indication for aortic valve repair or replacement. However, an end-systolic dimension >55 mm or an end-diastolic volume >30 mL/m$^2$ in the setting of normal left ventricular ejection fraction (LVEF) (>60%) is also an absolute indication. AR is a combined pressure and volume overload pathophysiology, has the highest end-systolic myocardial stress of any valvar lesion, and is generally well tolerated for decades, only becoming symptomatic after the myocardium has exhausted its ability to eccentrically and concentrically remodel

**FIGURE 9-8**  A series of steady state free precession (SSFP) images discerning the very nature of aortic regurgitation, and the potential for over- or underestimation if reliance is made on a single projection. Note the ability to discern the mechanism of the regurgitation, namely subtle failure of leaflet coaptation, is possible and best seen in bottom right panel (*arrow*).

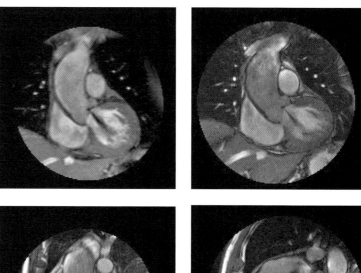
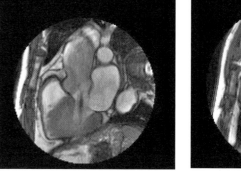

## TABLE 9-2

### Grading of Aortic Regurgitation

| AR Grade | Regurgitant Fraction |
|----------|----------------------|
| Trace | <10 |
| Mild | 10–20 |
| Moderate | 21–39 |
| Severe | >40 |

AR, aortic regurgitation.

through a combination of sarcomer addition in both parallel and in series. In that this period of relative compensation is not punctuated with heart failure symptoms until very late, gargantuan-sized left ventricles are often observed. LV ejection performance is frequently well preserved; however, at the first sign that ejection fraction (EF) is approximately 60% or has become <60%, this lesion should be corrected. Unlike aortic stenosis, where there is typically dramatic afterload mismatch and which is spectacularly reversible, despite markedly depressed LVEF, the dysfunction induced by AR is often irreversible once the LVEF has dropped below 60%. The American College of Cardiology/American Heart Association (ACC/AHA) guidelines also recommend aortic valve correction once the left ventricular end-diastolic dimension (LVEDD) is >75 mm, indicating that the lesion is generally well tolerated and that incipient volume overload telegraphs that occult LV dysfunction, if it has not already occurred, is imminent. Note should be made that the one-dimensional measurements derived from the literature are generated from men of a 70- to 80-kg stature, indicating that women of smaller habitus will benefit from earlier intervention. Indeed, awaiting the standard thresholds of a man is a grave disservice to

most women, and body surface area corrections should be aggressively adopted.

Because volumetric assessment is well performed by CMR, a common strategy adopted is to perform serial AR evaluations to measure the regurgitant fraction and LV volumetrics, gauging AR progression and myocardial deterioration. When the LV ejection performance is judged to be declining toward low normal, either immediate surgery, or careful, watchful, waiting strategies, with expectant surgical correction when the threshold is passed are employed.

The salient features of PVM of aortic valve for the evaluation and quantification of aortic stenosis (see Fig. 9-10) by CMR are as follows:

- Localization of aortic valve leaflets in a coronal plane
- Slice selection 10 mm superior to aortic valve leaflets at area of greatest dephasing artifact
- Phase velocity encoding (VENC) in three directions (X, Y, and Z)
- Set VENC sensitivity to an expected number in which the peak transvalvar gradient will not exceed this threshold.

Once the coronal images were obtained, the aortic valve plane and the aortic valve leaflets were localized as shown in this image (see Fig. 9-10). The slice selection was prescribed perpendicular to the jet approximately 10 to 15 mm superior to the aortic valve leaflets. At this slice, the phase VENC was applied in three directions to yield peak and mean velocity as well as velocity time integral (VTI).

*Analysis of PVM*

- Flow analysis can be performed using any of a number of ready vendor-made prototype commercial packages. We use MEDIS analytical package (Leiden,

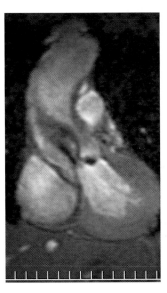
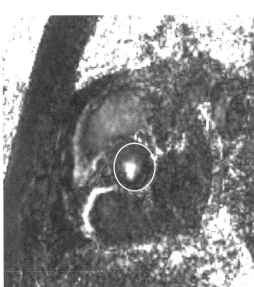

**FIGURE 9-10** Left panel: Gradient-recalled echo (GRE) image of severe aortic stenosis and the associated dephasing artifact in the shape of a systolic plume. Right panel demonstrates the use of phase velocity mapping to interrogate the extent of the aortic stenosis by quantitating the peak and mean velocities. The PVM generated plane is placed parallel to the aortic valve plane (perpendicular to the long-axis of the dephasing plume to generate the image in the right panel.)

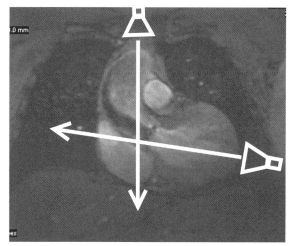

**FIGURE 9-11** A schematic demonstrating the lack of user-dependence ability for cardiovascular magnetic resonance (CMR) to define and interrogate velocities, independent of body habitus and geometric considerations. Notice that any plane can be selected that optimally interrogates velocities, as opposed to echocardiographic techniques (simulated) that rely on predefined manual acquisitions.

**TABLE 9-3**

Summary of characteristics and differences between conventional velocity measurements through Doppler and cardiovascular magnetic resonance phase velocity mapping

| Flow velocity by TTE | Flow velocity by CMR |
|---|---|
| Excellent temporal resolution | Modest temporal resolution |
| More accessible | Less accessible |
| Less labor intensive | Relatively labor intensive |
| User dependent | User independent |
| Inability to image flow in 3D | Ability to image flow in 3D |
| Cosine $\theta$ errors | Cosine $\theta$ errors uncommon |
| Limited by window | Not limited by window |

CMR, cardiovascular magnetic resonance; TTE, transthoracic echocardiography.

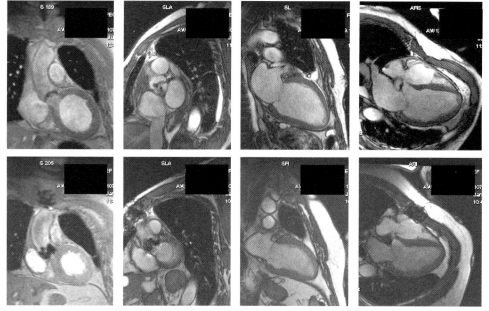

**FIGURE 9-12** Steady state free precession (SSFP) images. The top panel demonstrates a patient with severe compensated aortic stenosis with moderate left ventricular hypertrophy, and systolic dysfunction, not felt to be a candidate for aortic valve replacement. Note the heavily calcified aortic valve and dilated ventricle. Using phase velocity mapping (not shown) we demonstrated that the patient had myocardial reserve with severe afterload mismatch such that he underwent successful aortic valve replacement (bottom panel). These images were obtained 6 months post aortic valve replacement (AVR) in which his ejection fraction went from 19% to 52% confirming the capability for incredible myocardial recovery despite apparent prohibitive left ventricle (LV) dysfunction, if the primary pathology is pure aortic valve or stenosis. Images relate to case study 7.

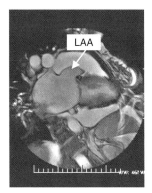 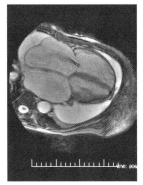 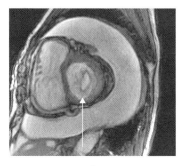

MVA = 1.4 cm² by planimetry

**FIGURE 9-13** Steady state free precession (SSFP) images. Left panel demonstrates the mitral valve with a large left atrial appendage (without obvious thrombus) and a large pericardial effusion. The middle panel demonstrates the dephasing artifact of tricuspid regurgitation and the large circumferential pericardial effusion, while the right panel depicts the restricted mitral valve leaflets, which by planimetry, reveals mild mitral stenosis. All images were obtained with the patient in atrial fibrillation at a rate of 98 beats/minute. Images relate to case study 8. LAA, left atrial appendage; MVA, mitral valve area.

The Netherlands) and/or MARISSA (Chase Medical, Dallas, Texas).

- Examination is done of entire 3D cross-section of aortic valve plane at level of maximum apparent gradient.
- Peak velocity is measured.
- Mean velocity is measured.
- VTI is calculated (if necessary).

In Fig. 9-10, right panel, the flow analysis was done offline using a semiautomatic MEDIS flow analytical package. Once the images were loaded onto this software, the region of interest was drawn encircling the whole cross-section of the aorta (see Fig. 9-10, right panel) and these contours were then automatically tracked to other images with minimal user input (correct the contours if required). This gave both the graphic as well as numerical time-resolved peak and mean velocities with the VTI. The post-processing time for CMR PVM was <2 minutes.

Interrogation of the aortic valve by CMR PVM incorporates several features that are characteristically quite different compared to standard echocardiographic measurements:

1. The entire jet in a cross-section is evaluated as compared to an "icepick" view, such that any velocity in that plane is detected. This is especially important for eccentric jets.
2. Any plane that can be envisioned in 3D space is acquirable by CMR; no user window or angle dependence is present in CMR (see Fig. 9-11)
3. The ability to interrogate in all three imaging planes (X, Y, and Z) is perhaps the chief advantage of CMR, permitting evaluation of flows and velocities that are in the plane orthogonal to the aortic valve, not

simply across it. This advantage is even more critical when it comes to evaluating intracardiac shunts, which frequently have nonperpendicular flow fields.

4. Exact location of the maximum velocity can be elucidated, as compared to continuous wave measurements by echocardiography whereby a peak velocity is obtained, but is not specifically related to an anatomic region.

In CMR there is no euphemistic term, *poor body habitus* or *poor acoustic window*. Further, the angulations frequently necessary to interrogate high velocity jets are not always optimally obtainable by either transthoracic echocardiography (TTE) or transesophageal echocardiography (TEE). This is emphasized in Fig. 9-11 diagrammatically, whereby the echocardiography probe may be unable to be aligned parallel to the direction of the maximum velocity. This eliminates cosine $\theta$ errors. These concepts are summarized in Table 9-3.

## CASE STUDIES

**Case Study 7.** A 76-year-old white man with a harsh systolic ejection murmur, referred for CMR (see Fig. 9-12, top panel). After convincing the surgeons this was an excellent case of afterload mismatch, while assuring them he would survive, he underwent AVR. The lower panel shows the patient 6 months' post AVR with an LVEF 55%, and a smaller LV with decreased LV mass, absent pleural effusion, and he is now mowing the lawn. Note the paramagnetic effect from the bioprosthetic aortic valve (left panel); not a contraindication for CMR (no prosthetic or bioprosthetic valves, including the pre-6,000 Star-Edwards, are contraindicated).

**Case Study 8.** A 63-year-old white woman with lupus who presents with progressive shortness of breath (SOB) (see Fig. 9-13). In addition to a large but nonhemodynamically significant pericardial effusion, she has evidence of mild (1+) mitral stenosis, mild aortic stenosis, and moderate (3+) tricuspid regurgitation. The short-axis (right panel) depicts mitral valve quantitation by planimetry. Direct visualization, as well as pressure half-time analysis, can be also be done. Evaluation of the left atrial appendage (LAA) (left panel) is also performed to evaluate for thrombus, should valvuloplasty be considered. Minimal MR is seen.

# CHAPTER 10

# Thoracic Magnetic Resonance Angiography

Robert W. W. Biederman

The study of thoracic angiography is chiefly concerned with evaluation of the aorta and its branch vessels. Cardiovascular magnetic resonance (CMR) has rapidly become a valuable modality for evaluation of both adult and pediatric aortic disease. The reason for this rapid acceptance of CMR is multifactorial: chiefly, the ability of CMR to image in a noninvasive manner, coupled with its intrinsic ability to image in any three-dimensional (3D) plane, makes it an ideal imaging tool, and the resolution that CMR provides for evaluation of the sometimes complex, perturbations that occur, adds another level of utility to this technique.

CMR has been shown to be the reference standard for the evaluation of aortic aneurysms (see Figs. 10-1 and 10-2), as well as having the highest sensitivity and specificity for the detection of aortic dissections (see Figs. 10-3, 10-4, and 10-5). When compared to transesophageal echocardiography (TEE) and x-ray angiography, CMR for the detection of aortic aneurysms, has been shown in multiple studies to have a sensitivity and specificity >98%. Particularly for aortic aneurysms, the ability to serially follow with high dimensional reproducibility allows optimal timing of surgical intervention. This issue has even greater relevance when nonaxial imaging is used. Reliance on axial imaging, frequently over- or underestimates dimensions compared to measurements made in nonorthogonal views. For instance, in the elderly population, as the descending aorta approaches the diaphragmatic hiatus, the lumen no longer travels perpendicular to the transversal plane, and the obliquity of the vessel results in overestimation of the lumen size. These features of CMR have an immediate clinical translation, avoiding inadvertent referral for surgery or worse still, actual surgical intervention. For this reason, CMR has been demonstrated to be the most appropriate modality, adding important surgical information, such as the presence of mural thrombus and other intraluminal perturbations, with near 100% accuracy.

More recently, the ability to add magnetic resonance angiography (MRA) to traditional magnetic resonance imaging (MRI) has further improved the capability of evaluating the aorta. Although older MRA data sets were acquired slice by slice, acquisitions were long and laborious, often taking 30 minutes of acquisition, and requiring extensive post-processing time. These acquisitions have been largely replaced with gadolinium contrast studies (see Figs. 10-6 and 10-7). The gadolinium agent is inert with almost no demonstrable side effects in patients with normal kidney function, and the increased T1 effect granted to the blood pool improves, not only the time of acquisition, but improves contrast, allowing increased fidelity of reconstruction. Three-dimensional reconstruction is now performed in an automated or semiautomated manner, and results in exquisite high-resolution surface and volume renderings. These images provide excellent roadmaps for planning surgical interventions (see Fig. 10-8).

The basis of CMR imaging for the thoracic vessels typically relies on double inversion recovery (DIR) and steady state free precession (SSFP) sequences, allowing diagnosis of aortic anatomy. Generally, non–breath-hold oblique images provide the necessary fidelity and resolution to allow assessment of intraluminal dimensions and morphologic features with high reproducibility. Flow-related enhancement (FRE) is a particularly important feature that must be accounted for in the determination of both luminal wall thickness and intraluminal pathology. Obtaining breath-hold images, reducing slice thickness, or changing the phase direction can improve image quality when considering flow-related artifacts. The SSFP sequence allows improved image contrast, to distinguishing between thrombus (dark) and normal blood (bright). On DIR images, slow-moving blood will not have had sufficient time to exit the imaging plane, and therefore may also be seen in these images (see Fig. 10-3). Direction of flow in antegrade or retrograde patterns is helpful in ascertaining the likelihood

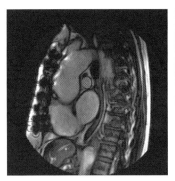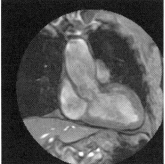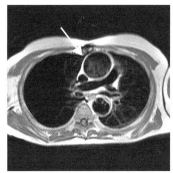

**FIGURE 10-1** Proximal ascending aortic aneurysm originating at the sinotubular junction sparing the sinus of Valsalva but distorting the aortic valve architecture with resultant mild (1+) aortic regurgitation. Note the prior sternal wires (left panel) from coronary artery bypass graft (CABG) surgery 10 years before distorting the anterior aorta, but minimally affecting the double inversion recovery (DIR) images (right panel) not precluding accurate measurements. The etiology of the aneurysm is not likely due to postoperative (iatrogenic) mechanism due to the symmetric nature and its involvement equilaterally around the sinotubular junction.

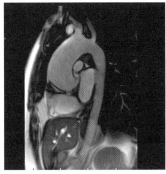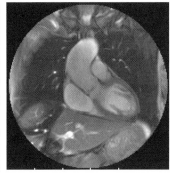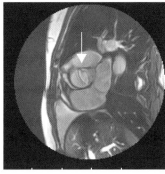

**FIGURE 10-2** The left panel demonstrates a moderately dilated proximal descending aortic aneurysm extending up to the distal descending aorta tapering at the arch. The middle panel further demonstrates mild sinotubular effacement and an asymmetric aortic valve. The right panel depicts a bicuspid aortic valve (*arrow*). Images relate to case study 1.

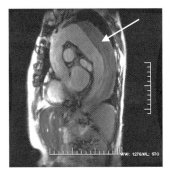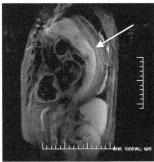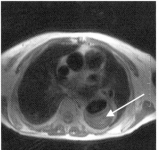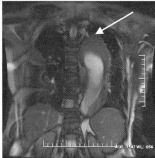

**FIGURE 10-3** Selected steady state free precession (SSFP) images (left panels) demonstrate a type B aortic dissection and what appears to be a large thrombosed false lumen. The right to left panels are selected double inversion recovery sequences, demonstrating the multiple layers of accumulated thrombus. Images relate to case study 2.

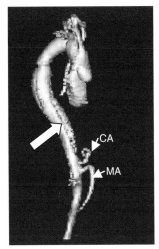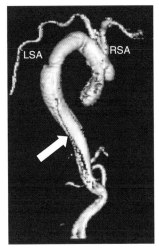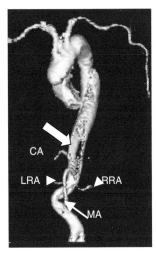

**FIGURE 10-4**  Rotating magnetic resonance angiography (MRA) of entire thoracic/abdominal aorta with a spiral type III dissection. Image acquisition was performed in 22 seconds. Note the spiral nature that is characteristic of a type III dissection as the aorta is rotated (*large arrow*). Other arteries are seen including the mesenteric artery (*MA*), celiac artery (*CA*), left and right and renal arteries (*LRA* and *RRA*) in the proximal and mid sections, as well as, large sections of the left and right subclavian arteries (*LSA* and *RSA*) arising from the true lumen.

for dissection propagation, as well as for detecting thrombus deposition. The pattern of blood flow within dissected lumens and aneurysms is well characterized by CMR using the SSFP sequence. The SSFP sequence represents a major improvement over the gradient-recalled echo (GRE) sequence for the determination of intraluminal pathology, because contrast is related to the intrinsic T2/T1 ratio of the tissue, and is not dominated by blood flow characteristics.

The use of MRA techniques involving a paramagnetic agent infused as a bolus (to reduce the blood T1) has resulted in high signal contrast of blood vessels, and

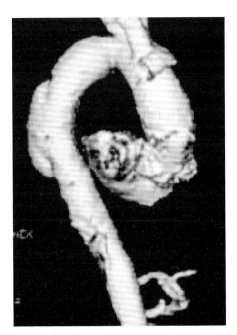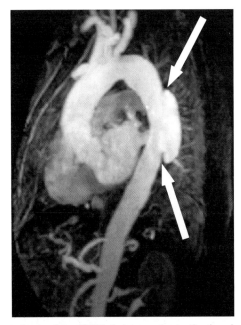

**FIGURE 10-5**  The two magnetic resonance angiographies(MRAs) demonstrate the focal Type Aortic III mushroom-shaped dissection of the mid thoracic descending aorta; however, the steady state free precession (SSFP) demonstrates the physiology of the dissection and suggests the etiology: a penetrating ulcer, arrowed. Images relate to case study 3.

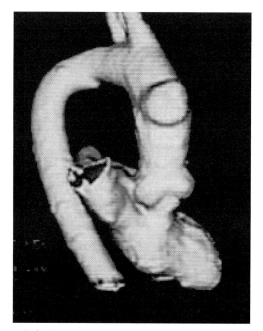
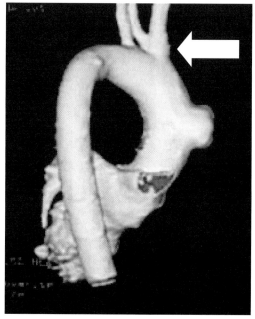

**FIGURE 10-6** Magnetic resonance angiography (MRA) depicts a focal, atypical aneurysm of the proximal ascending aorta. Note the bovine aorta (*arrow*). Images relate to case study 4.

in some cases coronary arteries or bypass grafts (see Fig. 10-9). In situations where either the DIR or SSFP sequences are not optimal, coordinated timing of contrast administration (using one of several approaches) permits rapid and reproducible vascular imaging. The fidelity of image acquisition allows vessels of submillimeter dimensions to be visualized. For instance, in a compliant patient, the intercostals vessels are often well seen in routine thoracic MRA. This has particular advantage for patients who have dissections, to allow an understanding of the need for an operation and for considering maintaining patency of the adjacent small vessels. Because acquisitions can be obtained in one to four table moves, the single bolus injection can be tracked as it passes through the aorta. Timed correctly, one can visualize the ascending aorta, arch, descending

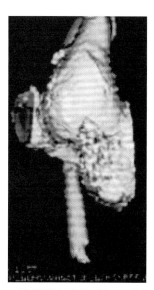
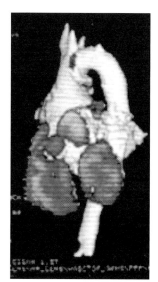
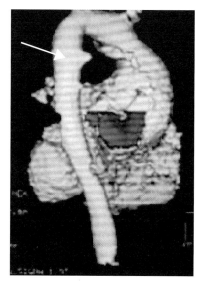

**FIGURE 10-7** Typical features of aneurysm with dissection. Note the penetrating ascending aortic ulcer seen as a small dimple on proximal descending aorta magnetic resonance angiography (MRA) (*arrow*). Images relate to case study 5.

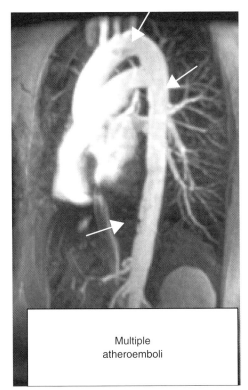
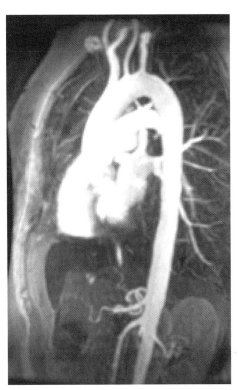

Multiple
atheroemboli

**FIGURE 10-8**   Cardiovascular magnetic resonance (CMR) was performed to evaluate for cardiac source of emboli, revealed multiple areas of atherosclerotic, as well as mobile plaque (left panel). The multiple location and sporadic nature of the plaques and mobile atheroma precluded surgical options, relegating her to coumadinization, for which a repeat magnetic resonance angiography (MRA) eight weeks later revealed resolution (right panel). Images relate to case study 6.

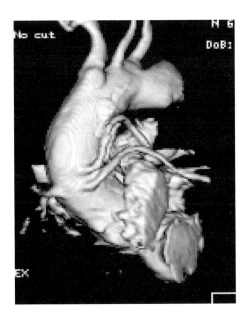
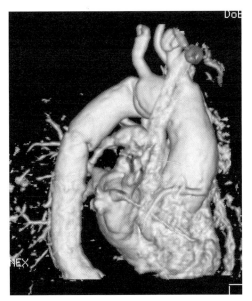

**FIGURE 10-9**   Cardiovascular magnetic resonance (CMR) of aorta, demonstrating no abnormality. Note also, the patency of three grafts. The saphenous vein graft (SVG) to left anterior descending (LAD) and SVG to obtuse marginal 1 (OM1) were both patent (left panel) as was the saphenous vein graft of the right coronary artery (SVG-RCA) (right panel). Images relate to case study 7.

aorta, abdominal aorta, iliac vessels, and finally the femoral and infrageniculate arteries.

## STRATEGIES FOR DETECTION OF AORTIC DISSECTIONS BY CARDIOVASCULAR MAGNETIC RESONANCE

It bears mentioning that the CMR magnet is generally not in close proximity to the emergency room or intensive care units. As a precaution, unstable patients have not been routinely imaged by CMR; however, careful screening of patients permits reasonably safe, accurate and relatively fast, high-quality images to be obtained in certain circumstances. For the intubated and paralyzed patient, paradoxically, CMR performs better, because it is much easier to manage breath-holding by manual control, permitting high-quality imaging in the patient who may otherwise have been uncomfortable. In our facility, we conduct a discussion with the patient when possible, to explain the details of the study to be performed, the breath-hold instructions to be followed, and the plan for contrast administration. All of this helps to reassure and relax the patient. Nonetheless, evaluation of the patient by the imaging clinician is important in cases of a patient *in extremis*. By evaluating each patient prescan, when believed to be in an emergent situation, we have been successful in imaging many patients who might not have been considered candidates for CMR, turning down only the rare patient who is severely hypotensive, coding, or actively infarcting. This adds a small element of a time penalty, but the benefit to the patient to have the optimal examination performed is far more beneficial than the added morbidity and mortality of other more invasive and, potentially less accurate, techniques.

Once in the scanner, a rapid series of non–breath-hold double axial inversion recovery (IR) images are first obtained, which quickly provide a large amount of information, allowing a preliminary working diagnoses to be formed. If breath-hold images are required, they are then conducted. A series of parasagittal and coronal SSFP images of the aorta serves as the major imaging strategy, providing a large amount of important clinical information relating to structure, flow direction and characteristics, lumen patency, and localization of pathology. Oftentimes, in the setting of aortic dissection, the ability to detect and characterize intrinsic intimal flap fenestrations helps to dictate the need for subsequent interventional protection of mesenteric, renal, and runoff vessels. Specifically, if a Type aortic III dissection is present (see Tables 10-1 and 10-2 for classifications), surgical correction of the

## CASE STUDIES

**Case Study 1.** A 45-year-old male presents with mild chest discomfort and is discovered to have a systolic ejection murmur. In Fig. 10-2, the left panel demonstrates a moderately dilated proximal descending aortic aneurysm extending up to the distal descending aorta tapering at the arch. The middle panel of Fig. 10-2 further demonstrates mild sinotubular effacement and an asymmetric aortic valve. The explanation for all is revealed in the third panel on the right panel of Fig. 10-2, which depicts a bicuspid aortic valve (*arrow*), which is strongly associated with ascending aortic dilatation.

**Case Study 2.** Presenting with severe back pain radiating to the abdomen and very different from his earlier myocardial infarction chest pain for which he underwent prior coronary artery bypass graft (CABG) years ago, this 72-year-old hypertensive man is emergently referred for CMR. Selected SSFP images (see Fig. 10-3, left panels) demonstrate a type B aortic dissection with what appears to be a largely thrombosed false lumen. Note the origination site in extremely close proximity to the left subclavian artery (LSA). Selected DIR images (see Fig. 10-3, right panels) demonstrate the multiple layers of accumulated thrombus. A combination of DIR and SSFP images helps to delineate whether this is sluggish flow or was truly a thrombosed false lumen. Thrombosed lumens can, and often do, appear similar to sluggish flow, but SSFP sequences demonstrate blood motion. This is critically important to the surgeon contemplating urgent repair. In this patient, CMR demonstrated a completely thrombosed false lumen, confirmed at surgery.

**Case Study 3.** An 88-year-old man with chronic back pain for more than 1 year worsening over recent weeks presents for CMR. The two MRAs demonstrate the focal type III mushroom dissection of the midthoracic descending aorta; however, the SSFP demonstrates the anatomy and physiology of the dissection and suggests the etiology: a penetrating ulcer (see Fig. 10-5). After medical management, a follow-up CMR was performed after 3 months, demonstrating relative stabilization. However, he again returned early one morning with acute back pain. A repeat CMR this time showed progression, for which he underwent surgical correction. Endoluminal stents were not available at the time of the CMR, negating this minimally invasive approach.

**Case Study 4.** A 67-year-old white man status post CABG 15 years ago has peculiar findings on routine CT scan, prompting a CMR. The MRA depicts a focal, atypical aneurysm of the proximal ascending aorta (see Fig. 10-6). Review of the surgical records shows early reoperation

**TABLE 10-1**

Aortic dissection classification (DeBakey)

| | |
|---|---|
| Type 1 | Dissection originates in the ascending aorta and extends to or beyond the arch |
| Type 2 | Dissection is contained within the ascending aorta |
| Type 3 | Dissection originates beyond the left subclavian artery and involves only the descending aorta |
| Type 3a | Dissection is contained within the thoracic aorta |
| Type 3b | Dissection extends into the abdomen |

ascending and arch aorta may be performed followed by balloon correction of aortic intimal flap fenestrations if they are not detected. In our laboratory, the evaluation of aortic pathology is not complete until the associated valvular and ventricular anatomy and physiology are defined. This entails evaluation of the aortic valve, sinus of Valsalva, and sinotubular junction, to detect the presence of aortic regurgitation. If present, the mechanism of valvular dysfunction is described, aiding in considerations for composite graft implantation. The extent, direction, and magnitude of the aortic regurgitation can be semiquantitatively assessed, and can be quantified by phase velocity mapping. SSFP images of the ventricle can be obtained to assess the impact of aortic regurgitation, left and right ventricular function, the presence of left ventricular hypertrophy, regional wall motion abnormalities, and left ventricle (LV) size. The presence of a pericardial effusion is an ominous sign, and should alert the interpreter that the dissection plane has extended through the pericardium. Generally, this means that there is occult dissection extending into the proximal ascending aorta. Given the large field of view (FOV) that CMR provides, the presence of a pleural effusion, especially a left pleural effusion, suggests that there has been extravasation of blood beyond the aortic wall and this is a major adverse cardiovascular prognostic sign.

Following standard SSFP imaging, dedicated segmental analysis is performed of regions in which earlier images have detected pathology. In these instances, evaluation of the dissection flap as it travels through

**TABLE 10-2**

Aortic dissection classification (Stanford)

| | |
|---|---|
| Type A | Dissection involves the ascending aorta |
| Type B | Dissection involves only the descending aorta |

<24 hours after CABG for bleeding. The most likely diagnosis is chronic contained rupture of aortic cannulation/deairing site with postoperative focal aneurysm. This was treated medically.

**Case Study 5.** A 69-year-old black man presents with chest and back pain for 1 year and a normal noncontrast CT scan at that time. After acute worsening, a CMR was performed demonstrating typical features of aneurysm with dissection (see Fig. 10-7). Note the penetrating ascending aortic ulcer seen as a small dimple on proximal descending aorta MRA (*arrow*), classic for an impending true dissection in a second location, the management of which is identical for both, that is, surgery. The mechanism for both locations is thought to be rupture of the vasa vasorum that progressively dilates and thromboses, only to eventually break through to the intima from which the forces of the cardiac contraction (dP/dT) propagate the rupture.

**Case Study 6.** A 59-year-old white woman status post abdominal pain was found to have multiple infarcts of a presumed embolic nature: splenic, renal, and left toe infarcts. A noncontrast, followed by a contrast, CMR was performed to evaluate for cardiac source of emboli (see Fig. 10-8). CMR revealed multiple areas of atherosclerotic, as well as mobile plaques. The multiple location and sporadic nature of the plaques and mobile atheroma precluded surgical options relegating her to coumadinization, for which a repeat MRA revealed resolution after just 8 weeks. A hypercoagulable state was investigated and revealed factor V Leiden deficiency, for which she was placed on life-long anticoagulation.

**Case Study 7.** A 63-year-old black man presents several weeks after his first CABG with atypical chest pain, prompting a CMR MRA to evaluate his aorta, which demonstrated no abnormality (see Fig. 10-9). Note the patency of his three coronary artery bypass grafts. The MRA as a 22-second, single-table move, examination was performed as the test of choice. His saphenous vein graft (SVG) to left anterior descending (LAD) and SVG to obtuse marginal 1 (OM1) were both patent (left) as was his saphenous vein graft of the right coronary artery (SVG-RCA) (right). This CMR prevented the need for a repeat cardiac catheterization.

**Case Study 8.** Dynamic 2D SSFP imaging yields a high amount of detail to differentiate between moving blood and thrombus (see Fig. 10-10). In the left and middle panels of Fig. 10-10, note the thrombosed false lumen that is barely noticeable in the MRA (right panel). This problem is true of any modality which is dependent on

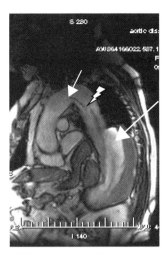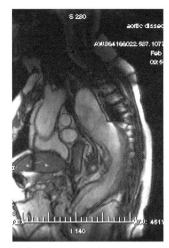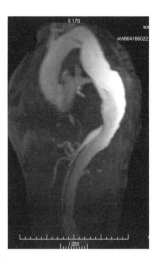

**FIGURE 10-10** Two-dimensional dynamic imaging yields a high amount of detail in this patient with a thrombosed false lumen (left panels), barely noticeable in the magnetic resonance angiography (MRA) (right panel). A type B dissection, with a small true and larger false lumen is present. Note the thrombosed false lumen (*largest arrow*), autocommunications between true and false lumen (*zigzag arrow*), and that the dissection continues into abdominal aorta (*smallest arrow*). Images relate to case study 8.

the mesenteric area is important to define the patency of the superior and inferior mesenteric arteries, as well as the celiac artery. Determination of whether the intimal flap affects the renal arteries is important. Defining whether the true lumen supplies both, one, or none of the renal arteries has major clinical implications and this can be performed by CMR with dedicated SSFP imaging.

Our philosophy is that all imaging of the aorta in the setting of either aneurysm or dissection should be complete or nearly complete *without* the need for MRA. This strategy far predated concerns for nephrogenic sclerosing fibrosis (NSF). We utilize MRA to further define the anatomy and course for the referring physician or surgeon, often employing endoluminal angiography (see Figs. 10-10 and 10-11). Primarily, contrast is used when the need to provide clarity in 3D for the computed tomography (CT) surgeon is indicated. An instance in which we employ MRA, almost without question, is when the patient has presented with signs and symptoms of an aortic dissection which are not visible by CMR. In this setting, the suspicion of a penetrating aortic ulcer is high (see Fig. 10-7). SSFP imaging, while allowing reasonably high resolution, may require a high degree of suspicion before a small or moderate size ulcer is visualized. Using gadolinium MRA, the entire aorta can be quickly analyzed, reconstructed, and interpreted for peculiar mushroom-shaped defects that extend beyond the aortic lumen (see Figs. 10-5 and 10-7). Interestingly, these generally small, aortic lesions present with a similar ripping, tearing sensation that is associated with a classic aortic dissection. Despite their relative innocuous appearance, a recent study demonstrated that they

contrast opacification of the lumen. A large type B dissection, with a small true, and larger, mostly thrombosed, false lumen is present, continuing into the abdominal aorta. Subtle autofenestrations are present (*zigzag arrow*) permitting for near symmetric flow between the true and false lumen, as confirmed by the similar signal intensity. The finding of autofenestrations is an important observation, because it will help delineate surgical or intervention strategies, specifically designed to surgically create fenestrations if they are not present (see Fig. 10-11). Creation of ducts between the true and false lumens allows for flow to mesenteric, renal, and intercostal arteries to be less compromised, and is generally a favorable prognostic sign.

**Case Study 9.** After a TEE, x-ray angiogram, and a CT scan failed to define fully the anatomy and pathology in this 68-year-old white man with multiple aneurysms and saccular outpocketings, he was referred for MRA before any surgical considerations (see Fig. 10-12). After SSFP imaging was performed (not shown), an MRA with a 22-second acquisition was performed. MRA is rendered as surface (left) and volume (right). Figure 10-13 demonstrates a "virtual luminal angiography" permitting traveling through the lumen and inspecting from inside the aorta, that is, not the conventional approach from outside the aorta. It was from this perspective that the diagnosis of multiple saccular aneurysms was made. The patient was deemed not to be a surgical candidate. A workup for an arteritis, fibrillin gene abnormality and Behçet disease was entertained.

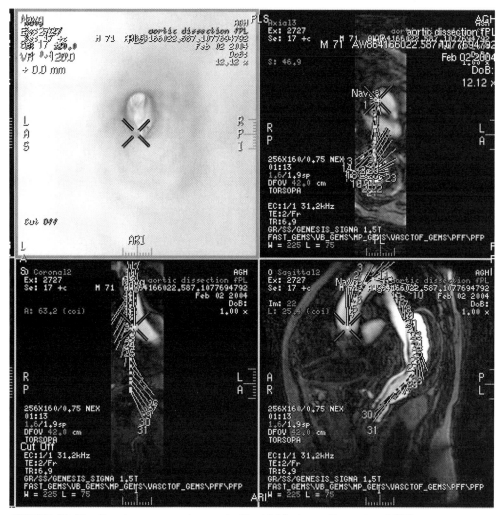

**FIGURE 10-11**   For the same patient as in Fig. 10-10: three-dimensional (3D) representation of multiple projections of the angiographic rendering (clockwise from top left: virtual rendering, axial, coronal, and sagittal views). Each point depicted provides virtual triangulation in 3D space as the aorta is traversed. The operator defined which lumen to travel through, and several autocommunications (fenestrations) are present between lumens. Images relate to case study 8.

should be treated as a *form fruste* of aortic dissection. Finally, intraluminal hematoma is an ominous harbinger for conversion to true aortic dissection. These are extraordinarily difficult to image by TEE or x-ray angiography because the lumen may not be deformed. Using CMR, careful evaluation for a crescent, thickened aortic wall, typically in the arch and descending aorta should be made in every aortic dissection presentation, especially in a patient presenting with signs and symptoms of dissection, but in whom none is seen on standard imaging. This can be performed using either the DIR sequence or the SSFP sequence, but the MRA is the most sensitive for this, sometimes elusive, pathology. The recognition of an intramural hematoma is a very important finding, because it has the same clinical implications as a true dissection. It is

**Case Study 10.** A 64-year-old man presents 9 months after a composite graft with chest pain. What is the abnormality depicted by the arrows in Fig. 10-14? (a) psuedoaneurysm (b) perigraft leak (c) endograft leak, or (d) loculated pericardial effusion The correct answer is a perigraft leak—note the heterogeneous high signal on the T2 images. This is most consistent with perigraft glue used more often in the last few years by the surgeons to limit bleeding and stabilize the graft. Note the MRA (upper middle panel) demonstrating no evidence of gadolinium extravasation.

**Case Study 11.** A middle-aged man in mild distress presents for evaluation of LV function after an equivocal

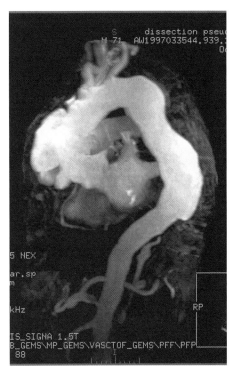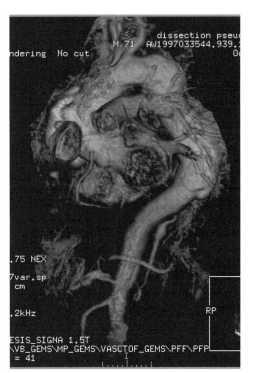

**FIGURE 10-12** Magnetic resonance angiography (MRA) showing multiple aneurysms and saccular outpocketings, rendered as surface (left) and volume (right). Images relate to case study 9.

been shown that most of the dissections have as their initial presentation, rupture of the small vasa vasorum with subsequent expansion to form thrombus within the intimal wall. As this expands, the intima eventually ruptures, forming the true dissection. Therefore, the observation of an intramural hematoma allows for medical or surgical therapy to proceed, recognizing that fully one third of all intramural hematomas will progress to frank dissection.

Preoperative assessment has been shown to be accurate for the often complex, aortic reconstructions that have been the hallmark of advanced cardiovascular surgical approaches over the recent decade (see Figs. 10-12 and 10-13). Composite grafts, interpositioned grafts, Bentall technique, hemiarch repairs, and "elephant trunk technique" are some of the creative surgical techniques employed in the field of aortic repair. Extensive aneurysmal changes involving the descending, arch, and descending thoracic aorta, or thoracoabdominal aorta can undergo a complex repair in which the descending aorta and aortic arch are repaired first with a graft segment left within the proximal descending thoracic aorta. In large descending aortic aneurysms, the aorta is transected and repaired with an interposed graft with replacement of any of the mesenteric intercostals and renal arteries as a button to the graft. More recently, aortic vascular endoluminal grafts can be placed in various positions within the aorta and limit the obligate

echocardiogram was performed for atypical chest pain. One of the advantages of CMR that often goes unrecognized is its large FOV, which in this case, demonstrated the ability to pick up critically important, pathology (see Fig. 10-15). While the MR angiogram (see Fig. 10-15 left panel) was performed after the SSFP 2D images (other panels), SSFP functional images revealed a descending type III dissection, prompting further CMR imaging.

**Case Study 12.** Thoracic MRA performed in an older patient with a complex spiral dissection seen on MRA (see Fig. 10-16). Straddling the proximal thoracic aorta is a partially thrombosed false lumen imaged late, permitting (partial) contrast opacification of the false lumen with the center panel depicting virtual angiography (best seen in the DVD). Visualization of the mesenteric and renal vessels provides assurance that the true lumen supplies all of the extra-aortic abdominal vasculature. Note that the left renal artery (LRA) arises at the junction between the visualized true lumen and the nonopacified false lumen. A measure of the symmetry of blood flow between the true and false lumen is intimated in that there is absent false lumen signal at the level of the abdominal aorta, indicating the sluggish, asymmetric blood flow to the false lumen.

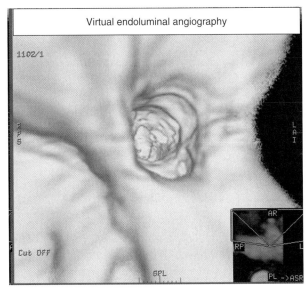

**FIGURE 10-13**  Magnetic resonance angiography (MRA) with Navigator General Electric (GE) reconstruction for same patient as in Fig. 10-12 showing virtual luminal angiography, which was performed to demonstrate marked aneurismal intraluminal defects through the entire ascending, arch and descending aorta. Image relates to case study 9.

**Case Study 13.** A question asked clinically is, can we perform virtual luminal angiography in the carotids? In a 65-year-old man who presented for evaluation of his thoracic aorta, sequentially timed MRA was performed to track, not only the thoracic aorta but also to acquire the carotid arteries. Virtual luminal angiography was performed in the carotids (see Fig. 10-17 right panel) with manual tracking of the contrast–intimal interface. Does it help for the evaluation of arch anatomy? MRAs in conjunction with virtual luminal angiography (see Fig. 10-17 right panel) are exceptional CMR methodologies to complement routine thoracic angiography. This has theoretic and practical advantages for the neurologist and vascular surgeon, when contemplating carotid endarterectomy or other carotid artery interventions.

**Case Study 14.** Using only SSFP sequences, a 60-year-old woman status post CABG 5 years who now reports progressive chest discomfort, radiating deep into her right chest with a ripping, tearing sensation completely different from her initial chest pain symptoms (that resulted in bypass surgery) undergoes CMR (see Fig. 10-18). Imaging demonstrates a complex, spiral dissection originating from the origin of, but not involving the ostium of the LSA extending throughout the entire thoracic aorta and deep into the abdominal aorta. A number of autofenestrations are visible, as well as evidence that the LRA is supplied by the true lumen. On other imaging (not shown), the right renal is derived from the false lumen. However, in that the flow characteristics of the descending aorta reveal nearly simultaneous signal intensity, it is reasonable to assume that flow is nearly simultaneous. The generally slightly brighter signal in the false lumen (right) as compared to the true lumen (left) denotes the *slightly* faster blood flow, again, likely not physiologically significant. There was no need for contrast MRA to be performed due to the high image quality of standard dynamic 2D imaging using SSFP sequences.

morbidity and mortality of an open surgical procedure. Especially for infrarenal aortic aneurysms, this procedure has become a standard in many institutions, for which CMR, with or without MRA, is extraordinarily helpful. Interventional techniques not requiring open incisions can be performed by either cardiologists in conjunction with cardiac surgeons or in the interventional radiology suite through a percutaneous iliac artery approach. Critical features that are important in decision making, include the accurate measurement of the neck of the aneurysm, accurate 2D and 3D measurements delineating the aneurysm in relationship to the often nearby or adjacent renal arteries, particularly for the often tortuous and ectatic abdominal aneurysms, nonaxial imaging incorporating coronal, parasagittal, or multioblique imaging often prevents over- or underestimation of the narrow neck and aneurismal anatomy.

Postoperative assessments by CMR are sometimes even more important, given the complexity of the aortic repair and replacement strategies available. Because image quality is high with CMR, with or without MRA, it is essential for the interpreting physician to have more than a passing knowledge of the surgical options available and the myriad of anatomic perturbations. The older grafts are generally circular, and appear as very dark signal voids on SSFP and GRE images, helping to distinguish them from the native aorta, which is generally much more irregular, and in this setting, typically atherosclerotic. More recently, perigraft accumulations

need to be identified either as graft leak, infection, or surgical glue. Formerly, a high T2 perigraft signal occurring weeks to months after surgery was considered to be an infection. However, with the advent of surgical glue to retard postoperative bleeding and limit leakage, as well as seal the graft to the native aorta, distinguishing between infection, blood, and glue is clinically necessary (see Fig. 10-14). Often, simple image characteristics are not helpful. Reliance on the operative note, and knowledge of the surgeon's general techniques is helpful. Generally, surgical glue gives a homogeneous T2 signal, whereas infection, although having a high T2 signal, is more heterogeneous and does not encircle

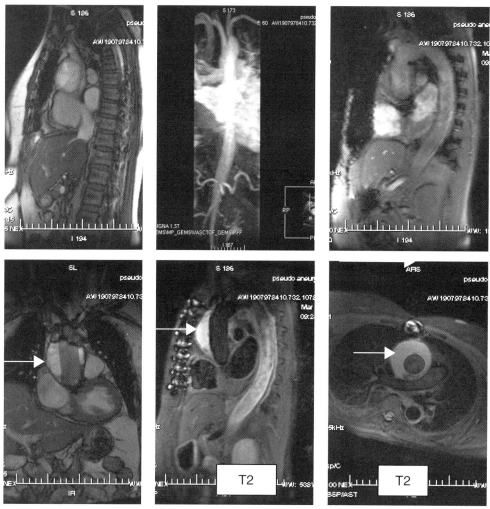

**FIGURE 10-14**   Perigraft leak. Note the heterogeneous high signal T2 images (lower panel). Note the magnetic resonance angiography (MRA), (upper middle panel) demonstrating no evidence of gadolinium extravasation. Images relate to case study 10.

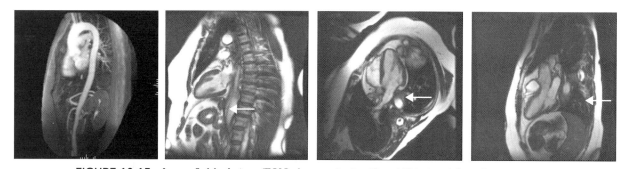

**FIGURE 10-15**   Large field of view (FOV) demonstrates the ability to pick up important, pathophysiology. Magnetic resonance angiography (MRA) (far left) shows aorta, and steady state free precession (SSFP) functional images (other panels) reveal a descending Type Aortic III dissection (*arrow*). Images relate to case study 11.

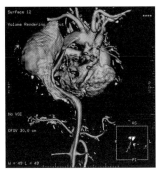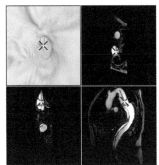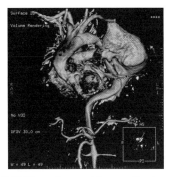

**FIGURE 10-16**    Thoracic magnetic resonance angiography (MRA) performed in a patient with a complex spiral dissection seen on MRA. The middle panel reveals virtual luminal angiography shown at a site of the intimal flap, matched by the site in the 3D angiogram. Images relate to case study 12.

the graft. Blood may have a very homogeneous signal, which is dependant on its age, can be dated, as well as seen to be free flowing on SSFP or GRE imaging. Endothelialization around the aortic graft can also be bright on T2-weighted images, but in the absence of a homogeneous signal, is usually related to surgical scar and collagen or fibrosis, and is a normal postsurgical finding. Some, but not all, aortic endografts are completely CMR compatible in that there is no or minimal paramagnetic effect. However, there are still a few that are non-CMR safe and require evaluation before imaging. By far, the industry direction is to make an increasing number of grafts (valves or any other prosthetic devices) magnetic resonance compatible.

The use of both MRA with CMR is helpful in evaluation of the patient with occult dissection (see Fig. 10-15), peculiar abnormalities of the visualized aorta (see Fig. 10-16), the adjunctive use in great vessel pathology (see Fig. 10-17), complex thoracoabdominal aortic dissections (see Fig. 10-18) in confirming or refuting suspicions other techniques have raised for aortic pathology (see Fig. 10-19) or atypical findings or presentations (see Fig. 10-20).

## AORTIC ARCH ANOMALIES

The ability to image the aorta and its great vessels is a great advantage for the CMR imager. Owing to the ability of CMR to image in multiple planes with a large FOV and with high spatial resolution, accurate demonstration of the vascular structures is possible without requiring contrast administration to achieve a high signal. Identification of related nonvascular structures such as the trachea, bronchi and branch bronchi,

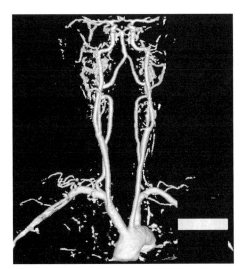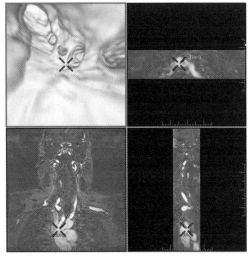

**FIGURE 10-17**    Sequentially timed magnetic resonance angiography (MRA) was performed to track, not only the thoracic aorta, but also to acquire the carotid arteries allowing virtual luminal angiography (right panel) and surface rendering (left panel). Images relate to case study 13.

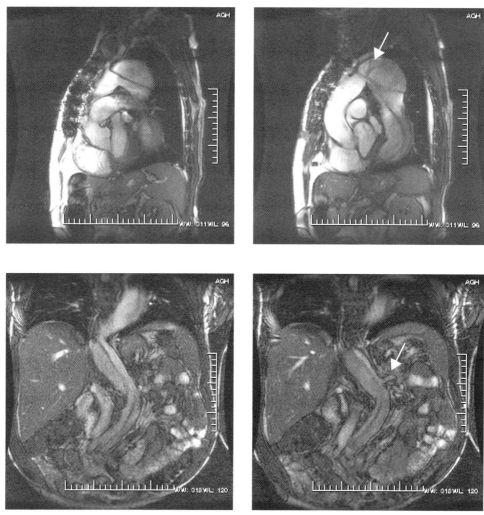

**FIGURE 10-18** Cardiovascular magnetic resonance (CMR) demonstrating a complex, spiral dissection with a number of autofenestrations visible (top panel *arrow*), as well as evidence that the left renal artery is supplied by the true lumen (lower panel *arrow*). Images relate to case study 14.

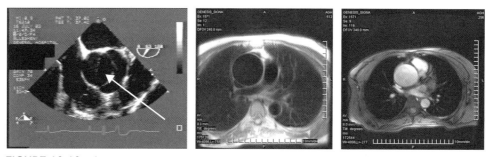

**FIGURE 10-19** A transesophageal echocardiogram was read as probable proximal aortic dissection (left panel). The cardiovascular magnetic resonance (CMR) was performed using double inversion recovery (DIR) and steady state free precession (SSFP) imaging to conclude that the diagnosing transesophageal echocardiography (TEE) results to be artifactual. Images relate to case study 15.

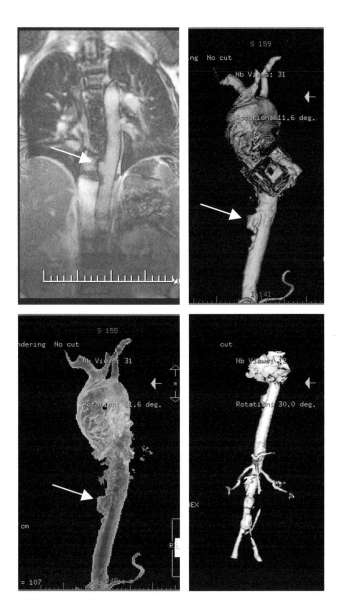

**FIGURE 10-20** Upper left panels show steady state free precession (SSFP) aortic wall defect, that in the clockwise magnetic resonance angiography (MRA) reconstruction (volume, surface, and transparent) reveals a large penetrating aortic ulcer with evidence for a localized dissection; the natural history of penetrating aortic ulcers. Images relate to case study 16.

**Case Study 15.** An anxious 40-year-old woman presents with sudden onset of sharp chest pain radiating to her back, with diaphoresis shortly vigorous exercise. A transesophageal echocardiogram was performed emergently at 5:30 AM, which was read as probable proximal aortic dissection. With $\beta$-blocker and anxiolytic therapy, the pain subsided. In that her presentation was peculiar and her physical examination did not corroborate with the TEE finding, a CMR was performed at 7 AM (see Fig. 10-19). Using DIR and SSFP imaging only, the 12-minute study conclusively found the TEE suspicions to be an artifact. No further clinical sequelae occurred over the next 2 days and on follow-up over the 1 year, she has had no further episodes of pain. Her acute presentation was likely precipitated by acute stress.

**Case Study 16.** A 75-year-old white woman with very severe back and unrelenting abdominal pain prompts a CMR examination (see Fig. 10-20) with a most unusual presentation, a penetrating aortic ulcer (*arrow*) reformatted by a transparent MRA technique and a standard 3D MRA.

**Case Study 17.** An unusual presentation for a middle-aged woman who presents with mild dysphagia and undergoes CMR with MRA after barium swallow revealed an abnormality (see Fig. 10-21). Formed by an abnormal congenital malformation (fourth brachial aortic arch anomaly) whereby the right subclavian artery arises as a separate aortic vessel and distal to the LSA but travels posterior to the aorta before emerging to supply the right arm, occasionally this abnormality (*arrow*) can be responsible for dysphagia. Occasionally, the ostial and proximal segment of the aberrant artery, lacking in neural crest cells, becomes very aneurismal, occasionally dilating to >8 cm; then it is known as a diverticulum of Kommerell. In this case an esophagogastroduodenoscopy (EGD) failed to demonstrate any physically significant obstruction.

esophagus, and other structures that are adjacent to the aorta, permits high-resolution visualization of many congenital aortic/arch anomalies. Again, the workhorse sequences are DIR, SSFP, with or without MRA. Generally, we utilize contrast enhancement for better display of the arch anomalies for the referring physician, as well as confirmation of the SSFP/DIR findings. Surface and volume rendering can be performed following a 15 to 20 seconds MRA with display to the interpreter provided within 1 minute. The most common arch anomaly is a bovine aorta in which there are only two supraaortic vessels. The right subclavian artery and right common carotid arise off a common origin with the left subclavian, slightly more distal, but arising generally in its correct location. This benign lesion is important when cross clamping or manipulation of the great vessels is considered.

Anomalies of the aortic arch are to be defined in three categories, as follows:

1. *Anomalies of the left aortic arch.* The left aortic arch with an apparent right subclavian artery is the most common anomaly of the aortic arch with an incidence of 1 of 250 people. It is usually an incidental finding

and is asymptomatic. It arises as a fourth branch from the aorta (just beyond the left subclavian artery [LSA]) and travels obliquely from right to left behind the esophagus, to supply blood flow to the right arm. The descending aorta is to the left of the spinal column. A second variant is the left aortic arch with a right descending thoracic aorta. In this case, the arch passes backwards and to the left of both the trachea and esophagus with the distal portion of the arch traveling on to the right side behind the esophagus to continue as a right descending aorta (to the right of the spinal column).

2. *Anomalies of the right aortic arch.* The right aortic arch is defined with the arch to the right of the trachea and esophagus and the descending thoracic aorta to the right of the spine. There are several subtypes of the right aortic arch.

a. Right aortic arch with aberrant LSA: This is the most common anomaly in patients with the right aortic arch. In this anomaly, the fourth branch arises in the aortic arch after being embryologically separated in the following manner—the left common carotid is first followed by the right common carotid and the right subclavian artery is in the place where the LSA should be, while the aberrant left subclavian is the most distal great vessel. An interesting association is when the proximal LSA arises from its anomalous position and becomes markedly dilated (see Fig. 10-21). The name given to this specific anatomic anomaly is a diverticulum of Kommeral. This can also happen in the setting of a right aortic arch and anomalous LSA formed by a congenital malformation

(fourth brachial arch) whereby the right subclavian artery arises as a separate aortic vessel and is distal to the LSA but travels posterior to the aorta before emerging to supply the right arm. Occasionally, this ostial and proximal segment of the aberrant artery, lacking in neural crest cells, becomes aneurismal, rarely dilating to >8 cm, and generating diagnostic confusion unless recognized. Typically, mild odynophagia is the presenting symptomotology.

b. Right aortic arch with mirror image branching: The first branch off the right aortic arch is the left brachiocephalic artery. The right common carotid artery and right subclavian artery follow. Other associated congenital diseases may be present.

c. A right aortic arch with less subclavian artery isolation: This is an interesting anomaly in which the LSA arises off the left pulmonary artery by way of a left ductus arteriosus which is preceded by the left common carotid, right common carotid, and right subclavian arteries (RSAs), in that order. This is a rare congenital anomaly, often associated with tetralogy of Fallot or other cardiac malformations. Occasionally mistaken for subclavian steal syndrome due to the discrepancy in arm cuff pressures, this rare diagnosis bears further evaluation if suspected.

## VIRTUAL LUMINAL ANGIOGRAPHY

Reconstruction of the rapidly acquired 3D MRA is performed using relatively sophisticated post-processing algorithms; many vendors have the ability to physically subtract the contrast that was acquired, leaving behind

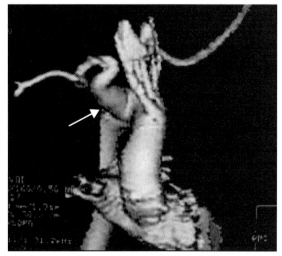
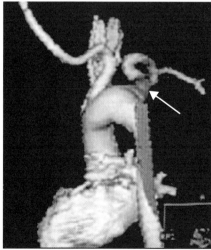

**FIGURE 10-21** The arrows point to the aberrant right subclavian takeoff with mild aneurysmal dilatation consistent with a small diverticulum of Kommerell. Images relate to case study 17.

only the nonluminal information (see Figs. 10-12 and 10-13). Essentially, the signal that remains is the interface between the intima/blood layer. While this requires manual reconstruction, the resulting images are breathtaking. Once reconstructed, the viewer is treated to a 3D trip through the aortic lumen and its associated vessels. Specifically, the imager no longer visualizes the vessel from the outside, but is transferred to the center of the structure and travels through it as if he is a single blood cell on a trip through the center of the aorta. This is analogous to "*The Fantastic Voyage,*" penned by Aldous Huxley many years ago. More than an imaging curiosity, this capability provides substantial information to the referring physician concerning the luminal topography. For instance, the surgeon now has an internal roadmap to understand where the area of greatest atherosclerotic debris resides before cross-clamping the aorta. Appreciating where the intimal flap arises from and assessing the extent of endogenous fenestrations is of critical importance to the cardiothoracic or vascular surgeon. Evaluation of vessels down to the size of 3 to 4 mm has been performed at our laboratory in coarctations with dissection flaps, to confirm the veracity of our standard MRA. Additionally, the spectacular presentation draws many a sigh from non–CMR personnel, exposing them to the wonders of CMR!

## CARDIOVASCULAR MAGNETIC RESONANCE ANGIOGRAPHY IN CONGENITAL HEART DISEASE

The use of MRA to evaluate patients with simple or complex congenital heart disease is a distinct advantage of CMR, especially in the pediatric population. A more detailed description of congenital heart disease will be covered in a later chapter.

# CHAPTER 11

# Extra Thoracic Magnetic Resonance Angiography

Robert W. W. Biederman

Generally, in discussions of cardiovascular magnetic resonance (CMR) most authors limit their discussions to supradiaphragmatic anatomic and pathologic vascular perturbations. We, however, believe that nonthoracic aortic vasculature should also be included. The purpose of this chapter is to emphasize to the clinician that the "C" in CMR stands for cardiovascular, and therefore includes the broader vasculature and is not limited to that adjacent to, or associated with, the small beating muscle in the center of the chest. The following will be a general discussion on the utility of CMR, with and without the use of magnetic resonance angiography (MRA), to understand peripheral angiography. Over the last decade, extensive research and investigations have demonstrated the utility, applicability, and reproducibility of noninvasive imaging of the peripheral vasculature using CMR. Many specialized textbooks are dedicated to that subject alone, and this single chapter will serve to summarize the capabilities of CMR. Specifically, it is not meant to be an exhaustive compendium of all that is known. In this chapter we will not focus on specific aortic disease as an individual entity, but only as related to conduits of the branches derived from the aorta with the exception of the carotid vessels, which are not included.

Many noninvasive assessments of peripheral vascular disease exist, including ultrasound which incorporates continuous wave, pulse wave Doppler, and two-dimensional imaging; exercise testing; impedance plethsmography; and magnetic resonance imaging (MRI)/MRA. Each of these noninvasive modalities has its own advantages and disadvantages. Before the development of MRA, the only suitable method to evaluate the peripheral vasculature was contrast arteriography. Now, virtually all vascular territories can be visualized by the use of, either in combination or individually, CMR and MRA. Although this chapter will be limited to arterial structure it should be noted that there is also a role for venous and lymphatic characterization by both anatomic and flow-related techniques.

As the population continues to age, the role atherosclerosis plays cannot be overstated. Beyond affecting the coronary bed, the aorta and the carotids, there is increasing recognition that impairment of the renal arteries and peripheral runoff vessels are major sources of morbidity and mortality. Unexplained hypertension affects a significant number of patients because of occlusion of one or more renal arteries. Claudication has been recently recognized by the National Institutes of Health (NIH) as one of the major morbidities facing our aging population, and strategies aimed at detecting its presence are in general under utilized by the internist, cardiologist, and the general surgeon. Historically, a major difficulty in this assessment was a lack of a suitable imaging strategy, placing the vascular surgeon, cardiologist, and interventionalist at a disadvantage when addressing this major disabling entity. With the recognition that diabetes plays a growing role in disease presentation, either due to its increase prevalence or better recognition, the search for occult atherosclerotic disease in this population has been recognized as being critically important by leading medical societies. Peripheral arterial disease is the most common cause of systematic obstruction in the major extracoronary arteries. For the most part, the pathophysiologic understanding of this disease process is identical to that of the coronary artery tree. The risk factors for atherosclerosis of the noncoronary arteries are identical to those of coronary artery disease patients. Detection by CMR follows a similar pathway to that utilized in invasive strategies, aiming to detect pathology that exceeds 50% obstruction. In general, as the disease process progresses, luminal encroachment graded as >70% is likely to be responsible for symptomotology. Claudication, whether it is of the lower extremity or upper extremity through effort related activity, is almost always the universal presenting symptom. Intermittent claudication can be mild, progressive, and debilitating and can wax and wane.

Because the therapies for peripheral arterial disease, while still in their infancy, have generally improved over the last decade, the CMR capability to detect disease has progressed rapidly. Despite these improved imaging strategies, detection of the disease does not always lead to optimized therapy for all vascular territories. For instance, the external iliac arteries, a source of substantial debilitating buttocks claudication, are rarely intervened upon. A chief therapeutic option remains adopting conservative measures, strongly focusing on preventing progression of disease, improving exercise capability with walking, conditioning exercises, and cessation of smoking. Several pharmocologic therapies are available but have not generally resulted in dramatic improvements in symptoms. The fall-back position for patients who have failed conservative therapy is interventional vascular or surgical therapies, which have shown great promise in reducing certain morbidities and mortalities. The characteristics of CMR are ideal in detecting atherosclerosis within the peripheral vascular bed; early experimental research suggesting this may be an important modality to risk-stratify atherosclerotic plaques.

## SPECIFIC CARDIAC MAGNETIC RESONANCE IMAGING TECHNIQUES

Utilizing both the double inversion recovery (DIR) and the steady state free precession (SSFP) sequence, the great majority of aortic iliac disease can be diagnosed. The SSFP sequence is an improvement over the older, flow-dependent, gradient recalled echo (GRE) sequence in that turbulent flow, which previously resulted in overestimation of disease state, is less problematic. Both axial and coronal images are ideal for this presentation. Utilizing a combination of SSFP and localized axial sequences to grade disease state more effectively, the territory of the ileofemoral and infrageniculate arteries can be defined. Compared to dynamic imaging, the addition of gadolinium-based MRA sequences offer substantial improvement in visualization, which leads to increased confidence in diagnostic interpretations. Therefore, in our laboratory all peripheral vascular studies, despite the level of confidence obtained with noncontrast imaging, are completed with MRA. Only in the rare instance in which the patient cannot undergo intravenous administration, will we attempt to utilize time of flight (TOF) imaging. This contrasts with examination of the aorta in which non-contrast imaging is often sufficient to not require MRA.

With three-dimensional (3-D) MRA, surface and volume rendering views are obtained, providing high-quality information rapidly (see Fig. 11-1). However, on occasion, reconstruction information is equivocal. In

## CASE STUDIES

**Case Study 1.** A 65-year-old man presents with left leg claudication, and on examination a left proximal iliac bruit is thought to be heard (see Fig. 11-2, top left panel). The patient is referred for CMR ileofemoral angiography. The distal abdominal aorta is well visualized, as is the right ileofemoral system. Arising at the ostial left iliac artery is a long 2.5-cm lesion with clean "cutoff" sign. A very faint "string sign" is also seen. The combination is indicative of a subtotal occlusion. The referring physician was notified and the patient was promptly sent for x-ray angiography with a plan for a left iliac angioplasty/stent. The following day I received a call from the angiographer stating, "There are widely patent bilateral iliac arteries. The site of the proximal right iliac stent is also widely patent!" Unbeknownst to all, the patient had earlier undergone implantation of one of the first iliac stents to be placed in the state. This is now a well-known artifact. It requires vigilance on the part of the interpreter, who may not necessarily be privy to all of the necessary information. The clean cutoff sign is now retrospectively, a clear indication of a nonanatomic stenosis associated with a stent paramagnetic artifact and due to the "shielding" effect of the stent.

**Case Study 2.** A 67-year-old man status post bilateral femoral artery conduits now with two symmetrical peculiar bilateral aneurysmal formations at the anastamosis to the native vessel, imaged with coronal SSFP (see Fig. 11-2, lower left panel) and confirmed by MRA (see Fig. 11-2, lower right panel). Note the prior aneurysm clips seen as paramagnetic artifact appearing to deform the bladder (filling with the T1-weighted contrast), Fig. 11-2, lower left panel. An additional SSFP (see Fig. 11-2, upper right panel) reveals a large mass in the abdomen that is a partially undigested heavy breakfast masquerading as a large mass.

**Case Study 3.** A 65-year-old white man presents with right leg and buttocks pain and claudication. An x-ray angiogram was not definitive in explaining the nature of the vascular problem despite digital subtraction angiography (DSA), mostly due to what appeared as a plethora of collaterals (see Fig. 11-3). A single-station runoff is performed which clearly demonstrates substantial epigastric to ileofemoral collaterals as well as external iliac stenosis. The patient underwent iliac to femoral bypass with improvement and reduction, but not complete elimination, of the right buttocks pain (presumably due to retrograde flow to the external iliac arteries).

**Case Study 4.** A 22-second breath-hold "stem-to-stern" MRA was performed in a 45-year-old man (see Fig. 11-4). One single large FOV acquisition was

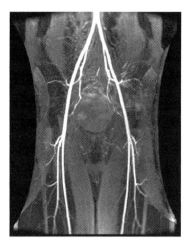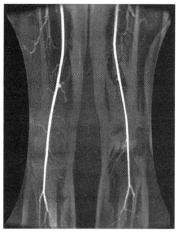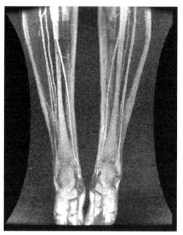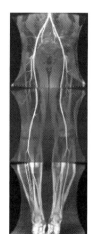

**FIGURE 11-1** Multiple station acquisition of ileofemorals with peripheral runoffs seen with a single bolus injection. Data were acquired using a bolus chasing technique and ordered sequentially. The composite reconstruction is displayed (far right), which facilitates diagnostic and interpretive abilities, as well serving as a roadmap for the interventionalist/vascular surgeon.

these cases, returning to the source images and scrolling through them serially is recommended. Interrogating the axial, sagittal, and coronal images as source data permits more accurate interpretation, because the data are not summated. The T1-weighted sequences with blood suppression produce images in which turbulent flow from highly stenotic jets is suppressed, and is therefore not a source of error in overestimation of the degree of stenosis. Importantly, the MRA reconstructions can be used as a source of "vascular roadmaps" for the interventionalist and for the surgeon. This is in addition to simple screening for aiding in decision making regarding interventional strategies (see Fig. 11-2). Perhaps the cardinal advantage of MRA is the ability to define arterial collateralization in a meaningful manner. Several studies have demonstrated the increased ability of MRA compared with angiography to detect collaterals that can be utilized in revascularization strategies (see Fig. 11-3). Additionally, studies have documented the ability of CMR to be performed in a painless and rapid manner as compared with x-ray angiography. The most rapidly growing section of CMR is in the area of peripheral angiographic evaluation (see Fig. 11-4), specifically for runoff vessels.

## CONTRAST MAGNETIC RESONANCE ANGIOGRAPHY ADVANTAGES

1. Gadolinium-inert, safe, fast
2. Nonionic
3. Non-nephrotoxic
4. Non–x-ray requiring
5. No arterial access

acquired, delineating nearly the entire thoracic aorta (only the cranial arch is not seen) extending throughout the descending thoracic aorta, entire abdominal aorta, and proximal ileofemoral vasculature. Note the ostial and proximal/mid superior mesenteric artery (SMA), inferior mesenteric artery (IMA), and renal arteries. Three-dimensional surface reconstruction was reformatted and selected images were displayed. By altering the signal intensity of the post-processing algorithm, increased or decreased visualization of the vasculature can be achieved.

**Case Study 5.** A 60-year-old woman status post coronary artery bypass graft (CABG) 5 years now reports progressive chest discomfort, radiating deep into her right chest with a ripping, tearing sensation completely different from her initial chest pain symptoms that resulted in bypass surgery. The CMR demonstrated a complex, spiral dissection originating from the origin of, but not directly involving, the left subclavian artery, extending throughout the entire thoracic aorta and deep into the abdominal aorta (see Fig. 11-5). A number of auto-fenestrations are visible (arrow), as well as evidence that the left renal artery is supplied by the true lumen (arrow). On other images (not shown), the right renal flow is seen to be derived from the false lumen. However, in that the flow characteristics of the descending aorta revealed nearly simultaneous signal intensity, it is reasonable to assume that flow is nearly simultaneous. The generally slightly brighter signal in the false lumen (right) as compared to the true lumen (left) denotes the slightly faster blood flow, likely not physiologically significant.

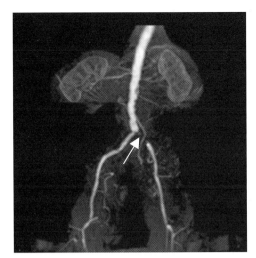

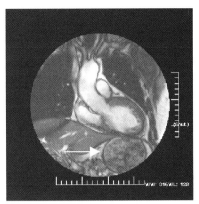

**FIGURE 11-2**  Top left panel, relating to case study 1, showing single ileofemoral station runoff with manual formatting. Other images relate to case study 2. Lower right, single-stage ileofemoral runoff with volume reformatting. Lower left, steady state free precession (SSFP) images highlighting signal void in vicinity of surgical clip. Top right, SSFP image of heart and stomach region.

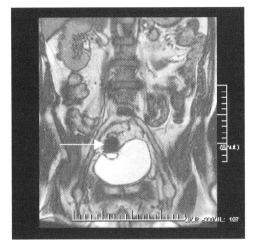

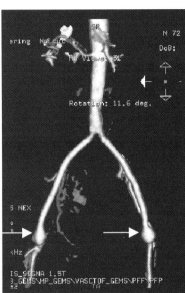

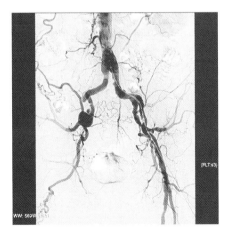

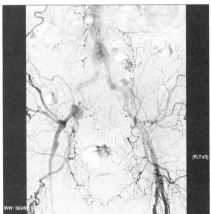

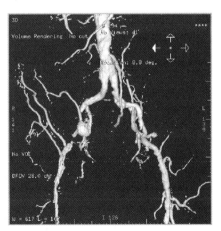

**FIGURE 11-3**  X-ray angiography as a digital subtraction (DSA) of the ileofemoral system (left and middle panels). Single-stage ileofemoral magnetic resonance angiography (MRA) (right panel) revealing a maze of collateral vessels and external iliac stenosis. Images relating to case study 3.

**FIGURE 11-4** A single 22-second 44-cm field of view (FOV) magnetic resonance angiography (MRA) acquisition nearly encompassing the entire vascular tree from the ascending aorta through to the iliac arteries. Images correspond to case study 4.

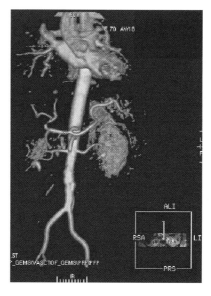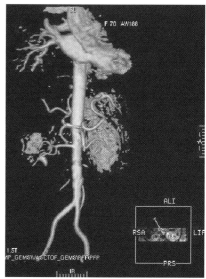

6. Fast (seconds to minutes)
7. Non-NPO required
8. Accurate, reproducible, favored
9. Delineation of collaterals
10. Time resolved
11. Multistation capability (bolus tracking)
12. Reliant on T1 reduction and not dependant on flow characteristics of blood
13. Allows integration of noncontrast techniques (e.g., SSFP, DIR, turbo-inversion-recovery [TIR] and phase velocity mapping [PVM]) (see Fig. 11-5)
14. Substantial rapid post-processing capabilities (see Fig. 11-6)

## CONTRAST MAGNETIC RESONANCE ANGIOGRAPHY DISADVANTAGES

1. Potential for claustrophobia (1% to 2% of general population)
2. Requires technologist familiarity with both anatomy and MRA methodologies

**Case Study 6.** Surface rendered MRA of a 9-second scan performed in a 51-year-old man presenting with chest and abdominal pain (see Fig. 11-6). In the upper right panel, a very subtle defect is seen, inferior to the ostium of the left renal artery. Using both DIR and SSFP imaging, in combination with the volume rendered MRA, no evidence of dissection is seen, although suspected in the SSFP sequence. Incorporating both contrast and noncontrast imaging demonstrates this is an atherosclerotic plaque, but not the likely source of the patient's pain. Note, also from the surface rendering angiogram in the middle panel that anatomic and arterial information from the right and left ventricle, as well as the mesenteric, renal, and ileofemoral system are well displayed. Even the vasculature supply to the small and large bowels is reasonably well depicted as is the right ureter. Note the high-fidelity resolution of the MRA reformatting possible with (left panel) and without (middle panel) the small vessel vasculature all dependant on the intensity leveling reformat chosen.

**FIGURE 11-5** Steady state free precession (SSFP) imaging alone to demonstrate flow characteristics of the true and false lumen. Images correspond to case study 5.

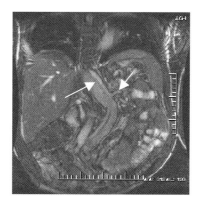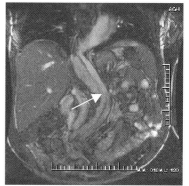

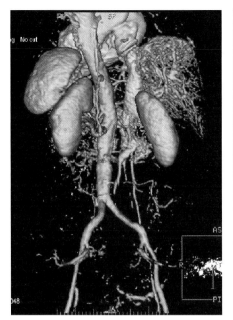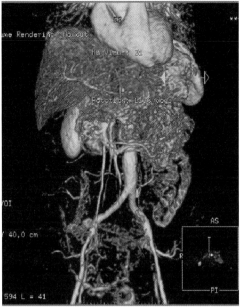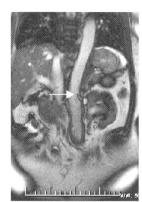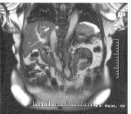

FIGURE 11-6   Surface rendered magnetic resonance angiography (MRA) is performed in 9 seconds with volume and surface reformatting. The right panel images are steady state free precession (SSFP) views depicting a subtle defect inferior to the ostium of the left renal artery. Note the localized dissection seen in MRAs in left and middle panels. Images correspond to case study 6.

3. Requires gadolinium intravenous injection
4. Requires a CMR physician, thoroughly acquainted with the pitfalls and artifacts customary to MRA
5. Potential for over-reliance on MRA given its high resolution, potentially minimizing noncontrast additive CMR techniques

Recently investigators from Cornell University have documented the addition of utilizing large blood pressure cuffs inflated to 30 and 60 mm Hg (subsystolic) to improve the ability to visualize the infrageniculate vessels. The theory is that there will be less washout of the gadolinium if the venous pressure is significantly elevated, thwarting return of contrast back to the heart. This has been demonstrated to significantly extend the resident time of the contrast, allowing improved visualization of collateral circulation and thereby positively impacting the primary goal of detecting suitable conduits for surgical anastamosis. The blood pressure cuffs are placed on the thigh as high as possible but are not inflated until just before the MRA acquisition to avoid patient discomfort. The blood pressure cuff retards early venous enhancement relative to the arterial enhancement and improves MRI, especially for smaller vessels such as infrapopliteal and plantar arteries.

For runoff vessels, dedicated peripheral vascular surface coils add higher signal-to-noise ratio (SNR) and contrast-to-noise ratio (CNR) compared with the body coil. This is particularly important for evaluation of the popliteal and infrageniculate vessels. More

**Case Study 7.** An abdominal aorta, mesenteric and renal artery MRA acquired as a staged 10-second bolus-tracking acquisition, demonstrating in fine detail the SMA, IMA, and renal arteries extending to the secondary and tertiary branches (see Fig. 11-7). The common iliac system is also visualized in this 40-year-old man referred for hypertension, and shown to have no evidence of renal artery stenosis.

**Case Study 8.** MRA of the renal artery with bilateral accessory arteries obtained in a 52-year-old woman referred for systemic hypertension (see Fig. 11-8). No evidence of renal artery stenosis is present. The MRA allows visualization of the vasculature deep into the renal cortical medullary territory. A renal cyst is also present as depicted by the lack of contrast uptake.

**Case Study 9.** An MRA with virtual luminal angiography performed, revealing the patency of the renal vasculature (left) (see Fig. 11-9). The "fly-through" technology (middle panel) confirms the patency of the vasculature down to the tertiary vessels (right panel) depicted by the two arrows delineating the bifurcation of the tertiary arteries (best seen in the DVD).

**Case Study 10.** While the focus of this chapter it is on extra thoracic, noncarotid vasculature imaging, it is clear that within the confines of cardiovascular imaging, recently, multichannel phase array coils have been used, permitting parallel imaging strategies to produce high-quality images in a reduced scan time. Multistation acquisitions can be performed, using either manual or automated table movement. The advantage of automated table movement is that it is fast, allowing single bolus chasing strategies to be employed.

Reconstruction algorithms for peripheral runoff vessels are similar to those previously described for aortic imaging. However, although large vessels such as the aorta are not critically dependent upon interpretation of small features, here heavy reliance on source images is mandatory, especially for the small vessels and evaluation of collaterals. Overestimation of percent stenosis is minimized by tracking source data in three dimensions. Additionally, some vendors permit off axial/oblique imaging to facilitate interpretation.

## MESENTERIC ARTERY EVALUATION

Similar to aortic and renal artery imaging, axial and coronal slices can be utilized to determine the anatomy and structural information of the mesenteric arteries. In this case, sagittal SSFP sequences are typically aligned such that the ostial, proximal, and mid vessels are well delineated. Generally, the celiac artery, superior mesenteric artery (SMA), and inferior mesenteric artery (IMA) are easily visible (see Fig. 11-7). Occasionally, the IMA is either absent or diminutive. As is common to any other vascular territory, MRA can be performed. When MRA is performed, owing to the limited abdominal

limited carotid artery information can be obtained (see Fig. 11-10). This 62-year-old patient was referred for routine MRA. Axial, para-axial, and coronal SSFP images (not shown) are obtained for routine evaluation and followed up with an MRA of the carotids for confirmation, and display. More than ever, evaluation of MRA carotids requires referral back to the source images in three planes for more careful scrutinization of the data, especially if stenoses are present. Virtual luminal angiography was also performed to evaluate the intimal surface and for documentation of vessel patency. Of interest, the right panel demonstrates the tracking of the left carotid artery distally up to the carotid foramen. It should also be noted that interrogation of the origin of the carotid arteries is important, in that arch disease extending into, and partially obstructing, the origin is important to distinguish, making clinical decision making more complete. Dual disease is not amenable to either carotid endarterectomy or angioplasty/stent therapy, but would require surgical intervention involving the arch. The knowledge of this *before* performing angioplasty or carotid artery endarterectomy has obvious ramifications.

**Case Study 11.** Carotid MRA is performed demonstrating vertebral and basilar artery vasculature (see Fig. 11-11). Since vertebral artery flow is often not symmetric and has arterial dominance, it is not unusual to see ipsilateral disproportionate arterial size. This does not necessarily indicate pathophysiology. Moreover, vertebral

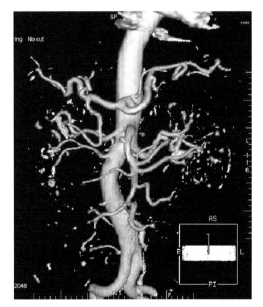
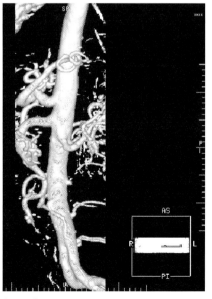

**FIGURE 11-7**   An abdominal aorta, mesenteric and renal artery magnetic resonance angiography (MRA) acquired as a staged, 10-second bolus-tracking acquisition. Images correspond to case study 7.

motion, typically, a large amount of arterial anatomy is generally seen. However, ostial and proximal disease is most often detected in the mesenteric arteries, with it being rare to find mid and distal mesenteric artery stenosis.

## RENAL VASCULATURE

Increased recognition of the role of renal vascular hypertension enters into the pathophysiology of atherosclerotic disease and has prompted an increased utilization of CMR to detect correctable forms of hypertension. Chiefly, renal artery stenosis is the key diagnosis to exclude. The finding of narrowing of the renal arteries by >70% has a high likelihood that it is causal to the hypertension. The coincident finding of moderate renal artery stenosis (50% to 70%) in an asymptomatic, normotensive patient, however, is not an indication for surgical intervention (see Fig. 11-8).

Several anatomic considerations are typically present in a patient with renal artery disease. Atherosclerotic plaques generally occur in the proximal one-third of the renal arteries. Additionally, atherosclerotic plaques within the intima of the aorta often encroach into, and partially obstruct, renal blood flow, resulting in an "effective" renal artery stenosis. Importantly, differentiation between ostial and proximal lesions is of critical importance due to their intrinsic differential response to percutaneous transluminal angioplasty (see Fig. 11-9). Generally, proximal lesions respond better to angioplasty whereas ostial lesions, initially responding

arterial flow is often not antegrade, such that the non-dominant vessel may have retrograde flow. This can be easily depicted on PVM, again not necessarily representing abnormal physiology. Note that the timing in both Figs. 11-10 and 11-11 has completely excluded jugular venous enhancement. Because venous efflux time is often very short, MRA requires careful synchronization. When using contrast injection techniques and timing is poor, post-processing is required to subtract venous structures. Commonly, 3-D TOF MRA before contrast is performed to limit the impact, should venous contamination be present. Virtual luminal angiography is performed (right panel) demonstrating the origin of the great vessels looking up at them from the greater curvature of the aorta from *inside* the aorta.

**Case Study 12.** A pulmonary MRA is shown (see Fig. 11-12) in a middle-aged woman who presents with chest discomfort and undergoes a "triple rule out" via CT scan. She is cleared from any abnormal radiographic findings but her chest discomfort persists over the ensuing 24 hours. She is referred for a CMR examination to evaluate the continued possibility of an aortic dissection. She is cleared for an aortic dissection, but on reconstruction of the temporally obtained images, a "cutoff" sign is seen along the left lower pulmonary artery (arrows). This is consistent with a pulmonary embolism. The D-dimer is also positive, making this a high post-test probability for pulmonary embolism. Review of the earlier obtained CT scan reveals only axial acquisitions

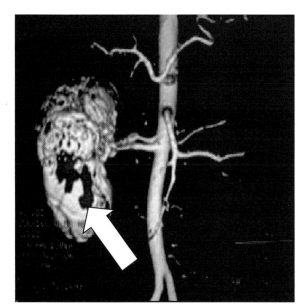
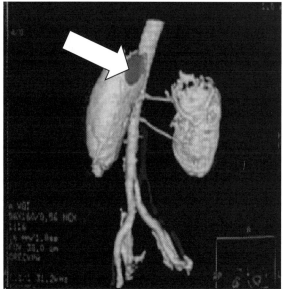

**FIGURE 11-8**   Magnetic resonance angiography (MRA) of the renal artery acquired in 13 seconds. Note the lack of T1 effect in the left renal parenchyma (arrows) due to failure of contrast uptake in a nonvascular area (renal cyst). Images correspond to case study 8.

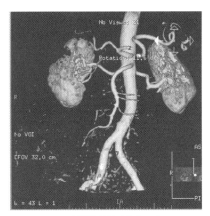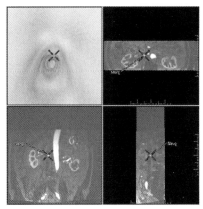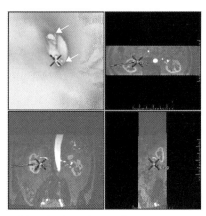

**FIGURE 11-9** A magnetic resonance angiography (MRA) with virtual luminal angiography (best seen in the DVD). Images correspond to case study 9.

favorably, have a higher rate of late restenosis. In young patients, fibromuscular dysplasia of the renal arteries is the most common source of renal vascular hypertension. Medial muscular fibroplasias is the most common variant in the adult, but is rare in children, and typically by MRA, produces a classical stringlike beaded appearance with alternating areas of medial thickening separated by any aneurysmal dilation. Takayasu arteritis is a very rare disease typically affecting young women, which can cause focal stenosis of the aorta and major branches, including the renal arteries. Classically defined in Asians, we and others have seen examples of this in whites.

The CMR study includes utilization of standard DIR sequences in axial and coronal projections followed by SSFP sequences in axial and coronal projections. When the renal arteries are in a single plane this approach works quite well for delineation and interpretation. Often, a coronal SSFP image completely depicts the ostial, proximal, mid, and distal arterial architecture deep into the renal parenchyma. However, as cases are referred primarily in older patients, multiple coronal and axial images are typically required. Our practice is to obtain as much diagnostic information as possible before confirmation with MRA. With sensitivities and specificities exceeding 90% in comparison with conventional angiography, this technique has found a wide referral basis. MRA with 3-D reconstruction can often be performed in seconds, including post-processing time. The accuracy of MRA compared with ultrasound imaging is significantly higher, with technical failures rarely being an issue for CMR. In the high-risk patient in whom hypertension, atherosclerosis, and diabetes is present, the serum creatinine may be elevated, making the use of iodinated contrast a relative contraindication. Further, invasive procedures have to navigate the tortuous and atherosclerosis ridden ileofemoral bed before selective engagement of the renal arteries, making this patient profile ideal for evaluation with CMR and MRA.

without a 3-D reconstruction post-processing algorithm, explaining the differences. The patient was placed on heparin and is presumed to have had prolonged venous stasis due to a cross-country flight.

**Case Study 13.** A 24-year-old woman with "copious and instantaneous left ventricle (LV) opacification upon saline contrast" seen on echocardiography. Separate imagings using SSFP and DIR sequences in axial and coronal projections reveal a sinus venosus defect. To better delineate the defect, an MRA was performed (see Fig. 11-13). Whereas typically there is a venous transpulmonary circuit time, a levophase early recirculation occurred due to the premature arterial flow into the left atrium from the anomalous right upper pulmonary vein, generating a rather striking pulmonary aortic angiogram. Generally, inclusion of pulmonary venous flow in an arteriogram would be ascribed to poor timing. This example highlights the abnormal physiology that can also account for such an observation, reminding the technologist and physician that not all MRA mistimings are erroneous; always consider the possibility that a rational pathophysiologic explanation may exist.

An added advantage of CMR is the ability to incorporate the physiologic estimations of the anatomic findings. PVM aligned in-plane with the stenosis allows co-localization of the anatomic stenosis with the maximum velocity. A stenosis in which velocities exceed 1.8 m per second suggests that the anatomic finding is clinically relevant. An additional PVM slice placed orthogonal to the prestenotic lesion allows comparison of velocities with the poststenotic velocity, and provides another way of detecting clinically relevant disease. An increase in velocity of >1 m per second is consistent with a significant stenosis.

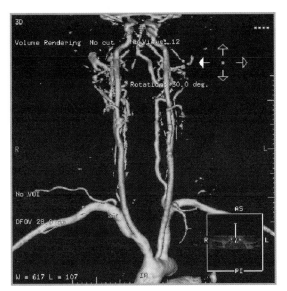
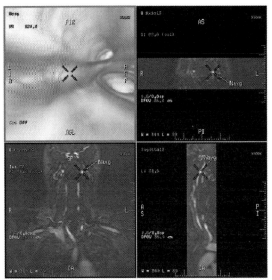

**FIGURE 11-10**   Routine magnetic resonance angiography (MRA) with virtual luminal angiography to depict vessel intimal pathology. Images correspond to case study 10.

A caveat concerning renal artery stents is warranted. The majority of stents placed are paramagnetic. Therefore, the paramagnetic artifact surrounding the stent is substantial and markedly limits the ability to detect in-stent stenosis. Contrast imaging overcomes some, but not all, of the paramagnetic effects due to its use of low echo-times (TEs). Similar to the physiologic imaging described earlier, velocities placed before and after the stent (or simply placed after the stent) can aid in detection of clinically relevant disease. In the latter case, generally, a velocity of >2 m per second after the stent is indicative of clinically relevant disease.

## CEREBRAL VESSELS

Although not truly under the purview of cardiovascular imaging, on occasion the cardiovascular CMR imager is asked to performing imaging of cerebral vessels. Figures 11-10 and 11-11 demonstrate the capability of CMR in this territory. Great care in interpretation of this territory should be taken; rigorous randomized multicenter studies such as the NASCET (North American Symptomatic Group Endarterectomy Trial) and European Carotid Surgery Trial (ESCT) have defined methodologies for interpretation. Interpretation

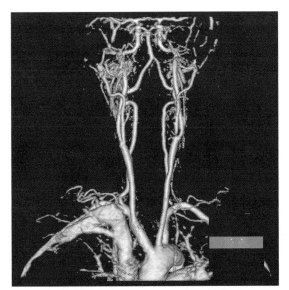
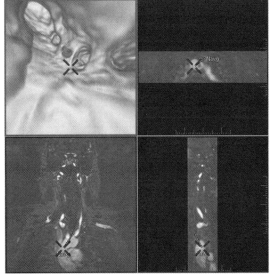

**FIGURE 11-11**   Carotid magnetic resonance angiography (MRA) is performed demonstrating vertebral and basilar artery vasculature. Virtual luminal angiography is in the right panel). Images correspond to case study 11.

of the vertebral-basilar system, likewise, has different implication for a perceived narrowing, as vertebral dominance is a normal finding. The interested reader is referred to general non-CMR texts for more information.

## PULMONARY ARTERY AND BRANCH PULMONARY ARTERY EVALUATION

### Pulmonary Embolism

Recently, the ability of CMR to image the pulmonary vasculature without the use of iodinated contrast, venous catheterization, or x-ray angiography has been accomplished with reasonable to high accuracy. Generally, the most common indication for CMR is for evaluation of pulmonary embolisms. Signs and symptoms suspicious for a pulmonary embolism warrant further evaluation, and currently less focus has been placed on the V/Q scan, given the availability of computed tomographic (CT) angiography. However, there are certain circumstances in which a patient is allergic to contrast, cannot undergo a V/Q scan, or when there is pulmonary parenchymal pathology where an alternative approach would be beneficial. The performance of a pulmonary MRA is not too dissimilar from an aortic MRA, requiring similar carefully timed contrast administration/image acquisition. Some centers favor a staged pulmonary angiogram in which the left and right pulmonary arteries are visualized by separate contrast injection with a larger field

of view (FOV) to define the subsegmental arteries more clearly. However, at our center, especially given the improved resolution of parallel imaging, we favor a single bolus administration with the FOV optimized for the entire pulmonary tree (see Fig. 11-12). One of the benefits of being able to apply post-processing algorithms is that the search for secondary and tertiary "cutoff" signs is facilitated. However, standard clinically important evidence seen on either surface or volume reconstructions is readily apparent and requires little more effort than the 15- to 22-second acquisition.

### Pulmonary Arteriovenous Fistula

Pulmonary arteriovenous fistulae are extraordinarily well defined by CMR MRA and are thought to be due to an embryological effect on the coronal capillary loops. An extracardiac right to left shunt is occasionally manifested by polycythemia with low arterial $P_{O_2}$. On the pulmonary angiogram, a small, medium, or large abnormality with very irregular borders and round circuitous vascular patterns is typically seen. The other finding is the striking normalcy of the unaffected pulmonary vascular territory with the exception of a large number of emptying vessels supplying the arteriovenous malformation (AVM) on the affected side. Occasionally, dermatologic manifestations are present that help raise or lower the clinical suspicion, because 50% are associated with Osler-Weber-Rendu syndrome (hereditary hemorrhagic telangiectasia).

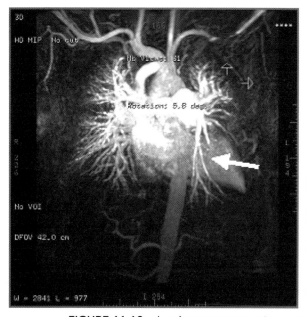
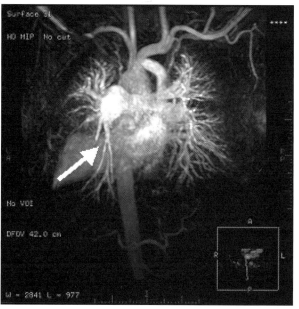

**FIGURE 11-12**   A pulmonary magnetic resonance angiography (MRA) performed as a single injection in the coronal projection. This acquisition was timed from a manual test dose of 3 mL to image at the point of main pulmonary artery contrast opacification. Images correspond to case study 12.

## Pulmonary Hypertension

In evaluating patients presenting with pulmonary hypertension, a characteristic finding that helps substantiate the diagnosis of primary pulmonary hypertension is the rapid tapering of segmental vessels, often referred to as *pruning*. While not necessary to affirm the diagnosis, the combination of axial and/or coronal imaging with SSFP/DIR sequences can raise or lower the post-test probability for this diagnosis, with MRA serving as a confirmation if necessary.

## Pulmonary Artery Aneurysms

Occasionally, pulmonary artery aneurysms, defined by a focal increase of >50% of the proximal main pulmonary artery, can be identified. These rare occurrences can be saccular, fusiform, or true aneurysms and are generally located proximally, but certainly can occur in the peripheral vasculature. In the former, pulmonary hypertension is the most likely etiology with a number of cases in our center measuring dilation to >60 mm. Paradoxically, these appear to be at low risk for rupture despite their often high associated pulmonary pressures, in contradistinction to aortic aneurysms. Occasionally, following repair for congenital heart disease, more peripheral pulmonary aneurysms are present, and CMR is an ideal approach to detect these. Especially, following Tetralogy of Fallot branch pulmonic stenosis is often present late after repair and can be easily visualized by MRA.

## Takayasu Arteritis and Behçet Disease

Pulmonary inflammation is rarely a presenting symptom, as can be seen with Takayasu arteritis, which also demonstrates brachiocephalic artery involvement. Behçet disease involves the pulmonary arteries, and on occasion is a vasculitis and should be suspected in patients with the typical dermatologic or mucosal findings. Most typically, aneurysms are present, and less frequently, stenosis is present.

## Follow-up

Follow-up for congenital heart disease (see Fig. 11-13), that is pulmonary embolism therapy or stent placement, can be performed well by CMR, either with or without MRA. It should be noted that if evaluation of patency of a stent is required, the paramagnetic effect from the stent will, at the current time, limit detection. We and others have demonstrated several ways of determining patency that obviates direct visualization of the stent. Using dimensional analysis, measurement of the either one or two dimensions or area present is compared with the poststent dimensions/area derived from MRA, and is helpful in assessing patency. Secondly, MRA in conjunction with PVM provides greater confidence. Specifically, quantitative prestent velocities are compared with poststent velocities and if they are <1.5 m per second, a high level of confidence is granted to support the patency of the stent.

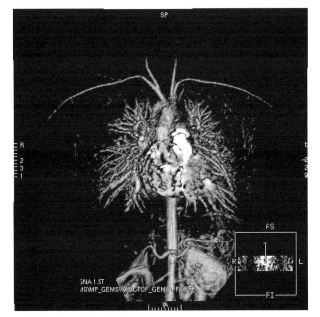 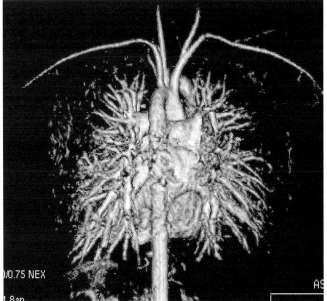

**FIGURE 11-13**   A pulmonary magnetic resonance angiography (MRA) is performed, but due to early recirculation from an intracardiac shunt (sinus venosus defect) there is opacification of both the venous and arterial vasculature; that is, this is not a contrast timing error but "normal" pathology which could easily be confused as venous contamination. Images correspond to case study 13.

Finally, using multiple table moves, the entire vasculature from the ascending aorta through the descending thoracic, abdominal aorta, ileofemoral, popliteal and infrageniculate arteries can be visualized.

## POST-PROCESSING

Generally, post-processing algorithms are somewhat standardized on most vendor platforms. Several optimization reconstruction schemas are possible. Obtaining a precontrast mask-image at all stations with subsequent subtraction allows for 'DSA-like' image generation. This additional step, which is minimally time intensive, is obtained just before the contrast acquisition stage. Again, source images demonstrate important insight into small details that might be obscured or misinterpreted if one solely relies on reconstructed maximal intensity projection (MIP) images.

## ARTIFACTS

As in most CMR images, metallic clips and implanted foreign devices will cause a susceptibility artifact. In most cases, however, when nonvascular structures are imaged, there is only minimal disruption of image features. In cases where intraluminal information is desired, this artifact can be devastating. However, by using extremely short TEs, generally near submillisecond, one can limit these susceptibility artifacts. While some signal-to-noise is lost, utilizing a wide bandwidth is helpful in achieving short TEs. Using fractional number of excitations (NEX) can also be helpful. Another strategy is to recognize that the stent mesh acts as if it were a small insulator, similar to a Faraday Cage. This effect limits the signal that is capable of penetrating the stent, effectively reducing the radio frequency (RF) flip angle within the stent. Increasing the flip angle above what would normally be necessary may be helpful. With very ectatic and tortuous vasculature, care must be taken to insure that the FOV completely incorporates the imaging volume, otherwise, a peculiar artifact of structure termination can be interpreted (in some views) as a high-grade stenosis. Therefore, it is important to rotate the post-processed images through 360 degrees. This generally occurs when either the anterior or posterior limits of the vasculature are inadvertently outside the desired matrix. MRA images require optimal contrast acquisition timing. Obtaining optimal contrast is critically dependant on the ordering of k-space relative to the contrast passage. Under most conditions, the center of k-space should be acquired during the maximum arterial contrast concentration. When the center of k-space is acquired too early, a characteristic "ringing" artifact is seen, in which ribbonlike streaks are seen aligned parallel to the lumen. The standard k-space acquisition is centric ordered, such that during the first 2 to 3 seconds of the acquisition, the central lines of k-space are acquired, determining the contrast conditions for the scan. The remainder of k-space is acquired during the latter part of the acquisition, adding to the high-resolution fine detail. However, there are alternative mechanisms of filling k-space such as elliptic or ellipto-centric, each with their own practical and theoretical benefits. Multiple techniques for timing of the contrast bolus exist. Each laboratory should become comfortable with its preferred technique, as each methodology offers advantages and disadvantages; we prefer the manual timing as described in Chapter 5.

## MAGNETIC RESONANCE ANGIOGRAPHY ARTIFACTS

1. Susceptibility artifact
2. Dephasing (intervoxel-phase dispersion)
3. Chemical shift artifact
4. Flow artifact
5. Flow-related enhancement
6. Ringing artifacts (acquisition of center lines of k-space prematurely or late)
7. Misinterpretation of lumen dimensions (due to thrombosis and hemorrhage)
8. Patient motion (bulk, respiratory, cardiac, bowel)
9. Metallic artifact (wires, prosthesis, artificial valves, stents, and surgical clips)
10. Arrhythmias
11. Wrap (fold over due to truncated FOV)
12. Truncated vasculature (desired image outside prescribed volume block)
13. Misinterpretation of normal (variant) anatomy

# CHAPTER 12

# Myocardial Perfusion and Viability

Robert W. W. Biederman

## MYOCARDIAL PERFUSION

Primarily, this chapter will focus on using cardiovascular magnetic resonance (CMR) to understand myocardial viability; that is the detection and distinction between scar and recoverable myocardium. We note that, myocardial perfusion strategies have predated the more recent use of delayed hyperenhancement (DHE). A considerable amount of data has been amassed concerning perfusion sequences designed to detect single, double, and triple vessel coronary artery disease (CAD) in a manner not dissimilar to current nuclear strategies. However, CMR differs strikingly from nuclear metabolic radionuclide tracer methods, because CMR perfusion strategies detects alterations in myocardial blood flow (typically related to epicardial vessels) whereas nuclear methods are sensitive to radiotracer interaction with a particular cellular domain, related to integrity of either cellular membranes or metabolism. Distinct differences exist chiefly in that CMR requires no radionuclide injection, has higher imaging resolution than current nuclear techniques, and retains the ability to detect subendocardial defects, and appears able to detect microvascular disease, especially in women, in the absence of epicardial disease.

CMR contrast agents, which are typically gadolinium based-chelates, generally have similar relaxivity rates, with the possible exception of for gadobenate dimeglumine (Gd-BOPTA), which produces approximately twice the 1/T1 effect. The critical action of contrast agents is that they increase the resident myocardial signal because of changing the T1-relaxation rate, and are generally safe in their pharmacokinetics and metabolism when cleared from the body by normally functioning kidneys.

Multiple methods for analyzing and processing CMR perfusion data exist. Typically, the first pass contrast kinetics are visually detectable, allowing comparison of rest and stress perfusion images. Alternatively, strategies exist to quantify myocardial uptake, using prototypic algorithms, most incorporating a measure of the input flow waveform to the myocardium, allowing normalization for underlying cardiac function. Typically, myocardial segmental analysis is performed on the slope of the time intensity curve. Myocardial segment time intensity curve metrics are compared for differences to determine the likelihood for territorial disease within the myocardium. More recently, attempts to improve the already reasonable sensitivity and specificity has led to considerations of double bolus strategies utilizing a low, followed by a high, dose contrast administration.

Paradoxically, low-dose gadolinium for detecting perfusion defects yields the best receiver-operator-characteristic (ROC) curve when using angiography as the "gold standard" for the detection of CAD. Therefore, doses of 0.5 mmol/kg are used to (a) maximize accuracy; (b) increase reproducibility among readers; (c) reduce susceptibility artifacts, which are a major source of error, especially at the interface between low and high regions of concentration of gadolinium such as those that exist along the intraventricular septum; (d) detect perfusion defects that exist at least 8 seconds after contrast injection in two or more contiguous slices, which has been shown to be a measure of maximum sensitivity in recent studies; and (e) detect microvascular disease.

CMR stress testing has now become an accepted protocol, with the following being the indications for stress testing:

1. Any suspicion for CAD
2. Inability for standard stress testing requiring exercise (treadmill)
3. Poor quality of other invasive or noninvasive study
4. Preoperative risk assessment

Contraindications for stress testing include the following:

1. Allergy to dobutamine or adenosine (or provoking agent)

2. Unstable angina
3. Uncontrolled arrhythmias
4. Severe aortic stenosis
5. Aortic dissection
6. Large (>55 mm) thoracic or (>45 mm) abdominal aortic aneurysm
7. Acute or subacute myocarditis
8. Acute or subacute pericarditis
9. Severe hypertension (>225 mm Hg or >120 mm Hg, systole or diastole, respectively)
10. Reactive airway disease (adenosine)
11. Bradycardia and/or advance arteriovenous (AV) block (>second degree Mobitz type II)
12. Myocardial infarction (MI) within last 3 days

Numerous protocols are available for stress testing:

1. Adenosine: IV infusion at 0.14 mg/kg/minute for 4 minutes and 1 to 2 minutes extra during imaging
2. Dipyridamole: Infusion of 0.56 mg/kg for 1 minute followed by a 4 minutes delay while endogenous levels of adenosine build up in the body
3. Dobutamine: Infusion at variable dose escalating strategies, generally 5, 1, 20, 30, and 40 μg/kg/minute for 3 minutes at each dose (atropine 0.25 mg to achieve age-predicted maximal heart rate (may repeat up to 4 times)

It is important to monitor the patient during stress testing to detect any untoward event:

1. Heart rate, blood pressure (BP), pulse oximetry, and electrocardiogram (ECG) (note: due to the magnetohydrodynamic effect marked blood flow–related changes render T-wave monitoring ineffective)
2. Constant contact with patient through visual video monitoring, cameras, and hand alarm (for patient to squeeze and alert imaging staff)
3. CMR monitoring for wall motion abnormalities
4. Keeping stocked crash cart nearby, and trained personnel ready to deal with the inevitable emergency that presents on stressing this intermediate- to high-risk group (ideally, a nurse is on standby during these cases, especially if risk is elevated) Typically, the code team are several minutes away from the CMR center, necessitating a high competency level with cardiopulmonary resuscitation (CPR) (advanced life support [ALS]). The physician in charge must have advanced and current basic cardiac life support (BCLS) training.

DHE imaging is often performed following perfusion imaging for viability evaluation. Gadolinium (see Fig. 12-1) is introduced that accumulates in infarcted tissue. The contrast agent is a chelate that decreases T1 of blood approximately threefold when administered IV with the following ideal characteristics:

1. Inert

## CASE STUDIES

**Case Study 1.**
DHE pre-percutaneous transluminal coronary angiography (PTCA) in a 56 year-old white man presenting with an acute anterior wall MI (see Fig. 12-1). The impact of a large type IV proximal left anterior descending artery (LAD) infarct is demonstrated with a large territory of nearly circumferential myocardial involvement.

**Case Study 2.** DHE in the same patient as in case study 1 at 6 months following PTCA, demonstrating marked improvement in the area of scar (see Fig. 12-2). The area at risk is substantially less in the very acute setting than in the 2 to 3 days post-MI. The impact of the acute revascularization intervention is demonstrated by comparison of the DHE regions pre- and post-MI.

**Case Study 3.** The integration of structure and function is easily performed by combining the steady state free precession (SSFP) and DHE images, taking less than 25 minutes to perform for both series in a 49-year-old woman with nausea and vomiting as her first presentation of this right coronary artery infarction (see Fig. 12-3). In the bottom right panel, note the mostly subendocardial infarction pattern of the basal and mid inferior wall that becomes more transmural at the inferior apex (chevron). This strongly supports a large amount of viable myocardium. The subendocardial extent (<25%) is best visualized in the lower right panel (arrow).

**Case Study 4.** A 39-year-old white man presents 1 year after a large MI, seeking a second opinion regarding consideration for undergoing a sixth PTCA for continued chest pain. A search for viability was performed (see Fig. 12-4). Perfusion imaging shown in lower left panel reveals a dense hypointense region, nearly perfectly superimposed on the region of DHE scar, suggesting little ischemia. The extent of scar was nearly transmural except for a small region in the mid-anterior and inferior septum, for which he had recently under gone several smaller vessel PTCA (posterior descending artery [PDA] and right ventricle [RV] marginal branches) with minimal resolution of his symptoms. No further interventions were recommended and the patient was placed on ranolazine, 500 mg (CVT) with complete relief of his symptoms in 6 weeks. He is chest pain free 2 years later.

**Case Study 5.** The ability to resolve subendocardial defects are substantially better with CMR than with nuclear imaging owing to the improvement in spatial resolution. As shown in this Fig. 12-5, this 41-year-old man with a 1-mm ST elevation MI 1 week previously,

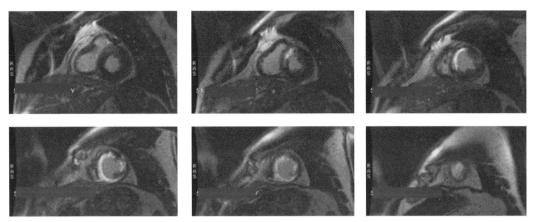

**FIGURE 12-1**    Delayed hyperenhancement short-axis images at 10 minutes post-injection of gadolinium (Magnevist, Schering, Princeton, NJ; 0.2 mmol/kg). Images are depicted from base to apex and from left to right and acquired in a series of single breath-hold acquisitions of 10 seconds each. Images relate to case study 1.

2. Safe, when cleared from the body by normal kidney function
3. Remains predominantly interstitial
4. High degree of discrimination between normal and infarct tissue
5. High degree of sensitivity and specificity (>98%) in detecting MI
6. Can image in less than 30 minutes
7. Can be combined with LV function analysis
8. Acute or chronic imaging
9. High reproducibility
10. Since 2003, the reference standard for viability

The mechanism of DHE is as follows:

1. A probe for cellular membrane integrity
2. Molecular size large enough to freely exist in the vascular space and rapidly distribute
3. Gadolinium decreases the T1, typically producing a bright signal in inversion recovery (IR) imaging
4. Gadolinium is excluded from myocardial cells with intact membranes
5. Signal attenuation depends on microheterogeneity of distribution in tissue because the media resides in extracellular not the intracellular space
6. Using IR prep, and a suitable imaging sequence, such as gradient recalled echo (GRE) or echo planar imaging (EPI), the volume of distribution ($Vol_d$) provides an index of the percentage of necrotic myocardial cells within a zone of ischemic injury
7. Indicator achieves a near equilibrium state due to the observed proportionality constant between the T1 relaxation rate of myocardium and the blood pool $Vol_d$
8. The interstitial space is slightly increased by $H_2O$ ($\approx$10%) but substantially increased (>70%) by loss of myocyte cellular integrity

and negative nuclear scan performed 1 day post-MI, has clear evidence for a lateral wall MI. This demonstration underscores the utility of CMR evaluation by DHE imaging to determine chest pain etiology in the absence of cardiac catheterization in certain populations.

**Case Study 6.** Direction of intervention services is depicted in this 64-year-old white woman with chest pain and two-vessel CAD, both with 80% proximal lesions. By perfusion imaging (see Fig. 12-6, lower right panel) only the PDA territory demonstrates hypoperfusion at rest, directing interventional efforts to that vessel, sparing the left circumflex artery, whereas both had by angiography, suitable indication. Note the extension of ischemia well beyond the scar, supporting the notion of intervention. The DHE imaging demonstrates that there will be a return of function given that <50% scar is present.

**Case Study 7.** A 65-year-old white woman with acute inferior wall MI, left ventricular ejection fraction (LVEF) of 25% by catheterization, and high-grade three-vessel disease, referred for viability assessment before performing a moderately high-risk coronary artery bypass graft (CABG) (see Fig. 12-7). The perfusion defect is in agreement with catheterization, in that there is high-grade resting hypoperfusion (worse in the inferior wall) indicating extensive CAD. The DHE images demonstrate a near transmural defect confined to the territory of the right coronary artery lesion, with otherwise viable myocardium. This is a very favorable pattern to support an excellent return of segmental function to a large amount of myocardium and substantial improvement of her postoperative ejection fraction (EF) at 6 weeks (EF 44%). Note the subtle RV sub endocardial infarct pattern curve.

9. Extent of enhancement represents the percentage of nonviable cells
10. Not accurate if the reactive oxygen intermediate (ROI) is subtended by a no-reflow zone (central core of necrotic cells), but after 20 to 40 minutes, this region typically attains an equilibrium concentration (note: if ROI includes a no-reflow zone, this area by definition is nonviable if imaged >2 hours postinfarct)

## INTERPRETATION OF DELAYED HYPERENHANCEMENT

1. The concept that "bright is dead" has been nearly universally recognized to require some modification. After pioneering work in the mid to late 1990s at our institution and others, it is clear that "timing is everything." Therefore, a key feature in infarct imaging, especially in the subacute setting (typically that period in which most imaging is performed) is to note that imaging be performed in a period after gadolinium has exited from the penumbra or peri-infarct region that is chiefly composed of edema. Present in the peri-infarct region are albumin and other proteins related to injury and healing which are strong binders of the gadolinium moiety. The optimum imaging period is $17 \pm 5$ minutes, therefore a time of 10 minutes has universally been adopted as the conventional time in which to initiate evaluation for a bright post-contrast pattern with high specificity for detection of infarct. If this pattern is seen, one can with high-accuracy gauge the presence of a MI *without* overestimating its extent (see Fig. 12-2).
2. The DHE pattern appears to be reasonably and clinically stable over the following 20 minutes,

**Case Study 8.** A 73-year-old black man with equivocal sestamibi perfusion read finally as negative, referred for evaluation by CMR (see Fig. 12-8). Following a markedly positive adenosine stress CMR test (lower panels) with clear evidence for a thin, but unmistakable, subendo-cardial rim of scar by DHE (top panels). This pattern demonstrates the importance of the high spatial resolution that CMR offers.

**Case Study 9.** A 63-year-old white man presents with cardiogenic shock. His catheterization shows subto-taled proximal LAD and minimal ancillary CAD. He underwent emergency PTCA. His nuclear viability test demonstrated no viability in the anterior, anteroseptum, and apical walls. CMR DHE confirmed the lack of significant viability sufficient to pursue intervention, based on the notion that he would not have meaningful recovery of function (see Fig. 12-9). He did not undergo CABG but required left ventricular assist device (LVAD) and was listed for cardiac transplantation.

**Case Study 10.** A 61-year-old black woman with a large MI by DHE imaging but with a region in the anteroapex that appears viable (see Fig. 12-10). The clinical suspicion was suggested that this might represent "paradoxical" viability—subendocardium viability with midwall and epicardial scar. It is known that the subendocardium is under the highest wall tension and greatest extravascular pressure, resulting in progressive compression of the tiny sub 200 micron vessels. Additionally, occlusion of the epicardial coronary arteries results in endocardial hypoperfusion, followed by epicardial hypoperfusion. Therefore, it would seem unlikely that this apparent "viable" subendocardial segment could

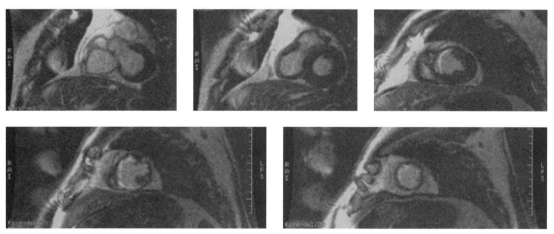

**FIGURE 12-2** Delayed hyperenhancement (DHE) images obtained in the same patient as in Fig. 12-2 showing selected short-axis slices obtained 6 months post percutaneous transluminal coronary angiography (PTCA). Images relate to case study 2.

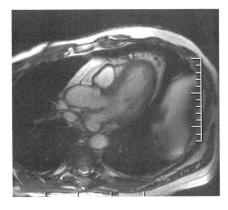
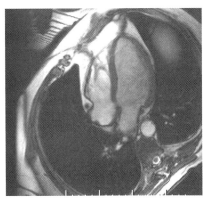
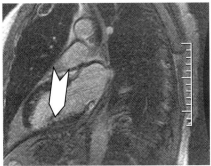
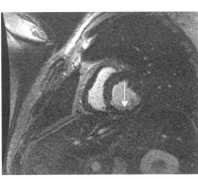

**FIGURE 12-3** Steady state free precession (SSFP) images (top row) and delayed hyperenhancement (DHE) images (bottom row) demonstrating integration of function, structure, and viability. *Arrow* points to subendocardial basal inferior wall infarct, and *chevron* points to more transmural extent of infarct at apex. Images relate to case study 3.

followed by an exponential decay curve, typically, complete (or asymptotically approaching zero) at 1 hour (see Fig. 12-3). Subsequent washout kinetics are somewhat dependent on wash-in kinetics. In general, there is little additional information to be gained by imaging past 15 minutes, except for one indication, which is addressed in the subsequent text.

3. The transmural pattern determines the extent of viable tissue. The general rule is that there is an *inverse relation between hyperenhancement and viability*, that is a lesser extent of the hyperenhancement region corresponds to greater extent of viable tissue, *and* the higher the likelihood, that upon *successful* revascularization, that myocardium subtended by nonenhanced tissue will have a return of segmental function of at least one functional grade.

a. Regions with <50% scar (bright) will have a high likelihood for return of segmental function upon successful revascularization

b. Regions with >50% scar (bright) will have a lower likelihood for return of segmental function, despite successful revascularization (see Fig. 12-4)

c. Tissues at either extreme will proportionately demonstrate the propensity to either improve or not, whereas those closer to 50% will have a variable performance. In the 50% regions, dobutamine provocation has been shown to help further discriminate, such that a positive myocardial response (augmented local contraction) will have a higher probability of improving

represent live muscle. Serial images over time demonstrate gradual regression of this dark region until it is nearly absent at 60 minutes. Because gadolinium is not a thrombin avid contrast agent (gadolinium moieties do not have affinity for thrombus), this confirms the diagnosis of severe microvascular disease (neither viable subendocardial rim nor small layered thrombus) with severe subendocardial hypoperfusion with subsequent retardation of contrast delivery to this territory. Over time, contrast molecules gradually enter this segment, confirming the lack of thrombus. Thrombus would retain this same dark signal, never dissipating until the myocardial pool of contrast has also washed out. The observation of severe microvascular disease, as seen here, has been recently shown to be an independent CMR adverse prognostic factor.

**Case Study 11.** A 59-year-old white woman with New York Heart Association's (NYHA) class IV symptoms was told, "all the heart is dead; nothing we can do". She was referred to CMR for viability assessment. Her nuclear perfusion scan (see Fig. 12-11, top panel) reveals a paucity of signal, chiefly in the septum, with the remainder giving almost negligible counts (read as no significant viability in any region). CMR confirmed the severe LV systolic dysfunction with a 3-D LVEF of 18%, and dilated, dysfunctional, thinning, and remodeled ventricle but preserved RV size and function. DHE was

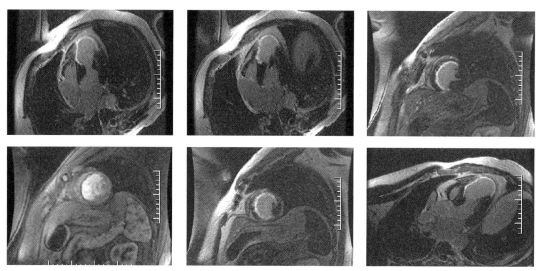

**FIGURE 12-4** Delayed hyperenhancement (DHE) imaging performed at 10 minutes post gadolinium (MultiHance, Bracco Diagnostics Inc., Princeton, NJ) at 0.1 mm/kg. Near complete transmural infarct pattern is present indicating no likelihood of significant improvement in segmental wall function (or chest pain) upon further angioplasty attempts. Note the dramatic discrimination between dead myocardium (white) and live myocardium (black). This is concordant with the dense full-thickness hypoperfusion defect seen in the entire septum (bottom left). Images relate to case study 4.

post-revascularization, thereby better defining viability (see Fig. 12-5).

The perfusion and DHE imaging information can be combined and clinically used in the following manner (see Figs. 12-6 to 12-9):

a. The segments that appear hypointense on first pass perfusion are a combination of ischemic *and* infarcted tissue
b. The segments that appear bright on DHE imaging are infarcted

concordant with nuclear imaging for the septum only. For the remainder of the LV, despite thinned walls, there were large areas of borderline DHE signal in the entire inferior, a large posterior, and lateral wall segments and a smaller apical zone. Many of these borderline segments were just above or at 50% viability, yet just at or below 5 mm in wall thickness. Older considerations by CMR would suggest that she was not a candidate for CABG, yet more recent experience, albeit with very

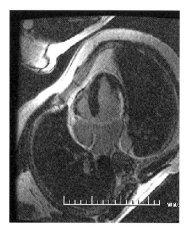 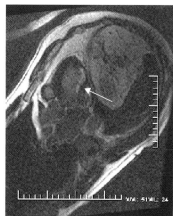 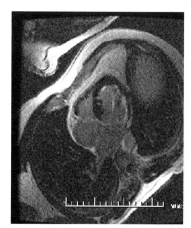

**FIGURE 12-5** Delayed hyperenhancement (DHE) imaging defining the level of resolution detectable; note the dual perfusion seen in the posterior-lateral papillary muscle (*arrow*) in this patient as depicted by discordant viability signal (one half alive, the other dead). Images relate to case study 5.

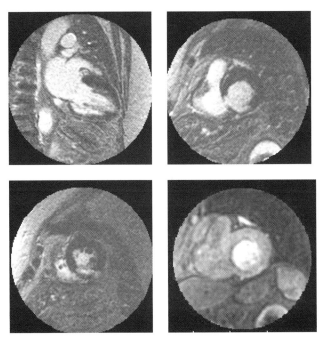

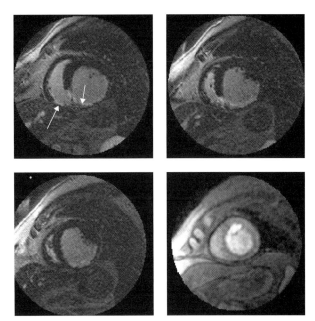

**FIGURE 12-6**   Delayed hyperenhancement (DHE) imaging demonstrating discriminate ability to define possible interventional strategies in a patient with two-vessel coronary artery disease (CAD) but one-vessel territory infarction pattern. Perfusion image shown in lower right panel. Images relate to case study 6.

**FIGURE 12-7**   Delayed hyperenhancement (DHE) imaging at 10 minutes post gadolinium injection. Note the subtle right ventricle endocardial and inferoseptal infarction pattern (*arrows*) with a pixel resolution of <1.5 mm. The perfusion image (lower right panel) depicts a defect far greater than the DHE imaging, indicating a large amount of high-grade resting hypoperfusion and a very high likelihood of return to normal function upon successful revascularization. Images relate to case study 7.

c. The difference between the two represents the my-ocardium that is defined as ischemic (and potentially salvageable)

$$\text{Therefore } a - b = c$$

One caveat is noted: Occasionally, in the acute or early subacute phase, **a** is dark, and a more central subsegment of **b** is *also* dark. This situation defines an area of necrosis and/or severe microvascular disease and is not to be confused with a central region of viable tissue. Pathophysiologically, the segment grossly represents tissue myocardial perfusion (TMP) score = 0 flow. This area is, by definition, nonviable myocardium (see Fig. 12-10).

The advantages of DHE are well described and include at a minimum the following features (see Table 12-1):

1. Inert agent
2. Can be combined with accurate measurements of function, structure, and perfusion
3. Very high resolution to resolve subendocardial infarcts (see Fig. 12-11). In one recent combined animal and human study CMR DHE detected 92% of all subendocardial defects whereas single photon emission computed tomography (SPECT) detected only 28%. Similarly, SPECT failed to detect 47% of

limited data sets, suggested that she might be a candidate for revascularization, especially because she had considerable LV remodeling. Therefore, after a long discussion with the patient and even longer one with the surgeon, she underwent a hybrid approach with PTCA to her LAD followed by three-vessel CABG. While her course was rocky; she was not extubated for 3 days, had a small postoperative bleed requiring exploration, remained on an LVAD for 4 days, she *walked* out of the hospital 2 weeks later. Her most recent LVEF was 35%.

**Case Study 12.** A 63-year-old black woman presented with chest pain. A very mild inferior wall hypokinetic zone was seen on functional imaging (not shown), but was not present in any other region. Two different perfusion sequences were used, the newer sequence using IR SSFP (see Fig. 12-12, upper right panel), demonstrating improved signal to noise ratio and contrast to noise, ratio showed a more global subendocardial defect, whereas the older sequence, employing IR fast gradient recalled echo (FGRE) (see Fig. 12-12, upper left panel) showed a more focal inferior/inferoseptal and anteroseptal defect corresponding to single or double vessel disease. Borderline LAD and left circumflex

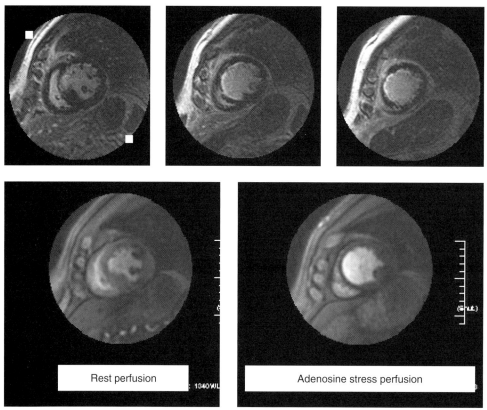

Rest perfusion

Adenosine stress perfusion

**FIGURE 12-8**    Delayed hyperenhancement (DHE) imaging 10 minutes post gadolinium (top row) with adenosine (0.14 mg/minute/kg) in the rest (bottom left) and stress (bottom right). Exact concordance between DHE and adenosine stress demonstrate the lack of reversible myocardium which should be considered before revascularization strategies. Images relate to case study 8.

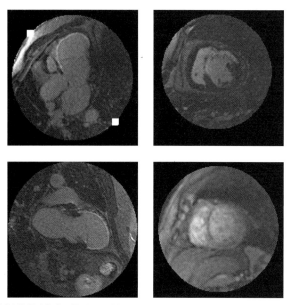

**FIGURE 12-9**    Delayed hyperenhancement (DHE) images 10 minutes following gadolinium infusion (top panel) with representative resting perfusion (lower right panel). Images relate to case study 9.

## TABLE 12-1

### Attributes Cross-Platform for Myocardial Infarction (MI) Imaging

| Characteristic | SPECT | ECHO | MRI |
|---|---|---|---|
| Spatial resolution | *** | ** | *** |
| Sensitivity | ** | * | *** |
| Specificity | * | * | *** |
| Quantification | * | * | *** |
| Speed | * | ** | *** |
| Cost-effectiveness | ** | * | *** |
| Platform availability | *** | *** | * |
| Claustrophobia | * | * | ** |
| Proven in MI | *** | * | ** |
| User-independent | * | * | *** |
| Reproducibility | ** | * | *** |
| Subendocardial imaging | | * | *** |
| Reproducibility | ** | * | *** |
| Viability | ** | * | *** |

SPECT, single photon emission computed tomography; ECHO, echocardiography; MRI, magnetic resonance imaging.

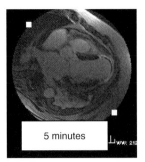 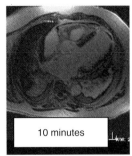 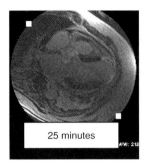 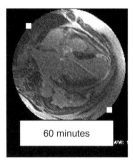

5 minutes    10 minutes    25 minutes    60 minutes

**FIGURE 12-10**    Delayed hyperenhancement (DHE) images taken serially over time to discriminate between viable myocardium versus thrombus versus severe microvascular obstruction. The late filling in versus late washout is conclusive of severe disease, representing severe microvascular obstruction which would correlate with thrombolysis in myocardial infarction (TIMI) flow 0 and tissue myocardial perfusion (TMP) flow 0 in the catheterization laboratory. Images relate to case study 10.

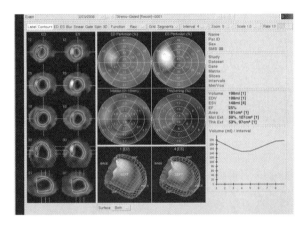

You make the call:
Alive or dead?
Operate or not?

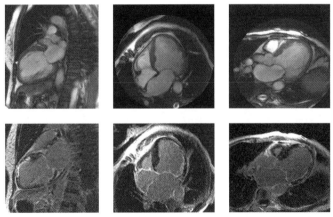 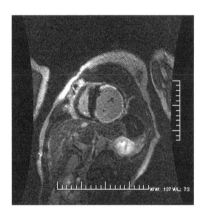

**FIGURE 12-11**    A Stress Thallium study (top panel) demonstrates lack of significant viability in most of the left ventricle in all segments but the septal wall with accompanying severe left ventricle (LV) systolic function, by single photon emission computed tomography (SPECT) imaging. Lower panel shows selected delayed hyperenhancement (DHE) images demonstrating the capability of cardiovascular magnetic resonance (CMR) to delineate with a higher spatial resolution that there is a modest, not overwhelming, amount of muscle that is viable, despite substantial LV remodeling, worthy of consideration for an interventional attempt in the setting of an left ventricular ejection fraction (LVEF) <20%. The ability to detect viable muscle in the myocardium in which the wall thickness is <6 mm is a key advantage of CMR due to its voxel resolution <2 mm, well below conventional radionuclide imaging modalities. This clinically translates into high negative and positive predictive values, and increased opportunities to intervene on those otherwise not considered as candidates for angioplasty or bypass strategies. Images relate to case study 11.

**FIGURE 12-12** A newer resting perfusion sequence using inversion recovery (IR) steady state free precession (SSFP) (right upper), demonstrating improved signal to noise ratio and contrast to noise ratio as compared to IR fast gradient recalled echo (FGRE) (left upper). Images relate to case study 12.

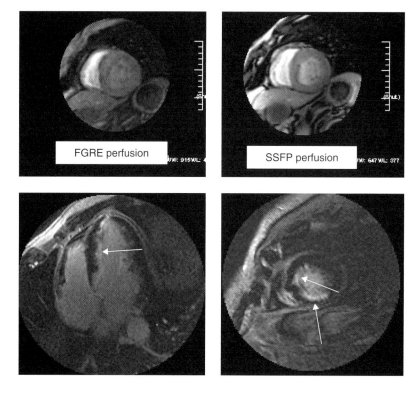

**FIGURE 12-13** A series of perfusion (left upper) and delayed hyperenhancement (DHE) images in a coronary artery bypass graft (CABG) patient with a peculiar midanterior wall transmural DHE signal. The spatial resolution on this sequence clearly demonstrates the ability to distinguish a transmural defect (*arrow*) from a subendocardial defect (inferior wall). Images relate to case study 13.

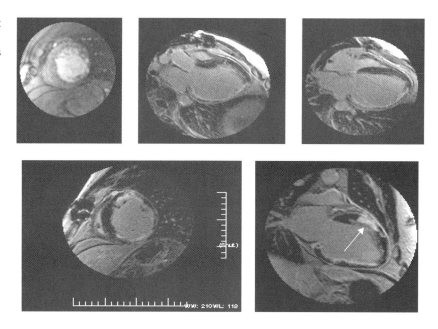

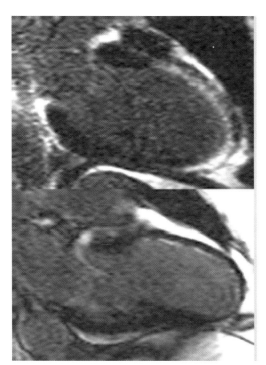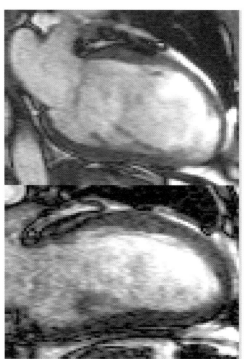

**FIGURE 12-14**   Delayed hyperenhancement (DHE) (left panels) and steady state free precession (SSFP) (right panels) images pre- (upper) and post- (lower) coronary artery bypass graft (CABG) in a very remodeled and thinned anterior wall that has only 5 mm epicardial rim of viability, yet demonstrates return to normal thickness after revascularization. Images relate to case study 14. Courtesy of Ronald Mikolich, MD, Youngstown, OH.

subendocardial infarcts in humans. This has immediate clinical translation—when a patient presents to the emergency room with chest pain and a "normal" SPECT study he/she is told that, "it is not your heart; it must be your esophagus, chest wall, or your imagination." This provides little solace to the patient, or to the referring physician, who is obliged to employ medical resources to uncover another suitable explanation for their symptoms. Yet, this has considerable socioeconomic impact, and unnecessarily burdens our hospitals and causes persistent angst to the patient. Effectively CMR negates this scenario.

4. Can be performed very quickly (<30 minutes)
5. The current "gold standard" for viability
6. Substantial binary interpretation, not reliant on differentiating subtle shades of signal intensity, in clinical images (black vs. white) (see Figs. 12-12 to 12-14)
7. May be used clinically to detect noninfarct pathology, discussed in Chapter 15

artery (LCX) disease were seen by catheterization (two 65% lesions) for which she underwent successful four-vessel CABG, not PTCA with stent to the inferior wall as suggested by the nuclear scan (and the FGRE scan). In addition to the inferior wall defect that was expected, both the perfusion and the DHE (lower panel) reveal additional involvement of the inferior and anterior septum, but there was only very limited, subtle perfusion defects (at rest) in any other territory. Here, a provocative CMR stress test might have detected the LAD and/or LCX moderate stenosis, but the detection of important CAD was enough to warrant a cardiac catheterization with strong pre-test probability for an interventional approach.

**Case Study 13.** A strange DHE pattern is seen in the lower left panel in a 52-year-old white man presenting with chest pain. While most DHE images, including the perfusion images, appear to be indicative of two-vessel territory disease, the midanterior trans-mural defect (see Fig. 12-13 arrow) with normal distal anteroapical segment defines an atypical coronary anatomy. In this patient with a three-vessel CABG, including a saphenous vein graft (SVG) to LAD, an alternative explanation is possible: his SVG-LAD graft could be occluded (as would be his SVG to D1 and SVG to PDA). However on catheterization, only his SGG-PDA was found to be occluded. The other grafts were all widely patent, raising a strong suspicion that he had perioperative infarction to his midanterior wall with subsequent spontaneous clot lysis and recanalization. This finding is often seen on DHE CMR.

**Case Study 14.** The threshold of 50% transmurality appears to be the conventional metric used to gauge the potential for recovery upon successful revascularization. However, despite considerable remodeling and thinning, such diseased myocardium may not have exhausted its ability to recover (see Fig. 12-14). The top panels show pre-revascularization images whereas the lower panels show post-revascularization images. Despite extensive thinning of the anterior wall (upper right panel), follow-up CMR using the SSFP sequences (lower right panel) demonstrates substantial improvement in wall thickness, suggesting that beneficial reverse remodeling has occurred.

# CHAPTER 13

# Cardiac and Extracardiac Tumors

Robert W. W. Biederman

The cardinal advantage that cardiovascular magnetic resonance (CMR) contributes to imaging of cardiac and paracardiac masses is surprisingly *not* its ability to visualize masses, but its ability to characterize tissue, potentially identifying the underlying histology and greatly enhancing the clinicians' ability to distinguish between benign and malignant masses. This is accomplished by virtue of the T1 and T2 relaxation properties of tissue. The combination of high spatial resolution and the large field of view provide an unparalleled ability to depict surrounding structures, making CMR an ideal technique to evaluate masses in context. The modality provides a virtual surgeon's view of masses and also serves as the pathologist's microscope. It is therefore clear why an increasing number of surgical decisions regarding "go or no go" are being made largely based on CMR data.

Details of specific characteristics of each of the different types of masses have been well described elsewhere and accordingly this chapter will provide examples of how CMR adds to the clinical armamentarium, or provides the correct diagnosis when combined with information from other imaging modalities. Specifically, cases in which malignant diagnoses were suggested by another modality and were confirmed to be benign (or *vice versa*) will be presented.

The general classification of cardiac tumors classically requires that a distinction be made between benign and malignant tumors. Certain key CMR features are very useful to differentiate malignant from benign tumors or paracardiac masses. Perhaps the most important observation is that most malignant tumors exhibit a signal that is isointense (or lower) with respect to the myocardium on T1-weighted images and high signal on T2-weighted sequences; whereas benign tumors generally exhibits isointense signal with respect to the myocardium in both T1- and T2-weighted sequences (see Fig. 13-1). In general, the tumor most commonly bright on both T1- and T2-weighted images is malignant melanoma (due to high melanin level), which is known to have a high predilection for metastasis to the heart (>60% likelihood). Pleural effusions ipsilaterally generally raise the suspicion that a tumor may be of malignant origin, especially if there is a concurrent pericardial effusion. Pericardial effusions in the setting of cardiac or paracardiac masses, counterintuitively, have only modest predictability for differentiating tumor etiology. The presence of infiltration is regarded as an ominous sign, portending malignancy. Malignancy is also indicated if the tumor is large (>5 cm) and bulky with central hypointensity on T1 weighting and a brighter central core on T2 weighting, suggesting a necrotic center, typically from the tumor outstripping its vascular supply and/or failure of neoangiogenesis. Heterogeneous tumor characteristics, except for myxoma or teratoma, strongly point towards malignancy. If the mass is heterogeneous, right sided, and there is a pericardial effusion, it is most often a malignant tumor (see Fig. 13-2) whereas if it is homogeneous, in the left heart, and there is no pericardial effusion, then the mass is almost always benign (see Figs. 13-3 to 13-7). Table 13-1 summarizes characteristics of several commonly encountered masses.

Contrast kinetics is very helpful in distinguishing malignant from benign masses. Contrast uptake is an ominous sign, indicating malignant potential. Most benign tumors do not have a well developed, nor needed, vascular supply. Myxomas may be an exception to this rule because they may have variable uptake with contrast administration. Radiofrequency (RF) tissue tagging is a technique that we have used extensively to help differentiate malignancy or "malignant" potential of benign tumors (see Figs. 13-1 and 13-8). The saturated bands of the tag excitation are applied in diastole across the myocardium and adjacent tumor. If there is no adherence or invasion, the tag lines should "slide" past each other during cardiac contraction, demonstrating freedom of attachment points. The pattern, when applied in orthogonal planes throughout the tumor/heart interface,

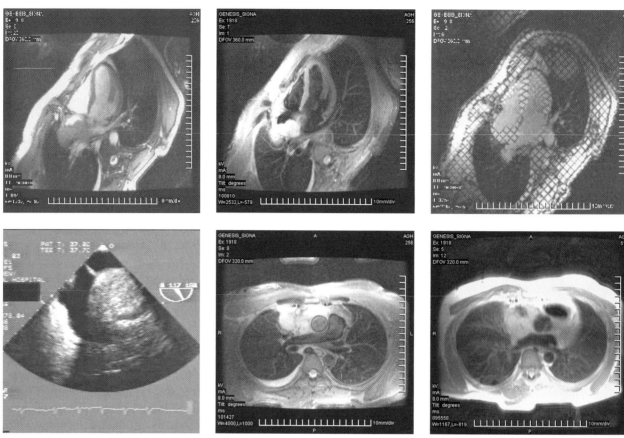

**FIGURE 13-1**   A collage illustrating the incorporation of several key sequences to interrogate location, structure and, most importantly, tissue characteristics of a retro-atrial (RA) mass. From top to bottom and left to right: triple inversion recovery (TIR), steady state free precession (SSFP), radiofrequency tissue tagging, a selected image (inner atrial septum) of the transesophageal echocardiogram (TEE), TIR demonstrating the superior extent of the mass, helping to absolutely exclude a myxoma, and a double inversion recovery sequence (DIR). Images relate to case study 1.

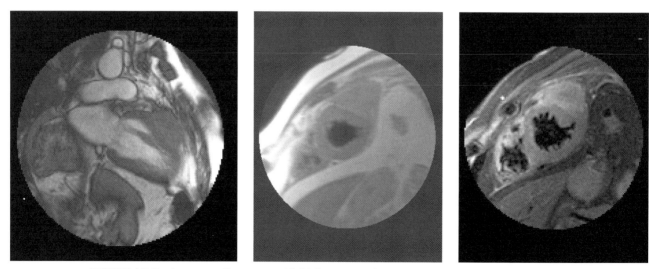

**FIGURE 13-2**   A paracardiac mass with high concern for invasion into the left ventricular (LV) myocardium. From top to bottom and left to right: two-chamber steady state free precession (SSFP), double inversion recovery (DIR), triple inversion recovery (TIR), perfusion, SSFP, and tagging. Images relate to case study 2.

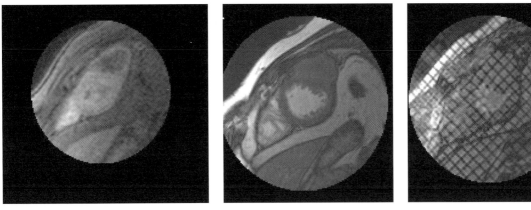

**FIGURE 13-2**    *(Continued)*

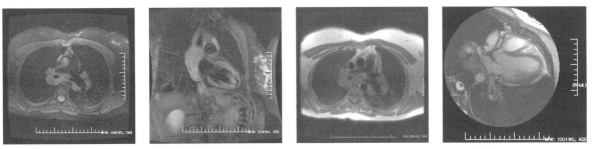

**FIGURE 13-3**    Sarcoidosis is demonstrated in these triple inversion recovery (TIR) sequences (left panels), double inversion recovery (DIR) (middle right), and steady state free precession (SSFP) (far right). Images relate to case study 3.

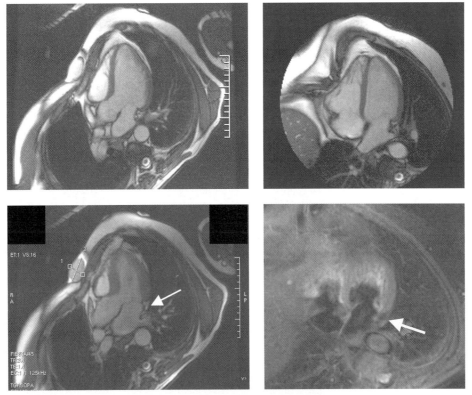

**FIGURE 13-4**    A series of steady state free precession (SSFP) sequences in the three- and four-chamber views with a triple inversion recovery (TIR) (lower right) demonstrating the mass to be that of an unusual intramyocardial lipoma (nulls on TIR). Images relate to case study 4.

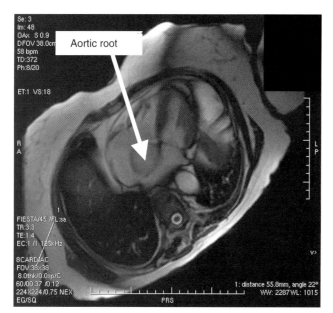

**FIGURE 13-5** A steady state free precession (SSFP) selected four-chamber view that demonstrates a peculiar shadow of an apparent mass. This is a partial volume effect of what was seen on echocardiography as a mass and shown to be a torturous aortic root in an elderly patient. The blood flow and morphology on orthogonal imaging confirms this as a normal variant, not a mass. Images relate to case study 5.

grants the imager a unique capability of assessing tumors, to predict before surgery whether a true surgical plane exists between heart and mass. This ability may be the second-most important feature that CMR renders to the oncologist and surgeon; the first being the ability

to perform "virtual histology" on many tumors, saving the patient from the morbidity and mortality obligate in most diagnostic confirmatory strategies that include biopsy.

The increased capability to detect benign variances of normal is illustrated. The understanding of gross cardiac anatomy has been relatively stable over the last 100 years, reliant on well-established autopsy findings. The days of Rokitansky and Virchow seem to have heralded the end of significant cardiac anatomy discoveries. However, the advent of dynamic imaging by CMR and computed tomography (CT) provides a new window to view anatomic features. In a small study performed at our laboratory, the insertion of the papillary muscle (PM) into the apical left ventricular (LV) myocardium was seen in 401 of 401 patients (100%). In 392 out of 401 patients (97.8%), the appearance of the PM was not a uniform appearing muscle arising from the inner face of the LV endocardium, but was a fingerlike series of long, rootlike slender trabeculae carneae traversing >1 cm before inserting into the main body of PM, challenging our previous understanding of LV PM anatomy (see Fig. 13-9). We termed this finding the "*cypress root*." Potential explanations accounting for the discord between autopsy and CMR include (a) the inability to see the fine detail by the naked eye during autopsy; (b) lack of belief that the PM was not a solid muscle; (c) even in live beating heart procedures such as open heart surgery, the true PM structure is not observable; and (d) myocardial systolic contracture at death (most often death occurs during systole *not* diastole). The capabilities of CMR to allow visualization of cardiac features *in vivo* afford

**FIGURE 13-6** Steady state free precession (SSFP) images (top) and triple inversion recovery (TIR) sequences (bottom) depicting a benign dense myocardial fibroma (*arrows*). Images relate to case study 6.

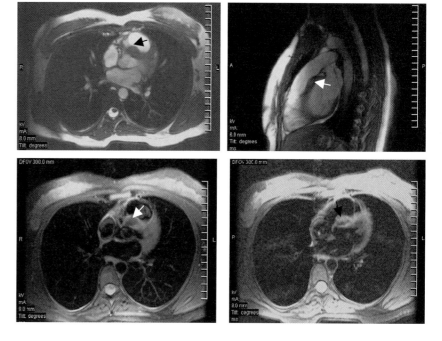

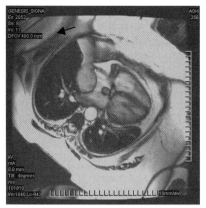 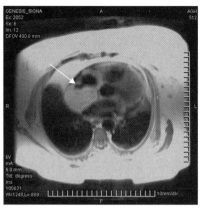 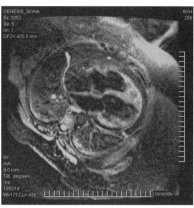

**FIGURE 13-7** Steady state free precession (SSFP) images of a large space-occupying mass in the retro atrium (RA) (left and mid panel, double inversion recovery [DIR]) with triple inversion recovery (TIR) sequences confirming nulling of fat and a diagnosis of inner atrial septal hypertrophy, not a mass as she was suspected of having. Images relate to case study 7.

a useful tool to study living cardiac anatomy. Unlike the widely accepted belief that PMs uniformly arise from the LV floor, they resolve into a "cypress tree" rootlike structure with multiple thin projections before coalescing into a thick muscle head. Such observations have far reaching clinical implications in areas such as mitral regurgitation, post-myocardial infarction (MI) remodeling, and electrical transmission of the His-Purkinje system, while challenging standard teachings. Additionally, they clearly demonstrate the additive utility of high-resolution CMR imaging.

The vast majority of cardiac masses are initially detected using transthoracic echocardiography (TTE), but typically cannot be unequivocally identified because of lack of differentiation of the echocardiographic signal. However, accurate mass identification is required before initiating therapy. In most centers, mass characterization is performed using a combination of transesophageal echocardiography (TEE), biopsy, catheterization, and CT scanning (see Figs. 13-10 to 13-19). CMR provides tissue contrast and permits flexible view selection sufficient for mass characterization. At our institution, from August 2002 to March 2005, CMR was performed using a gradient echo (GE) 1.5 T scanner in 76 patients referred for evaluation of cardiac masses detected by echocardiography. Contrast mechanisms exploiting intrinsic T1, T2, tissue relaxation properties, uptake kinetics of exogenous contrast agent, delayed hyperenhancement (DHE) and inversion contrast were used to identify fat and water signals to

## TABLE 13-1

Characteristics of cardiac neoplasms

| Mass | Location | T1 signal | T2 signal | Gad enhance | Features |
|------|----------|-----------|-----------|-------------|----------|
| Myxoma | LA | Isointense | High | ± | Pedunculated stalk |
| Fibroma | LV septum | Isointense/low intense | Low | ± | Well circumscribed |
| Lipoma | LA/RA | High intensity | Low | — | Older, obese females |
| Rhabdomyoma | LV = RV | Isointense | High | + | Intramyocardial |
| Papillary fibroelastoma | AV > MV > PV | Isointense | Isointense | — | Small, mobile on the valve |
| Angiosarcoma | RA, PA | Isointense | High | +++ | Cauliflower appearance |
| Hemangioma | LV | Isointense | High | +++ | Highly vascular |
| Paragangliomas | LA roof, spine | Low intensity | High | ± | Catecholamine producing |
| Pericardial mesothelioma | Pericardium | Isointense | High | + | On and distorts Pericardial |

LV, left ventricle; RV, right ventricle; LA, left atrium; RA, right atrium; Gad, gadolinium; AV, aortic valve; MV, mitral valve; PV, pulmonic valve; PA, pulmonary artery.

**FIGURE 13-8**  An unusual presentation in a highly symptomatic woman with radiofrequency (RF) tissue tagging on top left upper panel, steady state free precession (SSFP) on upper right panel, and delayed hyperenhancement (DHE) imaging early at 2 minutes (lower left) and at 5 minutes (right lower). Images relate to case study 8.

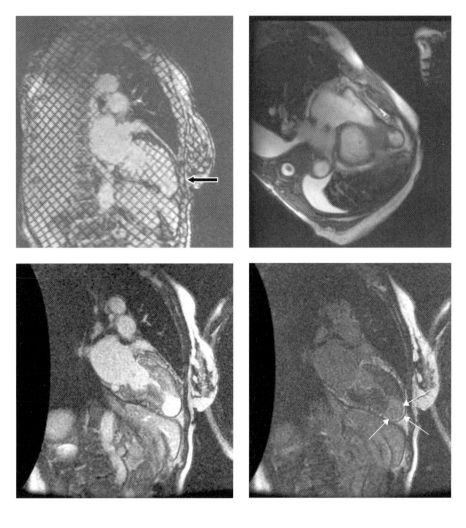

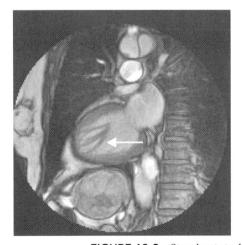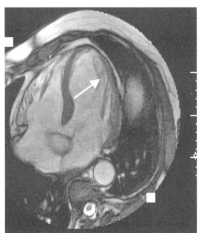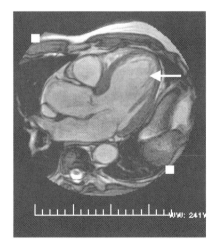

**FIGURE 13-9**  Steady state free precession (SSFP) images through this high-resolution imaging technique depicting anatomic information not seen in most imaging modalities, whereby the papillary muscles arise out of the floor of the left ventricular (LV) apex as a "cypress root" (*arrows*), not as a broad muscle. Images relate to case study 9.

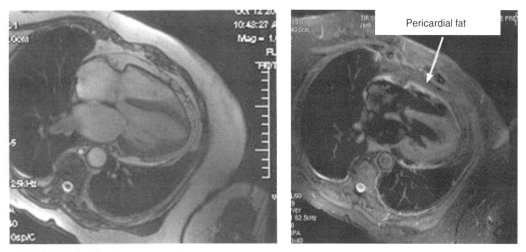

**FIGURE 13-10** Steady state free precession on left and triple inversion recovery (TIR) sequence depicting fat and its ability to be specifically characterized by cardiovascular magnetic resonance (CMR). Images relate to case study 10.

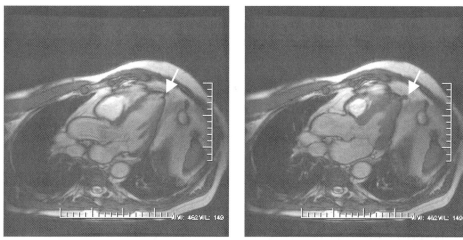

**FIGURE 13-11** Steady state free precession (SSFP) images in diastole (left) and systole (right) in a patient with a left ventricular (LV) apical diverticulum (*arrow*). Images relate to case study 11.

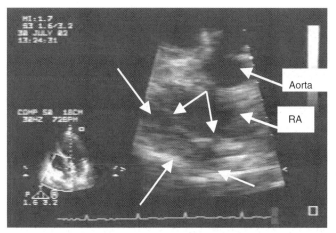
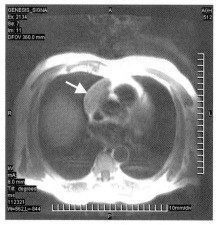

**FIGURE 13-12** Transthoracic echocardiographic imaging demonstrating a hypoechoic retro atrial (*RA*) mass with double inversion recovery (DIR) (upper right and lower left) and triple inversion recovery (TIR) on the lower right panel. Images relate to case study 12.

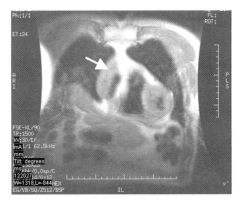
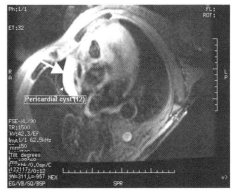

**FIGURE 13-12** *(Continued)*

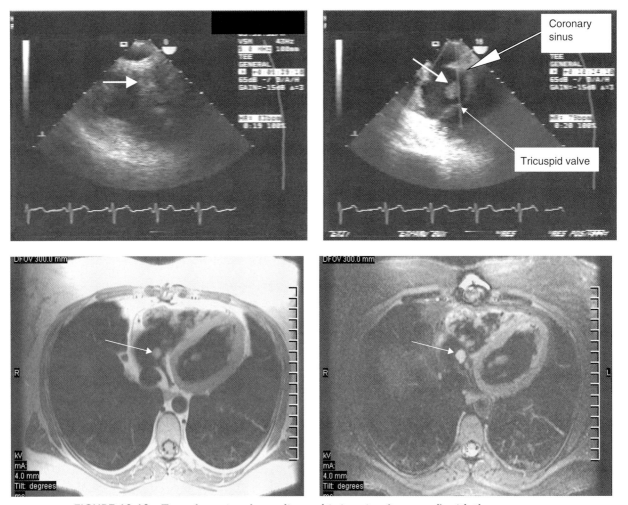

**FIGURE 13-13** Transthoracic echocardiographic imaging (top panel) with the upper right demonstrating a small mobile isointense mass. The bottom panels are cardiovascular magnetic resonance (CMR) double inversion recovery (DIR) (left) and triple inversion recovery (TIR) sequences (right). The *arrows* point to the mobile mass. Images relate to case study 13.

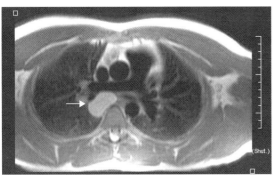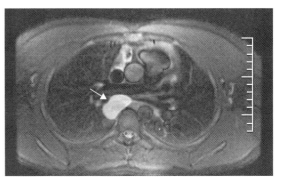

**FIGURE 13-14**   Double inversion recovery (DIR) (left) and triple inversion recovery (TIR) (right) of a bronchogenic cyst, highly proteinaceous giving rise to the bright T1 and T2 signal. Images relate to case study 14.

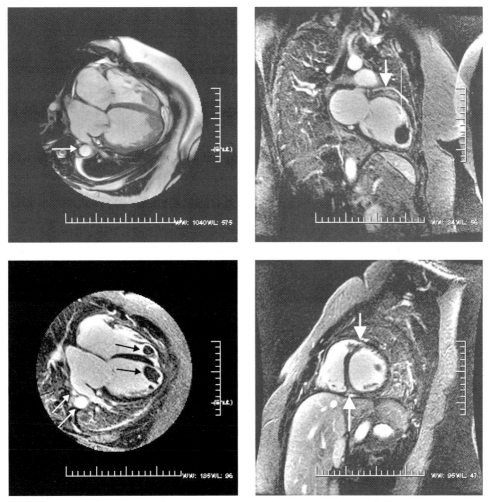

**FIGURE 13-15**   Steady state free precession (SSFP) sequence (upper left) demonstrating a hypointense signal in the right ventricular (RV) and left ventricular (LV) apices, moderately mobile and tricuspid and mitral regurgitation (best seen in the DVD). Delayed hyperenhancement (DHE) images depict the lack of contrast in the biventricular masses (*long arrows*) diagnostic in this setting of apical thrombi. Note the mid septal hinge point and mid anterior wall DHE signals (*small arrows*) likely indicative of prior viral cardiomyopathy as the etiology to her biventricular dysfunction. Images relate to case study 15.

**FIGURE 13-16** A 0.05 mmol/kg perfusion sequence (left) with an early (2 minute) delayed hyperenhancement (DHE) sequence (right) depicting a fortuitous contained dissection in this elderly man, hours after a motor vehicle accident. Note the accumulation of contrast outside the borders of the pericardium but in the admixture of irregular signal due to prior coronary artery bypass graft (CABG) graft pericardial and extracardial fibrosis. Images relate to case study 16.

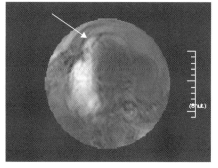
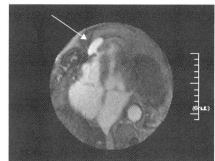

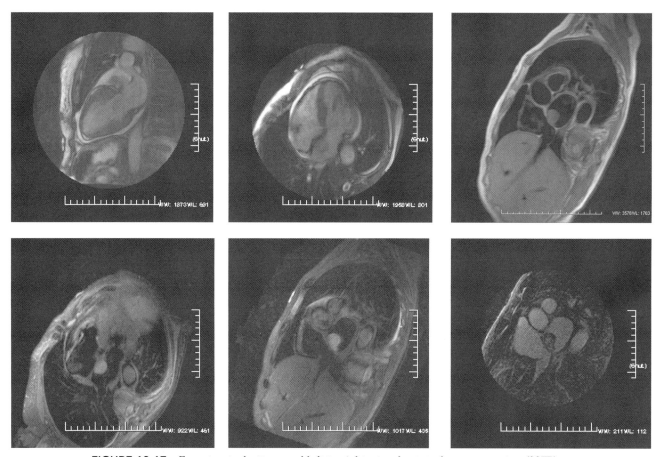

**FIGURE 13-17** From top to bottom and left to right: steady state free precession (SSFP), SSFP, double inversion recovery (DIR), triple inversion recovery (TIR), TIR, and delayed hyperenhancement (DHE) demonstrating a small left atrial (LA) myxoma. Note the variable enhancement pattern in this excision proved myxoma, a typical characteristic. However, it was atypical in that it was attached, broad based, without a pedunculated stalk. Images relate to case study 17.

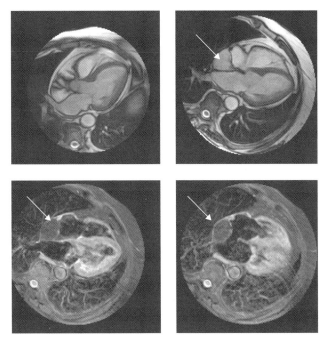

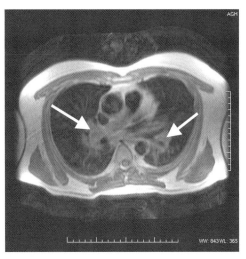

**FIGURE 13-18** Steady state free precession (SSFP) images (top) and triple inversion recovery (TIR) (lower) depicting a retro atrial (RA) lipoma (note capsule). Images relate to case study 18.

**FIGURE 13-20** Within 2 minutes of initiating imaging in this middle-aged man referred for arrhythmogenic right ventricular dysplasia (ARVD), this double inversion recovery (DIR) multislice axial image depicts extensive mediastinal adenopathy (*arrows*) refuting the referring diagnosis. Image relates to case study 20.

characterize masses. Of 76 patients studied, CMR was able to characterize 100% of masses into the following categories: 93.42% non-neoplastic, 6.57% malignant. Further breakdown was as follows: 38.15% (29 cases) as benign fat deposits, including lipomatous hypertrophy and epicardial fat; 5.26% were not masses but were normal variants, such as prominent crista terminalis (100%

of these were referred as echogenic material with a suspicion of thrombus, fat, or malignancy); 6.57% were diagnosed as myxoma; 7.89% thrombus. Of those diagnosed by CMR as malignant, verification was obtained by histopathology, and 80% were shown to be malignant and 20% benign (see Figs. 13-20 to 13-23). Of masses defined as nonmalignant, the clinical sequelae were consistent with the CMR diagnosis. We concluded that in cases with echocardiographic suspicion of a cardiac mass, the wide range of contrast mechanisms (intrinsic and

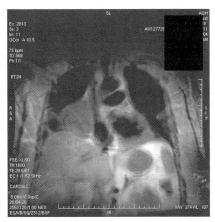
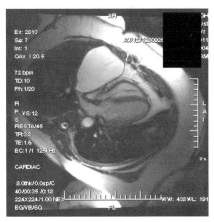
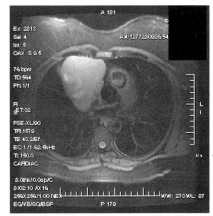

**FIGURE 13-19** Double inversion recovery (DIR) (left), steady state free precession (SSFP) (middle), and triple inversion recovery (TIR) (right) demonstrating the classic location, best seen on coronal left panel, nearly pathognomonic in its location alone, for a pericardial cyst, typically benign. However, middle panel demonstrates moderate retro atrial (RA) and right ventricular (RV) compression. The gelatinous nature of this proteinaceous cyst is extraordinarily well seen on the DVD where the reflections of the cardiac motion reverberate through the cyst. Images relate to case study 19.

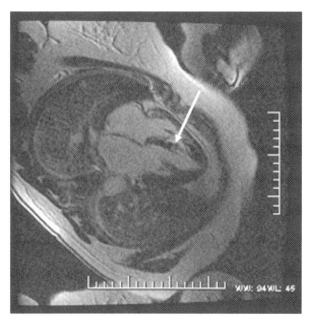 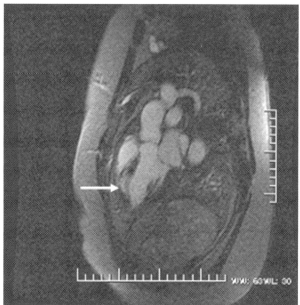

**FIGURE 13-21**    Delayed hyperenhancement (DHE) imaging demonstrating in the four- and three-chamber views (left and right) irregular midseptal enhancement strongly suggestive of myocardial sarcoidosis, which was proved by biopsy. Images relate to case study 21.

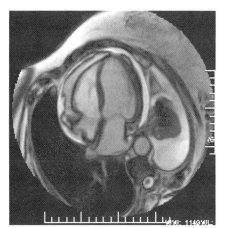 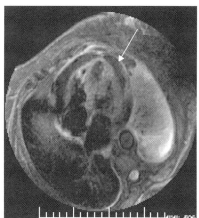 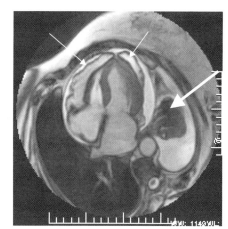

**FIGURE 13-22**    Cardiovascular magnetic resonance (CMR) steady state free precession (SSFP) demonstrates substantial accumulation of material in a small pericardial effusion. The tissue characteristics by SSFP, especially with the susceptibility (chemical shift, right panel) artifact at the border between the fat/pericardium are highly suggestive of a fat signal. Triple inversion recovery (TIR) images (middle) demonstrate marked nulling of the fat (*arrow*) with near superimposition with the SSFP (left) and are confirmatory that this is epicardial fat in a small pericardial effusion. The fat is a normal variant in a moderately obese woman. A small pleural effusion with atelectasis is also present (right panel, *thick arrow*). Images relate to case study 22.

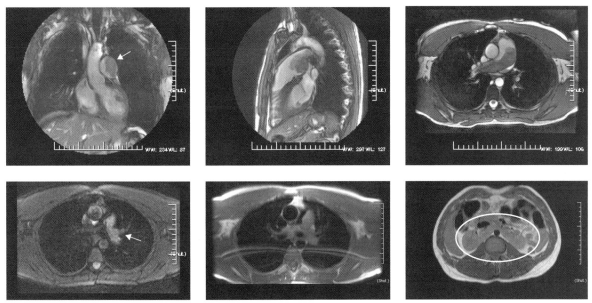

**FIGURE 13-23**    Selected steady state free precession (SSFP) (upper panel) in coronal, sagittal, and transverse views, and lower, triple inversion recovery (TIR) and double inversion recovery (DIR) of same view, and far right, DIR showing horse shoe kidney (*circled*). *Arrow* shows a large pulmonary mediastinal mass. The *arrow* points to the only region of local invasion as the remainder was easily sculpted out at surgery. Images relate to case study 23.

extrinsic) available to CMR permitted noninvasive characterization to be performed, differentiating with high specificity, non-neoplastic versus malignant lesions. These results suggest that CMR should be utilized following identification of cardiac masses to provide specificity and allowing the appropriate patient management.

## CASE STUDIES

**Case Study 1.** A 68-year-old white man presents for evaluation of a mass seen on TEE in the inner atrial septum, suggesting an atypical myxoma without a pedunculated stalk, a typical place for a left atrial (LA) myxoma to originate, Fig. 13-1. Surgical referral was made. The patient is referred for evaluation by CMR which demonstrates that the mass is atypical for a LA myxoma because it is predominantly in the retro atrium (RA), occupies the entire RA space, has an exceptionally broad base, and is large, irregular, and bulky. It is isointense with myocardium on T1 and very bright by T2, placing it within the realm of a malignant tumor. Evaluation of the extra-atrial tissue demonstrates substantial breach of the border, arising from outside the heart. In the upper right panel, the RF tissue tagging demonstrates lack of contractility as well as loss of the pericardial/cardiac border, indicating, as expected, lack of a surgical plane for resection. This man with a 45-year smoking history was

defined by CMR as having a bronchogenic carcinoma, which was confirmed the following day by open biopsy to be an undifferentiated sarcoma not amenable to surgery.

**Case Study 2.** A 69-year-old white man at an away Steelers football game suddenly collapses and passes out, Fig. 13-2. He is taken to a nearby hospital and x-ray and CT scan show a large mass in the vicinity of his left heart. When referred to our center, a CMR was performed. The mass was adjacent, and appears adherent, to a large territory of the LV as seen in the steady state free precession (SSFP) images. The perfusion sequence demonstrates gadolinium enhancement within the mass (except for a peripheral rim of contrast uptake) supporting a malignant process. The T1 and T2 sequences demonstrate a demarcation of the mass/LV borders, which indicates, especially in upper right panel, a surgical plane. The patient underwent aggressive mass debulking, and at surgery come the mass was demonstrated to have nearly clean margins, permitting widespread excision from the heart. The patient survived for nearly 3 years following the initial recommendations that he would not survive more than 1 month (because the mass was not deemed to be resectable). He made it to 2 more years of Pittsburgh Steelers games including their Super Bowl Championship.

**Case Study 3.** A 45-year-old woman presented with dyspnea on exertion, weight loss, and an abnormal chest x-ray causing concern for malignancy, Fig. 13-3. An echocardiogram raised suspicion for an extracardiac mass, prompting a CMR. Spin echo and T2 images reveal dense bulky masses adjacent to the right ventricle, superior vena cava, and RA. However, the first panel demonstrates a unifying diagnosis. Right paratracheal, para-aortic, and the nearly pathognomonic finding of esophageal-azygous lymphadenopathy is diagnostic for sarcoidosis. Note the characteristic lack of invasion, despite the bulk of the extracardiac mass. The patient underwent closed biopsy in which the diagnosis was confirmed.

**Case Study 4.** 65-year-old woman with slowly growing basal lateral wall mass around the posterior annular fibrous ring adjacent to the left circumflex artery, not amenable to closed biopsy, Fig. 13-4. Three-chamber and four-chamber views of the posterior-lateral wall region (see Fig. 13-4, arrow). The lower right frame confirms the ill-defined mass to be fat (arrow) by T2 sequence (triple inversion recovery [TIR]), an unusual intramyocardial lipoma.

**Case Study 5.** A routine echocardiogram seen on a four-chamber view performed on an 87-year-old man reveals a peculiar RA mass. CMR was performed, Fig. 13-5. SSFP imaging reveals an ectatic aortic root distorting the RA, masquerading as a large RA mass. This is a pseudotumor of the RA from a dilated aortic root.

**Case Study 6.** A right ventricular (RV) mass in a 24-year-old white woman seen by TTE. A CMR was performed revealing a well-circumscribed mass in the intraventricular septum that is homogeneous and isointense on the SSFP (see Fig. 13-6, upper panels), as well as isointense on the T2 sequence (see Fig. 13-6, lower panels). It is well circumscribed with no evidence of invasion, hemorrhage, or calcification, with mild protrusion into the cardiac chamber of no physiologic significance. Typically, little or no contrast enhancement is seen except for the peripheral capsule (rim), which is occasionally seen. In this young woman, a dense myocardial fibroma is characteristically shown here, typically seen in the septum, and requiring only routine following up with no need for biopsy or excision.

**Case Study 7.** A 65-year-old white woman presents with a peculiar finding on her TTE prompting CMR referral for probable invasive metastatic disease from a primary colon carcinoma which, by definition would place her as

having a stage IV non-resectable tumor. CMR demonstrates a large lesion >5 cm, but remarkably homogeneous, and by double inversion recovery (DIR) hyperintense and by TIR hypointense with respect to myocardium. There is near obliteration of the superior RA chamber. This is a classic case of lipomatous inner atrial septal hypertrophy, not a lipoma, as there is no capsule seen. Note the remarkable nulling by the T2-weighted sequence, which is of a similar intensity as the substantial cutaneous fat present. No evidence of metastatic disease was present, permitting colonic resection with colonic primary anastomosis and very long survival expected for stage I cancer. This pattern is not unusual in the elderly obese female population, and is a lesion for which CMR is often referred and it was gratifying to report the benign nature to both patient and referring physician.

**Case Study 8.** An unusual presentation of a 54-year-old white woman with dyspnea on exertion, early exercise fatigue, and a peculiar mass seen on an echocardiogram. CMR demonstrated a hyperdynamic LV with 3D ejection fraction (EF) of 80% and a moderate sized circular thin-walled apical mass with flow in it, Fig. 13-8. The limited differential diagnosis is LV aneurysm, LV pseudoaneurysm, or LV diverticulum or something else even rarer. She had no history of an MI, making the first option unlikely, but either of the first two as occult finding is possible. However, there is a narrow neck pointing toward either a pseudoaneurysm or an LV diverticulum. The RF tissue tagging (arrow) demonstrates no contraction to the apical region, negating the latter as the diagnosis. The upper right panel is a SSFP image, the remainder are DHE images (at 2 and 5 minutes) to evaluate for the presence of occult infarction, which is clearly demonstrated by CMR, shown best in bottom right panel (arrows) as a very thin, well delineated nearly transmural DHE signal. From this we concluded that this was a pseudoaneurysm, both by morphologic features of a narrow neck and through occult MI. As the patient was extremely symptomatic, she underwent surgery for excision, under the premise that her hyperdynamic state was exaggerated (or caused) by this lesion with high-velocity "to and fro" flow seen in the apical mass. Surgical pathology, however, demonstrated that this was a hamartoma. Embryologically, a hamartoma is of nearly the same structure as a muscle. This is a case where DHE cannot differentiate cardiac muscle versus a muscle-like structure, leading to an erroneous, but logical CMR conclusion. Review of the histology by this author did not completely negate the findings by CMR, because a layer of endocardial scar was clearly visible and hamartomas are *not* contractile. Apical resection did not cure her problem.

**Case Study 9.** A cypress root formation demonstrated by high-resolution CMR (see Fig. 13-9) whereby the apical myocardium gives rise to a rootlike structure *before* becoming a papillary muscle (PM). The apical myocardium forms an ever-growing lacy network of increasing coalescence of rootlike fibers to emerge as a finite and discrete homogeneous LV muscle (PM) only to again quickly divide into multiple branchlike fibers (chordae tendinea).

**Case Study 10.** An elderly obese white woman presents with a mass seen by echocardiography, seen in the pericardium by TTE. CMR reveals a small amount of pericardial fluid and on SSFP (see Fig. 13-10, left panel) a bright extrapericardial and epicardial signal that, by TIR (see Fig. 13-10, right panel), is confirmed to be fat, and not a pericardial tumor.

**Case Study 11.** An unusual apical defect was seen on cardiac catheterization. SSFP images demonstrate a contractile nonenhancing apical thin-walled structure (see Fig. 13-11), that is analogous to the earlier described diverticulum, because it is not specifically contractile (tethered by adjacent myocardium), it holds characteristics of a benign, but relatively rare, LV diverticulum (left panel is diastole, right panel is systole).

**Case Study 12.** An extracardiac hypoechoic mass is seen just outside and adjacent to the RA (see Fig. 13-12). CMR demonstrates the near classic location in the right costophrenic angle that by DIR is isointense-to-low intensity but homogeneous and hyperintense by TIR T2-weighted imaging, diagnostic of a benign pericardial cyst.

**Case Study 13.** A middle-aged man status post coronary artery bypass graft (CABG) several years presents with atypical chest pain for which a routine TTE reveals a mobile echodensity in his RA (top panel). CMR reveals the mass as a small circular lesion attached to the os of the coronary sinus but in the RA, atypical in location, with less than 10% found there. DIR (bottom left panel) images demonstrate the isointense nature whereas the TIR (see Fig. 13-13, bottom right) depicts the intermediate-to-hyperintense but homogeneous nature of the lesion. The pedunculated nature of the lesion is seen in the bottom right panel, at the coronary sinus os. The CMR tissue characteristics mentioned in the preceding text are indicative of a myxoma. As it was unusual, this was resected through a minimally invasive strategy, confirming the diagnosis.

**Case Study 14.** A mass in a 54-year-old black woman is seen on TEE as a single, discrete, well-defined structure. By CMR it is bright on both DIR (see Fig. 13-14, left) and TIR (see Fig. 13-14, right) with no evidence of invasion. Located in the typical extracardiac location with homogeneous signal, it is determined to be a benign bronchogenic cyst and requires no further evaluation.

**Case Study 15.** A 67-year-old black woman presents with 2 years of fatigue, shortness of breath (SOB), and weight gain and peculiar findings on echocardiography in the LV. CMR reveals a homogeneous echodensity in both apices of the RV and LV, biventricular failure, and dilation (see Fig. 13-15). SSFP images reveal two homogeneous broad-based lesions. DHE imaging suggests less of a broad-based lesion with a more pedunculated stalk but no contrast enhancement. Delayed enhancement imaging at 60 minutes fails to demonstrate any contrast uptake. Given the setting of global dysfunction, thinning and remodeling, pattern of DHE uptake, this is consistent with biventricular apical thrombi. Coumadinization was initiated with resolution of thrombus 6 weeks later by echocardiography.

**Case Study 16.** An 85-year-old man shortly after a motor vehicle accident: while everybody is watching a "peculiar" finding on echocardiography, he goes into ventricular tachycardia. Once he is stabilized, he is sent that afternoon for a CMR (see Fig. 13-16). Perfusion imaging (see Fig. 13-16, left) reveals a bright T1 signal outside the borders of the RV apical free wall. An early (30 second) postcontrast administration DHE sequence is obtained (see Fig. 13-16, right). A small mushroom shaped lesion is seen originating in the RV chamber with a small passageway leading through the apex into an oval "chamber" outside the RV free wall. The patient is 10 years status post CABG and now has a contained free wall rupture, with extravasation of contrast (blood) into a thickened, scarred pericardial/mediastinal fibrotic space, present due to the prior sternotomy. This scarring is fortunate, because he most likely would otherwise not have survived the free wall rupture into his mediastinum/pleural space and would have been exsanguinated. This contained rupture was electively followed up because he is believed to be protected by extensive pericardial adhesions (visible on CMR) and due to the high risk of sternotomy required RV repair. The patient does well under close follow-up for 5 days, is discharged, and at 1 year is still alive and driving.

**Case Study 17.** A 63-year-old white woman presents with a mass not well described on TTE. CMR reveals inner atrial septal mass (see Fig. 13-17); intermediate on

SSFP (T1) and bright on proton density and TIR (T2). The location and tissue characteristics are most consistent with a LA myxoma. The patient underwent an open excisional biopsy with surgical pathology confirming the LA myxoma. Note the heterogeneous signal on TIR (see Fig. 13-17, lower left), classic location, and tissue characteristic for a myxoma.

**Case Study 18.** A 48-year-old obese white woman is referred for CMR after a routine TTE demonstrated a large hyperechoic mass, partially obstructing the RA (see Fig. 13-18). CMR reveals the mass, but by TIR (see Fig. 13-18, lower panel) the tissue characteristics are that of fat. Notice the subtle capsule signifying a lipoma, and the not lipomatous inner atrial septal hypertrophy; both are benign lesions unless they become obstructive, then the term "malignant" is appropriate, but not to signify a carcinoma.

**Case Study 19.** This interesting presentation could potentially be one of several features in this 43-year-old woman (see Fig. 13-19): (a) invasive small cell; (b) hernia; (c) pericardial cyst; (d) mediastinal fat; (e) pericardial fat. The correct diagnosis is that it is a pericardial cyst.

**Case Study 20.** A 48-year-old white man referred for recurrent intrusive, refractory palpitations with high pre-test probability for arrhythmogenic right ventricular dysplasia (ARVD) was referred to CMR to confirm the diagnosis before implantable defibrillator placement. In Fig. 13-20, the DIR image demonstrates extensive adenopathy, including esophageal-azygous recess lymphadenopathy. This is nearly pathognomonic for sarcoidosis. The patient did not receive an automatic implantable cardiac defibrillator (AICD) but underwent a Wang biopsy, which is negative for sarcoidosis. An AICD is again planned but we insist that sarcoidosis is the most likely diagnosis. Therefore, a repeat biopsy is performed, which this time is positive for sarcoidosis. He is placed on steroids with remarkable abolishment of his palpitations, sparing him the defibrillator.

**Case Study 21.** A 55-year-old white woman was referred for known pulmonary sarcoidosis but had prolongation of her QRS and palpitations, raising concern for myocardial sarcoidosis (see Fig. 13-21). Using DHE postcontrast enhancement in exactly the same manner as for postinfarct imaging, except for a earlier post-contrast imaging (2–5 minutes) a definitive mid septal DHE signal is seen in a heterogeneous pattern, confirming the clinical suspicion of cardiac sarcoidosis. A biopsy easily confirmed the CMR diagnosis.

**Case Study 22.** A 45-year-old woman presents with an extracardiac mass seen on TTE. CMR SSFP demonstrates substantial accumulation of material in a small pericardial effusion (see Fig. 13-22). The tissue characteristics by SSFP, especially with the susceptibility (chemical shift) artifact at the border between the fat/pericardium, are highly suggestive of a fat signal. TIR images (see Fig. 13-22, middle panel) demonstrate marked nulling of the fat with near superimposition with the SSFP (see Fig. 13-22, left panel) and are confirmatory that this is epicardial fat in a small pericardial effusion. The fat is a normal variant in a moderately obese woman. A small pleural effusion with atelectasis is also present (see Fig. 13-22, right panel, arrow).

**Case Study 23.** A 32-year-old man returning from his honeymoon, experiences SOB while playing basketball. This worsens over 2 weeks. An echocardiogram was performed, which retrospectively was read as a possible density in main pulmonary artery (PA), for which heparin was initiated with no relief. CMR was performed (see Fig. 13-23). The left ventricular outflow tract view (see Fig. 13-23, upper left) reveals a large mass in the main PA, seen in subsequent views to be nearly occluding the PA and branch PAs. It is very distinct from the walls except for one small point of attachment seen in mid right PA branch (upper middle). A horseshoe kidney was detected on scout images (circled) raising the suspicion for a pulmonary angiosarcoma (although seen in 1 of 700 patients as a normal variant, it has an unusually strong association with angiosarcoma). The diagnosis was made as PA angiosarcoma by CMR. The patient underwent confirmatory biopsy in the catheterization laboratory and the diagnosis was changed to large pulmonary embolism given its coagulated blood appearance, and plans were made for reinstitution of heparin. When told of the diagnosis, we strongly suggested surgical pathologic confirmation. One hour later pathology revealed the mass to be a pulmonary angiosarcoma. He underwent radiation debulking and subsequent open resection followed by chemotherapy. He played basketball several months later with his young wife and newborn child.

# CHAPTER 14

# Congenital Heart Disease

Robert W. W. Biederman

The use of cardiovascular magnetic resonance (CMR) to evaluate congenital heart disease (CHD) has revolutionized the study and practice of CHD. It is almost as if CMR was developed primarily to assess CHD, with advantages for simple and complex, embryologically disparate disease processes in, typically younger, sick patients. Aspects that are ideal for this population include noninvasive, nonionizing radiation; no obligate need for contrast; ability to quantitate in highly accurate and reproducible manner both flow and velocity; visualization of ventriculoarterial conduits; assessing relationships between vascular structures that are typically not seen well on x-ray angiography; lack of requirement of acoustic window; and ability to visualize in any plane (see Fig. 14-1).

Hemodynamic assessment in a noninvasive manner is a key advantage that has been well recognized for detection and quantification of stenotic jets. Jets are characterized in terms of peak and mean gradient, and the temporal relationship of the jet to cardiac events can be assessed in a manner analogous to echocardiography, except that it can be done in an inherently three-dimensional manner. True quantitation of regurgitant jets, however, is not something that any other technique offers. CMR, through phase velocity mapping (PVM) allows calculation of the amount of blood flow crossing a selected plane, independent of relative orientation (see Fig. 14-2). For example, the same quantitation procedure can be performed in the setting of one valve possessing both a systolic stenotic jet and a diastolic regurgitant jet.

The ability to quantitate intracardiac shunts is well performed by CMR. Conventionally, echocardiographic measures cannot quantitate shunts well, and when attempted, these approaches are reliant on estimating velocity time integrals, which inherently assume that a parabolic flow is present. Similar arguments apply to the assessment of shunts in the catheterization suite where thermistor methods suffer in the presence of regurgitant lesions, whereas oximetry measurements suffer from a lack of specificity when there is >6% change in oxygen saturation levels. Fundamentally, this limits the ability to detect small shunts, which, although they may not be clinically significant, can become significant over time.

Typically, the CMR patient has been referred from a prior imaging modality in which the diagnosis was unclear. At our institution, echocardiography is the most often used test, followed by x-ray imaging and lastly, computed tomography (CT). Clarification of the disease process, relating an observation to the great vessels, evaluation of situs, evaluations of potential ventriculoarterial connection or intracardiac shunts are usually the indications to consider CMR (see Fig. 14-3).

A wide range of CMR imaging sequences are useful for patients with CHD. For a strategy that permits large amount information to be gleaned in a short time, to allow interpretation and permitting flexible planning, the double inversion recovery (DIR) sequence has proved to be very robust. When images are acquired in an axial view, anatomic relationships can be determined in a rapid manner, because the body is most commonly considered in this orientation. Relating the great vessels to the ventricles is easily performed in this plane, as is establishing the general relationships that exist between the atria and the ventricles, and additionally, some intracardiac communications can be assessed. The coronal view albeit less traditional, because it is not obtainable by conventional image modalities, reveals anatomic relationships in a superb manner, serving to delineate vascular and myocardial structures effectively in three dimensions (3D), when relating the series of 2D planes.

Defining situs is relatively easy when image quality is high. Situs solitus is the normal position, with the morphologic thin, smooth walled right atrium (RA) with its broad-based appendage and crista terminalis positioned to the right of the left atrium (LA), with its thin, miterlike, LA appendage. When reversed, the condition is referred

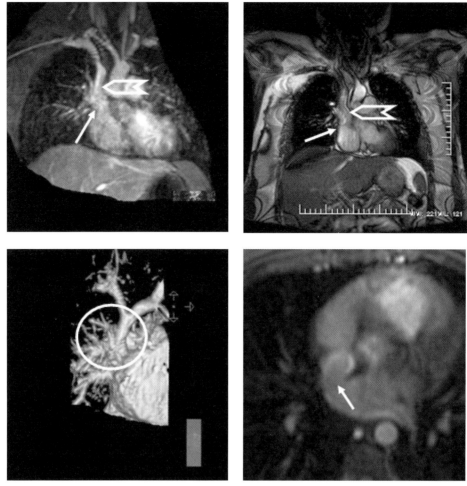

**FIGURE 14-1** Top panels show a limited region maximum intensity projection (MIP) (left). A steady state free precession (SSFP) (right) image acquired in the coronal projection at the level of the superior vena cava (SVC) demonstrates a confluence of the right upper and middle right pulmonary veins entering into the SVC/high right atrial (RA) junction. The lower panel images show a 3D surface rendition (left panel) of the magnetic resonance angiography (MRA) for the defect, demonstrating in the surface reconstructed view manually timed for the main pulmonary artery. The right panel shows the "broken ring" sign depicted by the *arrow* as the classic axial image that is diagnostic of a communication between the SVC and RA with a defect in the posterior inner atrial system. Images relate to case study 1.

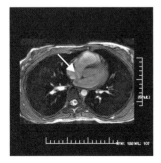 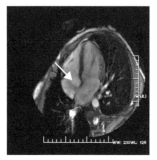 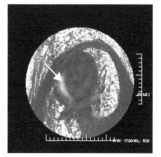 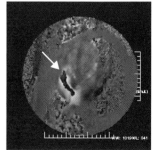

**FIGURE 14-2** A selected multislice steady state free precession (SSFP) sequence and a four-chamber view of an ostium secundum defect (far left and left) with phase velocity mapping (PVM) set low to a Venc of 50 cm/second shown in the left-to-right and anterior-to-posterior direction (right and far right) demonstrating the "Doppler-like" capability of cardiovascular magnetic resonance (CMR) with PVM. Quantitation was also performed to noninvasively determine the intracardiac shunt (Qp:Qs). Images relate to case study 2.

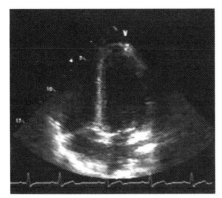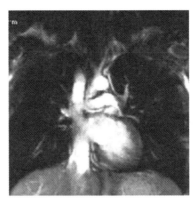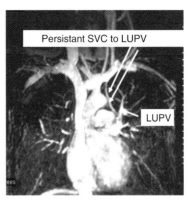

**FIGURE 14-3** Transthoracic imaging just before near simultaneous opacification of the right ventricular (RV) and left ventricular (LV) chambers by saline contrast (left). Middle image shows a single steady state free precession (SSFP) slice hinting at anomalous connection to the left upper pulmonary vein (*LUPV*)and confirmed by a temporal acquired maximum intensity projection (MIP) (*arrows*) (right). SVC, superior vena cava. Images relate to case study 3. (Best seen on DVD.)

to as situs inversus, and when ambiguous, it is referred to as atrial isomerism. This latter condition is associated with the visceral heterotaxy syndromes (see Fig. 14-4). Describing bronchial anatomy to identify the right and left bronchi is also quite helpful, especially when the lung isomerism is present. Right isomerism is associated with asplenia, whereas left isomerism is associated with polysplenia. Each condition has many associated atrioventricular (AV) connections. See Chapter 7 for more details.

Evaluation of pulmonary vein drainage is exceptionally well defined by CMR, as many combinations and anatomic normal variants are increasingly being recognized as clinically important (see Fig. 14-5). The axial plane generally allows recognition of the insertion point of the veins into the posterior LA. Usually, acquisition of a coronal plane permits unequivocal detection of the veins, and more importantly, when aberrant drainage is suspected, this plane permits delineation of a number of insertions into other vascular territories, including

## CASE STUDIES

**Case Study 1.** A persistent left superior vena cava (SVC) is visualized in a 46-year-old woman with shortness of breath (SOB), suggesting the possibility of a previously unrecognized unroofed coronary sinus atrial septal defects (ASD). However, a confluence of right upper pulmonary veins entering the high right atrium/proximal right SVC is seen (see Fig. 14-1), consistent with a sinus venosum defect. The sinus venosum defect is seen in a coronal image depicting the entry site into the RA (arrow) and right SVC (chevron). The bottom left image is a 3D surface from the magnetic resonance angiography (MRA) of a 29-year-old woman in whom a murmur was heard and an echocardiography was performed demonstrating right ventricular (RV) enlargement, which prompted the CMR. A sinus venosus defect was seen for which she underwent surgical baffle from the SVC/RA to the LA redirecting pulmonary flow to the LA and venous return to the RA.

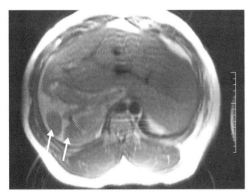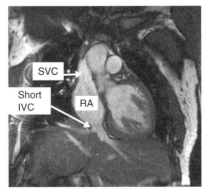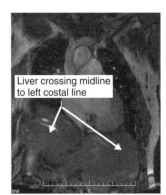

**FIGURE 14-4** Double inversion recovery (DIR) on left with steady state free precession (SSFP) in coronal projections demonstrating the heterotaxy syndrome. IVC, inferior vena cava; SVC, superior vena cava; RA, right atrium. Images relate to case study 4.

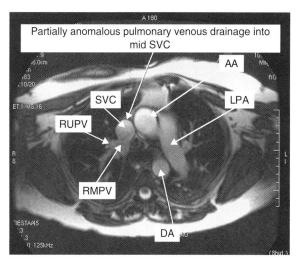
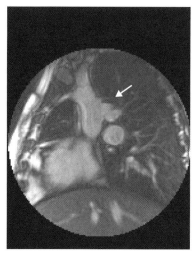

**FIGURE 14-5** Steady state free precession (SSFP) acquisitions in the axial (left) and parasagittal (right) demonstrating the anomalous insertion of right upper and middle pulmonary veins. SVC, superior vena cava; RUPV, right upper pulmonary venous; RMPV, right middle pulmonary vein; DA, descending aorta; LPA, left pulmonary artery; AA, ascending aorta. Images relate to case study 5.

infradiaphragmatic drainage, which is generally not detectable by other imaging modalities. In many cases in which right ventricular (RV) dilation is present, as seen on transthoracic echocardiography (TTE), and despite referral for transesophageal echocardiography (TEE) in which, "all four pulmonary veins are identified and enter into LA" CMR often detects a third right pulmonary vein (expected in many cases due to the smaller right middle pulmonary vein position that can be mistaken for the right lower pulmonary vein or right upper pulmonary vein). In these cases, often a sinus venosum defect is seen on axial DIR images, which easily detects a "broken ring sign" in which the posterior superior vena cava (SVC) is not completely closed and a defect is seen where the right upper pulmonary vein drains into the junction between the SVC and RA (see Fig. 14-1). Anomalous return, either partial in adults, or total in young children has been quite well described by CMR.

## ATRIOVENTRICULAR CONNECTIONS

The characterization of AV connections has been well described. We shall deal here with the use of CMR to aid in the distinguishing of morphologic ventricles, independent of their anatomic position within the mediastinum. As in contradistinction to echocardiography, the RV is easily identified. Perhaps the most distinguishing feature that indisputably identifies the RV is the presence of the moderator band, followed by the presence of trabeculations. These two features reliably identify the morphologic ventricle 100% of the time, allowing at a minimum, identification of the LV by default. Secondly,

**Case Study 2.** A 35-year-old woman presents with SOB. A CMR demonstrates a moderate-sized ostium secundum ASD (see Fig. 14-2). Various PVMs convincingly demonstrate the magnitude of the shunt which was measured as a Qp:Qs = 2.1 : 1 for which she underwent percutaneous placement of a closure device. SSFP and PVM were all that was necessary to accurately define the physiology. If an intracardiac shunt is suspected by SSFP imaging, confirmation can be obtained by switching to a gradient-recalled echo (GRE) sequence and increasing the echo time (TE) to 8.5 to 10 milliseconds. Further confirmation and quantification can be obtained using PVM as shown in the right panels. Often, a more dramatic visualization can be demonstrated through PVM than can be achieved by a dephasing artifact.

**Case Study 3.** An 18-year-old black male football player presents with SOB. Routine echocardiography reveals markedly positive bubble study (left arm IV). TEE performed demonstrates no bubbles crossing. Repeat TTE performed again show copious bubble immediately crossing from the RA to the LA. Unknown diagnosis prompts CMR (see Fig. 14-3). On the basis of presentation, a coronal SSFP was performed (mid panel) and suggested the diagnosis. Temporal MRA from the left arm shows two mechanisms of venous return into the heart. Note the exquisite anatomic detail depicted, demonstrating both anatomy and physiology with the transit of contrast over time and space. This is diagnostic of a very rare anomalous left upper pulmonary vein draining into the cardinal vein ("Partially Partial Anomalous").

the AV valves always stay with the appropriate ventricle regardless of placement of the ventricles. By CMR, the inner atrioventricular septum can be identified from a properly positioned four-chamber view. The tricuspid valve (TV) is displaced apically, whereas the mitral valve remains in the AV groove. The high resolution obtainable using CMR also permits unequivocal identification of the position and concordance of the atrioventricular relationships. Concordance defines normal atrioventricular relation; that is, RA connected to RV, LA connected to LV whereas discordance defines misplacement; that is, the RA connected to the LV and the LA connected to the RV. The valve apparatus is also important to define independent of the concordance, because valvar anatomy can be perturbed, requiring careful evaluation for the type and number of AV connections. These are typically best seen using dynamic steady state free precession (SSFP) imaging (see Fig. 14-6).

## VENTRICULOARTERIAL CONNECTIONS

Ventriculoarterial (VA) connections describe the relation between the morphologic ventricle and the great vessels. When the morphologic RV, as defined in the preceding text, inserts into the pulmonary artery (PA) and the morphologic LV inserts into the aorta, the VA connection is concordant. When the RV connects to the aorta and the LV connects to the PA there is VA discordance. Importantly, the definition, as in AV connections is independent of the spatial position of the chambers, and is dependant on the morphologic features, which are used to define the pathology (see Fig. 14-7). The CMR imaging views used to define PA and aortic anatomy are typically axial and coronal planes, but any obliquity can be prescribed, permitting clarification of the anatomic definitions. Both DIR and SSFP imaging are the workhorse sequences that are most beneficial for evaluation and diagnosis. When PVM is added, the vast majority of evaluations can be completed.

## EVALUATION OF INTRACARDIAC SHUNTS

Multiple levels of intracardiac communication (shunt) are possible and are detectable by CMR. In conjunction with an anatomic description, obtaining an understanding of the physiologic importance of a visualized anatomic defect is an added capability provided by CMR. CMR provides the ability to quantify shunts pre or post surgery, and may spare the patient from receiving an invasive procedure.

**Case Study 4.** This 32-year-old woman presents for evaluation of dyspnea. Routine CMR reveals an incidental finding of an interrupted inferior vena cava (IVC) (see Fig. 14-4). Note the multiple circular densities (see Fig. 14-4, left panel, arrows) indicative polysplenia, an often associated finding. This can be part of the Heterotaxy syndrome. Note the large SVC (middle panel) from the rerouted azygous return through which the mesenteric venous flow destined for the RA is rerouted. This is a benign variant for which, in the absence of imaging, she would be oblivious to her anomaly.

**Case Study 5.** Axial–SSFP images revealing anomalous right upper pulmonary venous (RUPV) drainage into the mid SVC in a 41-year-old woman with palpitations and mild dyspnea on exertion (DOE) (see Fig. 14-5). A sinus venosus anomaly is differentiated, as the RUPV drains into the junction of the high RA and low SVC. Note the confluence of two pulmonary veins into SVC; which are very important for complete surgical repair, in addition to identification of any and all anomalous drainage into the SVC because the surgeon may only be expecting to correct one vein.

**Case Study 6.** A 41-year-old white man with diagnosis of l-transposition since a child, and told he would never be normal. Multiple subsequent angiograms and TTEs and TEEs had been performed over the ensuing years, each reinforcing the last, saying that he had congenitally corrected transposition and eventually his heart would fail. Referred to us almost by accident, he underwent CMR (see Fig. 14-6). The RV moderator band is on the rightward and anterior trabeculated ventricle, whereas the leftward nontrabeculated ventricle AV valve plane is displaced atrially relative to the right AV valve plane (upper panels). There is no AV concordance (nor VA concordance). Although the *cardia* is markedly malrotated and superiorly displaced there is *no* transposition anatomy. The mother and son ask if they could hear the results of the study, stating how the grave diagnosis had affected her, her husband's, and her son's life, and how they wondered each day if they would wake up to see their son dead, day after day, year after year, and how it affected his grades, his plans for the future, and his relationships with others including his ability to marry as he got older. Is good news bad here? Indeed, good news can be catastrophic because they both realized how very different the last 41 years might have been.

**Case Study 7.** A 27-year-old black woman status post Jatene arterial switch for d-transposition of the great vessels referred for evaluation of right ventricle morphology and function (see Fig. 14-7). Instead of a Senning or Mustard atrial baffle or reconstruction technique,

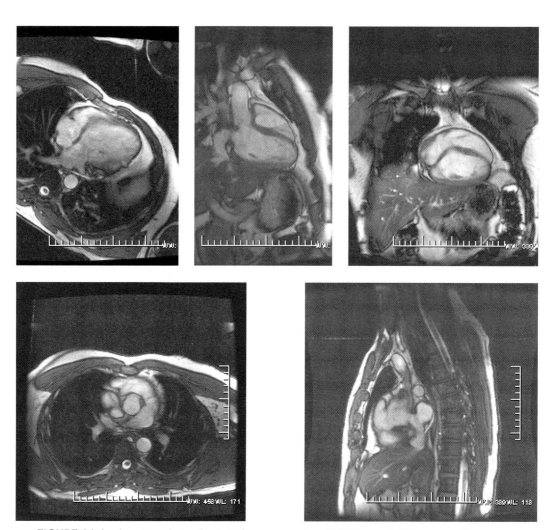

**FIGURE 14-6**   A series of steady state free precession (SSFP) acquisitions revealing malrotation of the LV and right ventricle (RV) but without evidence for an l-transposition morphology. Images relate to case study 6.

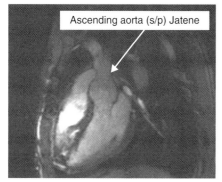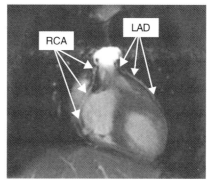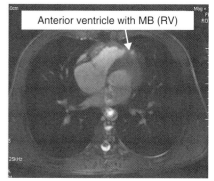

**FIGURE 14-7**   A series of steady state free precession (SSFP) images depict the ability of noninvasive delineation of the coronary buttons in a patient with Jatene arterial switch. The right panel demonstrates the moderator band in this d-transposition patient indicating the morphologic right ventricle. RCA, right coronary artery; LAD, left anterior descending artery; MB, moderator band; RV, right ventricle. Images relate to case study 7.

## Specific Shunts

### Atrial Septal Defects

There are four types of atrial septal defects (ASDs):

1. *Ostium secundum*: This is the most common ASD encountered, located in the middle of the interatrial septum, generally in the vicinity of the fossa ovalis. The four-chamber view depicts this lesion well, as does the axial view (see Fig. 14-2). However, caution must be heeded when using the DIR sequence, because partial volume errors frequently overestimate the defect or cause an apparent defect to be present when by SSFP sequences it is absent.

2. *Ostium primum*: This defect is located in the most caudal portion of the interatrial septum and it is frequently associated with other congenital defects, including ventricular septal defects. Often seen in conjunction with endocardial cushion defects, the mitral valve is frequently cleft, with resultant mitral regurgitation. The four-chamber and axial views are ideally suitable for assessing this anomaly, which is particularly well characterized by the common AV valve plane, with failure to demonstrate an inner atrioventricular septum.

3. *Sinus venosus*: This defect is associated with anomalous right upper pulmonary vein insertion into the junction of the low SVC/high RA junction. This defect is easily appreciated on axial DIR or SSFP images as a "broken ring sign" in which the posterior normally circular SVC is interrupted by the insertion of the anomalous vein. Of all the ASDs, this defect is the most frequently undetected lesion by standard imaging modalities because of its relative extracardiac location. Conversely, CMR, because of its large field of view (FOV) has been shown to be the technique of choice (see Fig. 14-1).

4. *Coronary sinus (coronary solitaris)*: This uncommon defect is characterized by an absent roof of the coronary sinus as it crosses inferior to the LA wall. Generally, this is seen from persistent left SVC dumping into the LA and on either two-chamber view or a caudal four-chamber view, the coronary sinus is absent. Sometimes this can be recognized by the absence of the coronary sinus os.

5. Sometimes referred to a mythical defect, a Gerbode defect is defined when there is a communication in the inner atrioventricular septum permitting, ostensibly, flow from the LV through this common membrane into the RA. This author has never seen such a lesion but it is speculated that it can exist anatomically.

The direction of shunt flow can be appreciated from observation of the origination of the defect with a combination of SSFP imaging, to give qualitative assessment and, in those cases in which the defect is small or equivocal, an addition of a the patient underwent the arterial switch (Jatene) surgery. In the left panel, arrow points to the reinsertion of the coronary arteries as a button graft from the native pulmonary artery (PA), as well as the anterior positioned RV with its moderator band delineating the morphologic RV as the original systemic ventricle.

**Case Study 8.** A 45-year-old woman with known ventricular septal defect (VSD) diagnosed at early childhood. After many years being lost to follow-up she is referred for CMR (see Fig. 14-8). Her examination no longer reveals a murmur of VSD but a harsh systolic ejection sound with loss of $P_2$ and a prominent RV $S_4$. Examination reveals hypertrophied RV free wall without VSD. In its place there is a prominent RV high septal muscle band creating dramatic subpulmonic stenosis (right panel) with a high velocity jet radiating into and across the pulmonic valve without frank pulmonic valvar stenosis. Spontaneous closure of VSDs has been shown to occur by several means, one of which is hypertrophy of the adjacent myocardial tissue, but on occasion is overzealous converting a volume overload situation into a pressure overload state, as in this case. The patient underwent myotomy with relief of the 98 mm Hg gradient and relief of symptoms.

**Case Study 9.** Standard SSFP images performed in a 32-year-old woman referred for reasons unrelated to her final diagnosis. In Fig. 14-9 left panel, standard two-chamber view provides the rationale for why the large FOV is a valuable commodity for CMR, where a moderate-sized patent ductus arteriosum is seen. Using PVM, the Qp:Qs was quantified as 1.3:1 and she underwent uneventful percutaneous coil closure and went home the following day.

**Case Study 10.** A 35-year-old man presents with a harsh pan-cyclic murmur, heard most prominently along his back, with symmetric pulse in his upper extremities but diminished pulses bilaterally in his lower extremities. A coarctation was suspected, as confirmed on the 20-second MRA acquisition (see Fig. 14-10, arrow). Note the severe coarctation and poststenotic dilatation. Additionally, an indication of the collateral circulation to the lower extremities can be gleaned from the widely dilated right internal mammary artery (chevron).

**Case Study 11.** A 36-year-old man with a history of Tetralogy of Fallot and large left bronchial collaterals has undergone several repairs since age of 6 years. He presents with a 6-day history of chest pain and progressive dyspnea on exertion. His admitting electrocardiogram (ECG) reveals a right bundle branch block, and negative cardiac enzymes. The patient continued

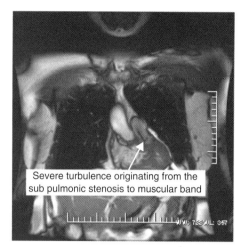 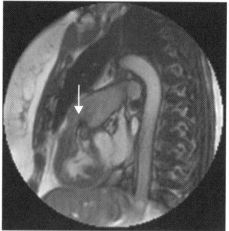

Severe turbulence originating from the sub pulmonic stenosis to muscular band

**FIGURE 14-8** Steady state free precession (SSFP) sequence in a coronal and sagittal projection with a dephasing artifact (left, *arrow*) and the severe subvalvar infundibular muscle band well depicted (right, *arrow*). Images relate to case study 8.

gradient-recalled echo (GRE) sequence with a longer TE (8.5–10 milliseconds) can increase the intervoxel dephasing artifact and thereby enhancing the flow turbulence. Previously, we and others, have shown a high degree of correlation in qualitative assessments between Doppler and GRE.

### *Ventricular Septal Defect*

There are four types of VSDs:

1. *Perimembranous*: This is the most common defect and occurs at the most cephalad location of the

to deteriorate, requiring mechanical ventilation, whereupon a transesophageal echocardiography was performed which suggested an ascending aortic aneurysm with possible focal dissection and normal left and right sized ventricle. To further delineate the anatomy, a CMR was performed which revealed gargantuan left and right ventricles measuring 98 mm and 54 mm in end-diastole, respectively (see Fig. 14-11). The left ventricle was extensively compressed from the right ventricle, resulting in severe distortion in the superior–inferior

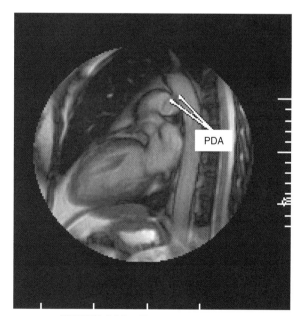 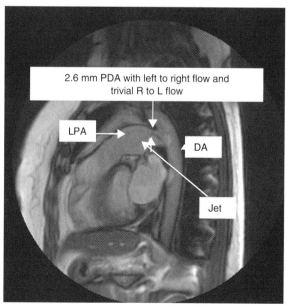

PDA

2.6 mm PDA with left to right flow and trivial R to L flow

LPA        DA

Jet

**FIGURE 14-9** Two steady state free precession (SSFP) sequences revealing the subtle but important dephasing artifact arising from the aorta and entering into the left pulmonary artery, indicative of a small patent ductus arteriosum (PDA). LPA, left pulmonary artery; DA, descending aorta. Images relate to case study 9.

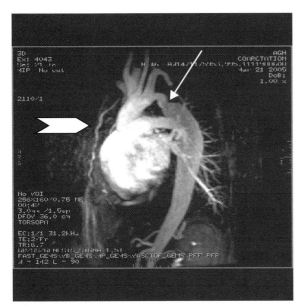

**FIGURE 14-10**　Selected image from an magnetic resonance angiography (MRA) acquired as a manually timed 3-mL test dose in a 20-second breath-hold. The maximum intensity projection (MIP) image demonstrates a slightly early acquisition of k-space, whereby the left ventricle (LV) and ascending aorta are preferentially opacified compared to the mid and distal ascending aorta. Images relate to case study 10.

ventricular septum, best seen in the four-chamber view.

2. *Muscular*: This is the second most common VSD and is defined by the complete enclosure of the defect by a rim of septal muscle, best seen in either the three- or four-chamber views (see Fig. 14-8).

3. *Apical*: This is a variant of the muscular defect and is located at or near the apex, best seen in the three or four-chamber views.

4. *Supracristal*: This defect is located in the subpulmonic area and is the most rare of the VSDs. It requires a high index of suspicion and is best seen in the RV out flow track view and confirmed in the paraxial view, typically as a small high velocity jet originating from just below the right coronary cusp entering into the high medial infundibulum.

The VSDs can be further classified into restrictive or nonrestrictive types.

As mentioned in the preceding text, and described in Chapter 30, quantitative assessment can be obtained in several manners. In that the quantitation of flow should be performed distal to the regurgitant lesion, the most accurate and reproducible technique is to quantitate flow at the proximal aorta and PA, obtained in a slice perpendicular to the long axis of the great vessel. When quantified in this manner, stroke volume can be used for calculation of Qp:Qs. The second method relies on

direction. The left atrium was markedly dilated and tubular, due to marked posterior dilation and displacement of the ascending aortic aneurysm. The right ventricle was markedly dilated and hypertrophied with severe pulmonic, tricuspid, and AR. The sinus of Valsalva was markedly dilated measuring 61 mm whereas the proximal ascending aorta formed a gigantic aneurysm measuring 93 × 83 mm, terminating cranially into a nearly normal size aortic arch. Most importantly, there was a focal dissection in the anterior and right lateral wall of the aortic aneurysm. Additionally, several aorta-to-pulmonary (bronchial) collaterals were seen, with many communicating directly with the left atrium.

**Case Study 12.** A 41-year-old woman who is status post Tetralogy of Fallot repair as a child now presents with SOB and a high-pitched systolic murmur radiating to her back. A 22-second 3D MRA demonstrates a severe proximal left PA branch stenosis (see Fig. 14-12), not an uncommon finding several years after the repair. Using PVM, there was a 42 mm Hg peak gradient across the stenosis. Balloon angioplasty with wall stent was placed with reduction of the gradient post catheterization to 6 mm Hg, elimination of murmur, and relief of symptoms.

**Case Study 13.** A male patient presents with palpitations and several episodes of syncope presenting with prodrome of palpitations and "heart racing." Enlarged RV seen on echocardiogram prompting CMR: four-chamber (see Fig. 14-13, left) and axial images (see Fig. 14-13, right) reveal marked atrialization of the TV with apical displacement of the septal leaflet of the TV. A strong association of Wolf-Parkinson-White syndrome with a septal bypass tract is present in 25% of cases presenting with Ebstein anomaly, as this young patient had.

**Case Study 14.** A 45-year-old white woman with mild chest pain (CP) and equivocal nuclear perfusion test underwent left heart catheterization with indeterminate course off a single coronary ostium. In Fig. 14-14, CMR reveals the left main arises off of a single right coronary artery (RCA) ostia, traveling posteriorly before emerging in usual coronary trajectory (benign nonintra-arterial course).

**Case Study 15.** A 48-year-old presents with a most unusual finding on a routine cardiac catheterization in which the trajectory of the normally arising left anterior descending artery (LAD) was seen to travel anterior with vessels arising from it to form a circuitous looping vascular bed of unknown emptying chamber (as described at cardiac catheterization). Seen in Fig. 14-15 are several serpentine loops, which when

**FIGURE 14-11** A series of multislice-axial steady state free precession (SSFP) images and one two-chamber SSFP sequence delineating with high resolution the grossly distorted anatomy and physiology including the first aortic dissection described in this a patient with Tetralogy of Fallot. AV, aortic valve; MV, mitral valve. Images relate to case study 11.

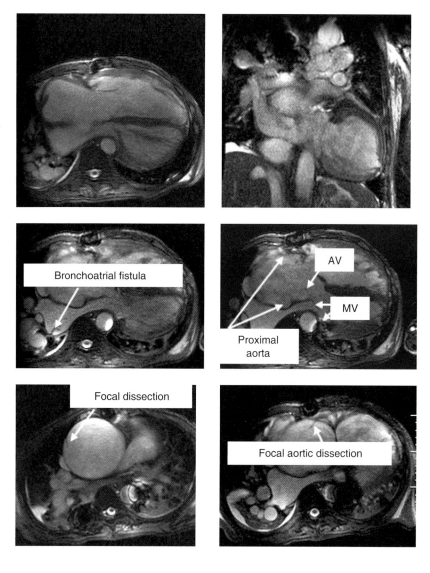

3D quantitation of the volumetric derived stroke (VDS) volumes and their subsequent comparison to produce Qp:Qs. We note that the volumetric Qp:Qs is inaccurate in the setting of any appreciable valvular regurgitation. In the absence of regurgitation, the two methods should correlate within 5% of each other. When using the PVM technique, we and others have shown exceptionally high accuracy and reproducibility when compared to flow phantom models ("r" values >0.95). Therefore, extraordinarily low degrees of shunting are relatively easily detected, which are often substantially smaller than can be appreciated by conventional imaging techniques.

### Patent Ductus Arteriosum

A patent ductus arteriosum (PDA) is a relatively common, but underappreciated form of CHD, most likely stemming from the difficulty in imaging this extracardiac defect. This defect is a communication between the great vessels, typically seen as a jet

followed carefully, were shown to be small arteries emptying into the anterior PA, diagnostic of an LAD to PA fistula.

**Case Study 16.** A 38-year-old presents with "bizarre" catheterization finding (see Fig. 14-16). Is it: (a) coronary fistula, (b) anomalous pulmonary vein, (c) ectatic left internal mammary artery (LIMA) graft, (d) cameral fistula, or (e) persistent left superior caval vein (LSVC)? The correct answer is (a) coronary artery fistula draining into the high infundibulum.

**Case Study 17.** CMR can often add valuable information in patients with cardiac or pericardial masses, even in settings where a CT has already been performed. A 74-year-old man with a 10-week history of increasing SOB and chest pressure sought evaluation. Coronary angiography and a chest CT were performed, with the

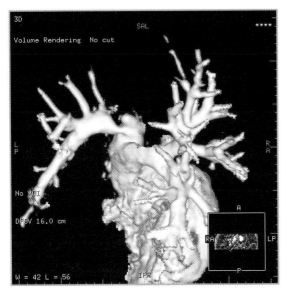

**FIGURE 14-12**  A 3D reconstructed surface rendered image of the main pulmonary and branch pulmonary vessels acquired in a 22-second breath-hold with manual timing at the level of the proximal right ventricular outflow tract (RVOT). Image relates to case study 12.

originating from the isthmus of the aorta, entering as a high velocity jet into the proximal left PA (left to right). Best seen in either a parasagittal or coronal view, the area of communication can be as simple as a small conduit or nearly adjacent great vessels with no or minimal communicating tissue (see Fig. 14-9). In the early and mid stages of this lesion, a near pan-cyclic high velocity dephasing jet is seen entering the PA. As the PA pressures increase, the duration of the jet shortens, until aortic and PA pressures equilibrate, when the jet essentially disappears. This is followed by a biphasic pattern, and as Eisenmenger syndrome ensues, PA to aortic flow occurs (right to left). Although semiquantitative estimation of severity is possible, again formal quantitation is the preferred technique. PVMs can be acquired using two techniques: (a) measuring proximal PA flow and distal aorta flow with comparison to produce Qp:Qs and (b) a more accurate but difficult technique, assuming the PDA is postductal, measurement of flow pre- and post-PDA is performed and when subtracted provides the amount of shunt in milliliters per beat.

## Aortic Coarctation

Aortic coarctation is another common defect. This lesion is an under-recognized, correctable, source of hypertension that arises as a fibrotic, often calcified, irregular stricture around the aorta, typically at the or near the isthmus formed as a remnant of the *ligamentum arteriosum*. Located at or just beyond the left subclavian artery (unless preductal), the defect is best seen in

finding of a large bilobed anterior mediastinal mass. He was transferred for further evaluation (see Fig. 14-17). Using as older FastCINE (GRE) pulse sequence, the CMR demonstrated that the mass was a $7 \times 9 \times 9$ cm aneurysm of the RCA. The aneurysm partially compressed the right ventricle. He was taken to surgery, and the aneurysm was resected. The patient recovered well.

**Case Study 18.** A 58-year-old man with atrial fibrillation was referred for CMR mapping of the pulmonary vein anatomy in preparation for possible pulmonary vein isolation. Shown here in Fig. 14-18, the 3D volume rendering MRA is the LA anatomy and associated pulmonary veins. A total of seven pulmonary veins were isolated (arrows) with four on the right side including a right middle vein and three on the left. Standard electrophysiological mapping would have identified only four (two on left and two on right) and likely, only they would have been ablated. However, if the source of the arrhythmia was in one of the other three veins (43% chance), the rhythm would have returned. This acquisition is accomplished easily on 20-second breath-hold and is rendered in 3D in an additional minute.

**Case Study 19.** A 50-year-old white man presents with positive stress test and ventricular tachycardia at conclusion of test, prompting emergency catheterization. Left heart catheterization (LHC) reveals anomalous LAD off RCA but course is unknown. The patient was STAT transferred for CMR (see Fig. 14-19). CMR axial image demonstrating a normal take-off off the RCA from the right sinus of Valsalva, and an adjacent left main artery arising from the same cusp traveling between the right ventricular outflow tract (RVOT)/PA and the aorta. This patient had dynamic compression from the intra-arterial course, a potentially lethal and often overlooked congenital anomaly. The intrinsic value of CMR in this indication is not due to its high resolution relative to cardiac catheterization, but due its ability to depict the proximal course of the coronaries with reasonable quality, and due its intrinsic capability to represent a large FOV with extracoronary anatomy *along with* the coronaries. This study was performed with the following characteristics and magnetic resonance imaging (MRI) study parameters:

1. Imaging time to detection of lethal anomaly: 8 minutes
2. Amount of nephrotoxic contrast: 0 mL
3. Amount of MRI contrast: 0 mL
4. Amount of x-ray radiation: 0 Sgy
5. Number of IVs needed: zero
6. Time of NPO: 0 minute
7. Number of minutes holding his groin: 0

**FIGURE 14-13** Gradient-recalled echo (GRE) images of a four-chamber and two multislice-axial projections in a patient with Ebstein anomaly. Images relate to case study 13.

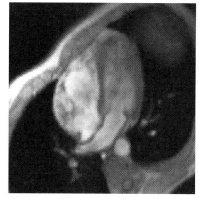
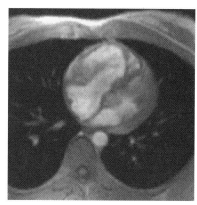

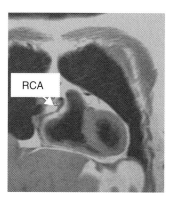
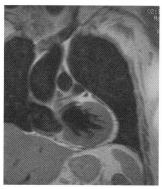
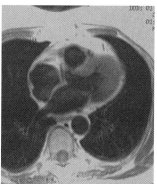

**FIGURE 14-14** A series of double inversion recovery (DIR) images depicting noninvasive evaluation of single-slice acquisitions of anomalous coronary artery anatomy. RCA, right coronary artery. Images relate to case study 14.

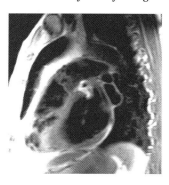
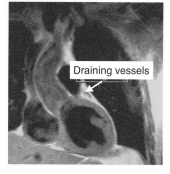
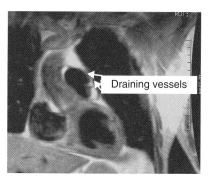

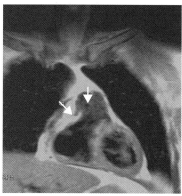
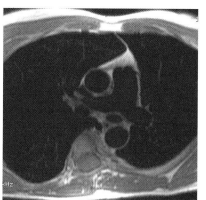

**FIGURE 14-15** A series of double inversion recovery (DIR) images depicting noninvasive evaluation of anomalous coronary artery anatomy in multiple views and the draining arteries. Images relate to case study 15.

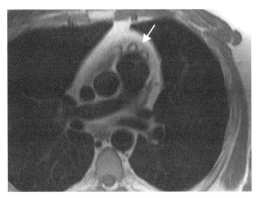 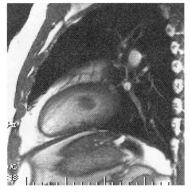 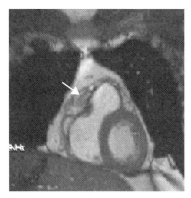

**FIGURE 14-16** Double inversion recovery (DIR) on left with steady state free precession (SSFP) in middle and right revealing a serpentine coronary fistula to the right ventricular outflow tract (RVOT). Images relate to case study 16.

either the parasagittal or the coronal view but can be suspected by a defect on axial DIR imaging performed at the level of the proximal descending aorta. The degree of systolic and diastolic turbulence directed into the descending aorta grants a semiquantitative measure of the severity, as does the degree of poststenotic dilation (see Fig. 14-10). Numerous associated lesions can be present, and form part of the *forme fruste* of the same defect. Transverse arch hypoplasia and descending arch hypoplasia can be seen, and are important features when considering surgery. The finding of a coarct should trigger a search for a bicuspid aorta, and proximal ascending aortic dilation. While seemingly unrelated, this triad forms an embryologically logical defect when there is believed to be a defect in neural

**Case Study 20.** A 54-year-old white woman presents with markedly abnormal chest x-ray (CXR) read as severe congenital heart disease, undefined. Echocardiogram relates markedly displaced cardiac structures but is unable to offer a definitive diagnosis. The first clue is that the heart is shifted strikingly to the left, more so than any congenital malformation should be (see Fig. 14-19). The absence of any distinct pericardial tissue confirms the patient as having generally benign course, rarely presenting with general strangulation of the LV or RV and even less frequently epicardial coronary artery constriction. This is diagnostic for a congenitally absent pericardium.

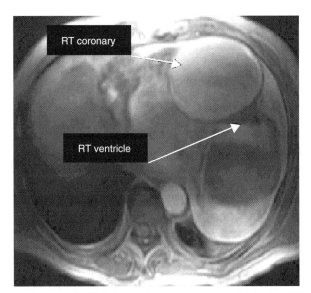 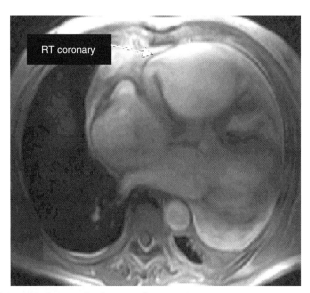

RT coronary

RT ventricle

RT coronary

**FIGURE 14-17** Gradient-recalled echo (GRE) images in a multislice-axial projection defining two near contiguous abnormal formations anterior to the right ventricular (RV) free wall that was an aneurysmal right coronary artery. Images relate to case study 17. (Courtesy of Tony Fuisz, MD, Washington Hospital Center.)

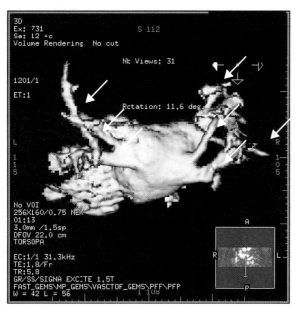

**FIGURE 14-18** 3D reconstruction of a 20-mL gadolinium (MultiHance, Bracco Diagnostics Inc., Princeton, NJ) injection for pulmonary vein anatomy timed off the main pulmonary artery with a manual timing 3-mL pre-scan. Image relates to case study 18.

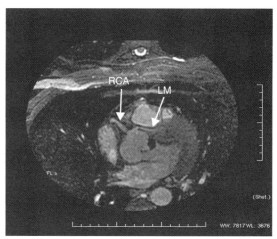

**FIGURE 14-19** A representative slice from a 3D volume acquisition of anomalous coronary arteries demonstrating, not the high resolution of cardiovascular magnetic resonance (CMR) in this case, but the ability of CMR to define anatomic structures (coronary arteries) relative to other structures (aorta and pulmonary artery) providing unequivocal capability to define anomalies. CMR is regarded as the "gold standard" in these cases. RCA, right coronary artery; LM, left main artery. Image relates to case study 19.

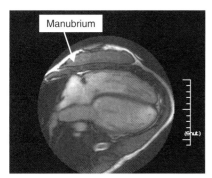 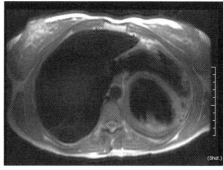 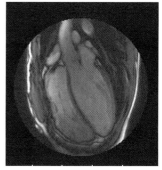

**FIGURE 14-20** A double inversion recovery (DIR) sequence sandwiched by two steady state free precession (SSFP) images. Despite the sequences showing epicardial fat (bright), there is no pericardial fat by either sequence. No evidence of pericardium (typically gray) is seen. Note the marked leftward displacement in each sequence, very atypical for any other congenital defect. Images relate to case study 20.

**FIGURE 14-21** A 3D reconstructed surface rendered aorta and arch vessels seen in the anterior (left) and posterior position (right) manually timed from the proximal ascending aorta. Note, the injection is slightly early but even so, clearly shows the pulmonary present. Images relate to case study 21.

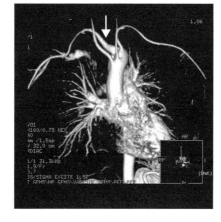 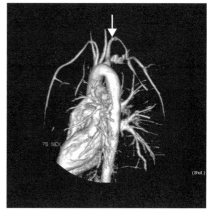

crest cells resulting in failure of elements of the media muscularis layer containing elements of collagen and fibrillin, resulting in loss of tensile strength of the aorta and subsequent dilation. Failure of leaflet formation is related, resulting in one of many leaflet anomalies, all generally characterized by the term *bicuspid aortic valve.* As discussed in the chapters on valvular disease and quantification, quantitation of associated aortic regurgitation (AR) and/or aortic stenosis (AS) can be made by PVM.

### Atrioventricular Defects

Abnormalities of the endocardial cushions result, invariably, in the ostium primum, with a superior VSD on a common plane with the AV valve, which is an associated pathognomonic feature. The SSFP four-chamber view is best used to define this lesion as well as the associated mitral regurgitation, which is invariably present. CMR is also ideally suited to describe the size and functionality of the related ventricles.

### Supravalvar, Infravalvar, and Valvar Stenosis

Previously, it was often noted that the pulmonic valve was not well delineated by CMR. However, when using the SSFP sequence, it can now be appreciated that this valve is well visualized. Additionally, the trileaflet pulmonic valves and its associated regurgitant or stenotic lesion can be carefully described and quantitated by using PVM. The associated infundibular and RV free wall hypertrophy can be seen and measured. Infundibular or subpulmonic valvar stenosis can be seen, quantified, and planes can be defined for the surgeon to use as roadmaps (see Fig. 14-8). Suprapulmonic stenosis, rare and typically in an "applecore" pattern, are easily seen on right ventricular outflow tract (RVOT) and axial views using the SSFP sequence. Again PVM aids in assessing the clinical significance, sparing invasive, often traumatic attempts to cross the lesion through catheterization. A word of caution is warranted. Often, the sinotubular ridge of the pulmonic valve, just above the pulmonary sinuses (analogous to the Sinuses of Valsalva of the aorta), is regarded in the catheterization suite as evidence for supravalvar stenosis. While not generally described as such, there is a pulmonic sinotubular junction which is normal and naturally smaller than the sinus of Valsalva, but unless constricted more than the proximal PA, is normal.

Supravalvar AS is a rare lesion, seen most often in the pediatric population and is generally a fibromuscular, sometimes calcified ring, generating high turbulence into the ascending aorta. The extent of the physiologic ramifications for the affected LV can be discerned by the extent of left ventricular hypertrophy (LVH). Subaortic stenosis, most often defined by the presence of a membrane, partially or completely, encircling

> **Case Study 21.** Left arch aorta and anomalous right subclavian (fourth brachial artery anomaly, shown with arrow in Fig. 14-19) traveling posterior to the trachea and the esophagus without evidence of dysphagia by real time imaging (not shown) in a patient presenting with atypical chest pain. No other associated congenital disease. No evidence of a diverticulum of Kommerell.

the left ventricular outflow tract (LVOT), most often arising from the anterior septum can be seen by, dedicated SSFP, DIR sequences applied with careful breath-holding. Often, image optimization is required and steps such as increasing the matrix or using two or three number of excitations (NEX) are required to bring out this subtle lesion. Occasionally, the membrane will be more typical of a muscular ridge or outpocketing. Demonstrating the anatomic location and distance from the related aortic valve leaflet is extremely helpful for surgical correction, which typically takes the form of resection or limited myotomy. Details of less discrete obstructive LVOT lesions, such as hypertrophic obstructive cardiomyopathy (HOCM), asymmetric subtype will be discussed elsewhere.

### Tetralogy of Fallot

This fairly common lesion is heralded by:

1. A perimembranous VSD
2. Overriding aorta
3. Infundibular pulmonary stenosis
4. Associated RV hypertrophy

CMR is exceptionally useful for the study of Tetralogy of Fallot (TOF) in that the complex lesion can be seen in many planes, the details of the aortic override and its relation to the VSD can be seen, measured, and a roadmap provided for surgical management. Often, patch closure and redirection of flow is not sufficient to relieve the outflow tract obstruction, necessitating LVOT enlarging (see Fig. 14-11). More importantly, the often present PA stenosis, either at diagnosis or as a late manifestation years later, is very well delineated by CMR and is especially helpful as the child develops into adulthood, when branch PA hypoplasia or frank stenosis occurs (see Fig. 14-12). Coronary artery anomalies are well defined by CMR and are important to identify before attempting a thoracotomy. Follow-up of palliative surgeries with established conduits such a Blalock-Taussig shunts, whereby the right subclavian artery is anastomosed to the right branch PA to increase pulmonary flow, are easily evaluated using both SSFP and PVM, aligned either parallel or perpendicular to the shunt.

## Tricuspid Atresia

Defined as the absence or severe hypoplasia of the TV, truncus arteriosus (TA) is typically associated with both AV and VA concordance and flow destined for the systemic circulation is routed through a VSD and an associated ASD or patent foramen ovale (PFO). Dimension and functionality of the RV depend on the extent of pulmonary flow, which is directly related to the presence of infundibular stenosis or valvular pulmonic stenosis. This sometime complex lesion has a myriad of anatomic variants that can be present: (a) AV concordance with VA discordance, (b) AV concordance with VA discordance with double outlet RV and usually adjacent atrial appendages, (c) associated pulmonary atresia with aorta derived from the LV, which is less frequent. CMR in axial and coronal planes well defines the anatomy. The axial plane usually depicts a normal to large sized LV with a small, remnant anterior positioned appendagelike structure that is the morphologic RV, sometime appearing as if there is open communication with the LV (through a VSD). It is important to recognize that the TV may be falsely identified as atretic if only axial images are obtained. The addition of coronal and para-axial oblique views using SSFP imaging clarifies the presence or absence of the TV, which may be off axis and underestimated if only axial images are acquired. The presence, following surgery, of conduits such as Fontan, modified Fontans, Hemi-Fontans, or Rastelli conduits are well performed by CMR and, most experts believe that CMR is the imaging modality of choice to define these postoperative modifications, permitting an understanding of their effectiveness and patency.

## Truncus Arteriosum

This very complex disorder has several types, all consisting of effectively a single ventricle over a large VSD out of which both the aorta and PA arise as a large, single great artery (truncus). The crucial issue by CMR is, in addition to establishing the diagnosis, defining the extensive and variable PA anatomy. Again, standard imaging fails to delineate, in the detail necessary, the varied presentation of PA originations. Because extensive aortopulmonary collaterals (APC) exist (bronchial) as endogenous attempts to improve pulmonary circulation, localization and defining the extent of their contribution to flow is essential. Often, these become extensive and overload the pulmonary circuit, requiring embolization. CMR exquisitely depicts their location for surgical or interventional strategies. Both axial and coronal imagings of the descending aorta are useful to describe the bronchial circulation. This approach is also used to describe one of the variants of TA, including TA type IV, in which the PA is atretic with a large VSD (now defined on its own as TA with VSD). This latter variant has dramatic APCs, some derived from the subclavian arteries as well to provide necessary pulmonary flow.

## Transposition of the Great Vessels

The complex CHD can be defined as two types:

1. d-transposition: In this anomaly, there is AV concordance but VA discordance with the pulmonary ventricle on the LV as a large valve (larger then the standard aortic valve) and with a characteristic large muscular valvular support. The coronaries arise from the PA; if they do not arise off the PA, suspect an alternate diagnosis (see Fig. 14-7). A Senning or Mustard repair of the atria was the standard; now a Jatene arterial switch is the favored surgical correction with an obligatory coronary artery switch. The coronaries are implanted typically as large buttons in which coronal images appear as large ears arising off the proximal ascending aorta.
2. l-transposition: In this form there is double discordance—VA discordance and AV discordance—but because the errors are equal, they offset. This is also referred to as congenitally corrected transposition of the great arteries. The RV and LV are switched, and otherwise the atria are in the normal anatomic position. On axial imaging, the aorta is anterior and rightward to the leftward PA. The coronary artery can be reversed (see Fig. 14-7).

# CHAPTER 15

# Alternative Uses for Contrast Imaging

Robert W. W. Biederman

Standard clinical uses for contrast imaging by cardiovascular magnetic resonance (CMR) have been described in the earlier chapters. Generally, these pertain to the use of the vascular imaging, including aortic runoffs, and mesenteric and renal imaging. More recently, the use of contrast administration for the understanding of myocardial properties has shown major advantages. Historically, T1- and T2-weighted sequences, or variations on them, provided all of the contrast weighting possible. In Chapter 12 concerning the late hyperenhancement sequence, delayed uptake within the myocardium was demonstrated to accurately detect myocardial infarctions (MI's). In this chapter, we will detail some of the more creative uses of contrast imaging for the identification of vascular, nonvascular, and myocardial properties.

## MYOCARDITIS

Recently, the evaluation of myocarditis by CMR has become an important tool in nonischemic cardiomyopathies. In patients presenting with signs and symptoms of heart failure, but without demonstrable evidence of coronary artery disease (CAD), the search for a nonischemic mechanism is possible using CMR. The pattern of late hyperenhancement in these patients is distinctly different from the pattern characteristic of MI (see Fig. 15-1). Importantly, in cases of myocarditis it has been stated that late hyperenhancement is sensitive, but not specific. We note that the phenotype of the delay hyperenhancement distribution with relation to the myocardium gives clues concerning the underlying etiology. Whereas a MI always originates in the subendocardium, extending toward the midwall, and finally, if large enough, become completely transmural, myocarditis patterns are generally much more heterogeneous (see Fig. 15-2). Specifically, myocarditis patterns are generally less focal, much more patchy with

skip lesions and, by definition, do not involve a coronary artery distribution (see Fig. 15-3). In some cases, the presentation of myocarditis can provide information about the long-term prognosis. This work is still maturing, but in general, larger, more focal patterns correspond with regional wall motion abnormalities, which will only marginally improve at 6 weeks, with residual contrast still present. Smaller lesions that are patchy or more diffuse, typically in concert with the clinical presentation, resolve in 6 weeks with a parallel improvement in left ventricular wall motion.

Most recently, several authors, including us, have made the interesting observation that the delayed hyperenhancement (DHE) signal in viral cardiomyopathy may demonstrate a linear stripe through the midwall of the myocardium with moderate signal intensity, which is generally a less intense signal than a DHE defined infarct (see Figs. 15-4 and 15-5). This pattern, sparing the epicardial and endocardial layers, may or may not involve more than one segment of the myocardium. Some investigators have performed electron microscopy and viral cultures, and have demonstrated a pattern that may, by purely imaging techniques, identify the offending pathogen. If the linear stripe occurs in the mid anterior and anteroseptal segment, there is a high likelihood that the agent is human herpesvirus 6 (HHV-6), whereas if it occurs in the posterior lateral wall (see Fig. 15-6) the agent is likely to be a parvovirus. CMR appears to be able to aid further in the clinical translation of this diagnostic strategy, because there have been limited observations that the septal pattern has a more ominous prognosis in that there is more left ventricular dysfunction, both globally and segmentally, whereas the posterior pattern has a more benign presentation with less deleterious impact on segmental function. Finally, depending on the location of the pattern, a prediction of interim left ventricular function can be made in that the septal pattern demonstrates limited recovery at several months after infection, whereas

**FIGURE 15-1** Delayed hyperenhancement (DHE) taken at 2 minutes after contrast injection, revealing focal high T1 signal of myocardium. Images relate to case study 1.

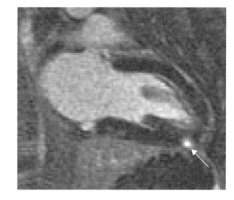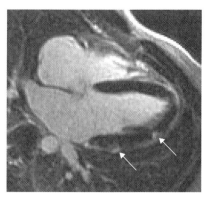

**FIGURE 15-2** Delayed hyperenhancement (DHE) taken at 2 minutes after contrast injection, revealing focal high T1 signal of myocardium in the two-, four-, and three-chamber views taken 1 week apart. Images relate to case study 2.

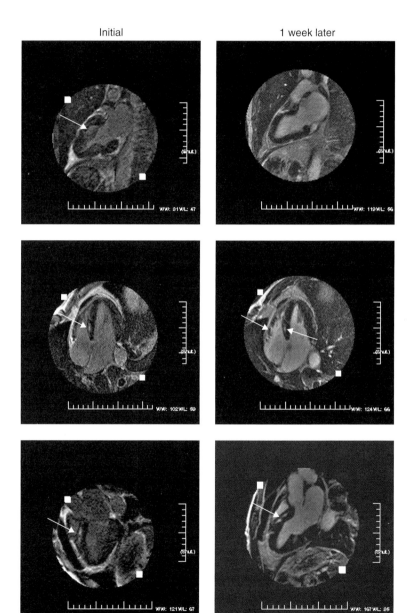

Initial        1 week later

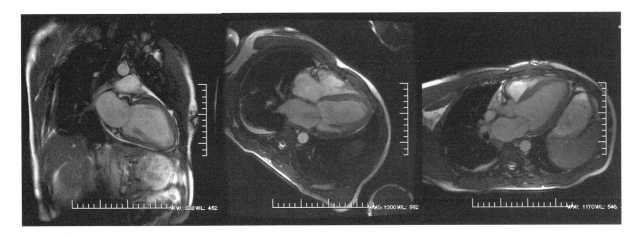

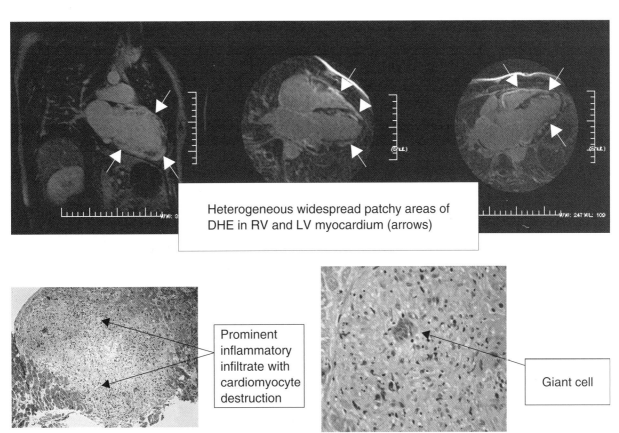

Heterogeneous widespread patchy areas of DHE in RV and LV myocardium (arrows)

Prominent inflammatory infiltrate with cardiomyocyte destruction

Giant cell

**FIGURE 15-3** Steady state free precession (SSFP) sequences (top panel) and matching delayed hyperenhancement (DHE) images (lower panel). Histology slides (right panel) demonstrating evidence of granulomatous formation with a giant cell (*arrow*). Images relate to case study 3.

the posterior pattern generally correlates with considerable improvement in left ventricular function (see Fig. 15-7).

Finally, in the absence of a CAD etiology, a finding of any one of the preceding patterns appears to be very helpful in explaining the etiology of the nonischemic cardiomyopathy. Upward of 40% of viral cardiomyopathies appear to have either a midwall stripe and/or a heterogeneous pattern, whereas 15% present with a bright pattern in the right ventricular septal insertion points. Therefore, when a nonischemic patient presents with a viral cardiomyopathy, there is a 50% chance of formally defining, or strongly indicating, the etiology. However, it should be noted that in fully 100% of this population, providing volumetric and left ventricular functional metrics is beneficial.

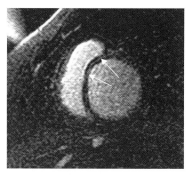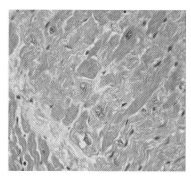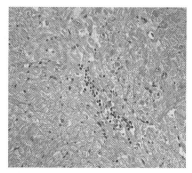

FIGURE 15-4  Delayed hyperenhancement (DHE) images in the short-axis acquisition (left) with histology images middle and right, demonstrating hypertrophy of myocytes but no myocyte destruction or cellular inflammation. Images relate to case study 4.

The finding of the midwall stripe has been proposed to be pathognomonic for a viral cardiomyopathy. However, we have recently seen several cases in which biopsy showed that the midwall stripe to be a *forme fruste* of idiopathic cardiomyopathy (see Fig. 15-4) and in another case a fatty pattern was seen. Early data supports that a finding of this pattern by itself may denote an adverse cardiovascular prognostic finding.

## CASE STUDIES

**Case Study 1.** A 30-year-old man presents with sudden onset of chest pain (CP) that had grown from mild to extraordinarily painful over the preceding 6 hours. His electrocardiogram (ECG), echocardiogram, and a subsequent coronary catheterization were all normal. He underwent CMR for evaluation of an etiology for his

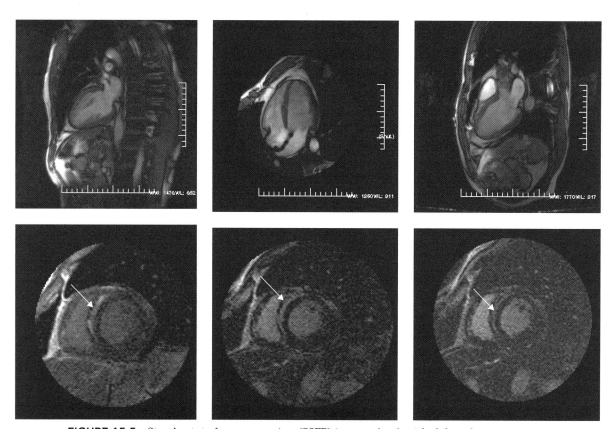

FIGURE 15-5  Steady state free precession (SSFP) images (top) with delayed hyperenhancement (DHE) images (bottom) showing a striking midwall septal hyperenhancement pattern not typical for infarct or myocarditis. Images were obtained at 2 to 5 minutes post–contrast administration. Images relate to case study 5.

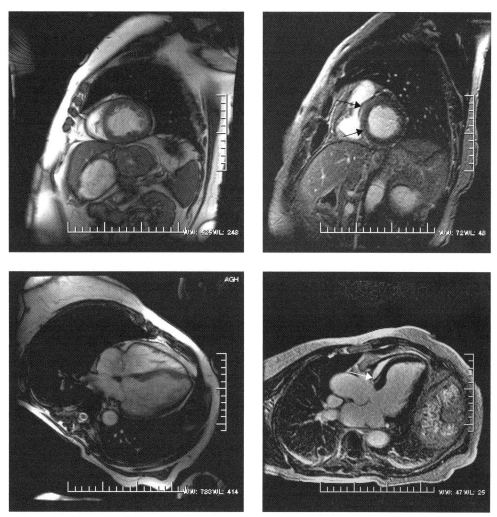

**FIGURE 15-6**   Collage of steady state free precession (SSFP) (left) and delayed hyperenhancement (DHE) (right) with midseptal myocardial enhancement in a linear homogeneous pattern. Images relate to case study 6.

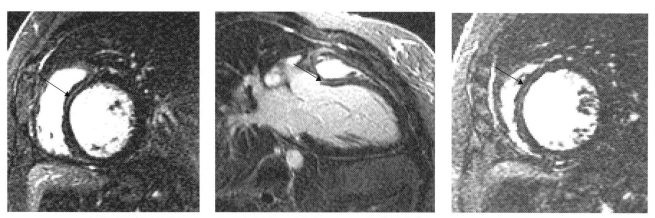

**FIGURE 15-7**   Delayed hyperenhancement (DHE) in the mid septal wall in a markedly dilated and remodeled ventricle. Images relate to case study 7.

## LEFT VENTRICULAR THROMBUS

The evaluation of masses, particularly apical masses, by echocardiography and x-ray angiography is sometimes difficult. The image resolution is limited by the inability to distinguish between myocardial and nonmyocardial structures. Particularly with x-ray angiography, a filling defect on ventricular angiography raises suspicion for a thrombus, but does not confirm it because other pathologies can be responsible for this observation. Typically, echocardiography is able to visualize abnormalities within the LV, but differentiation between a prominent trabecular pattern, aberrant papillary muscle, or left ventricular thrombus, may be difficult. Often, these patients are referred for transesophageal echocardiography. However this is an invasive procedure, generally requiring sedatives, and is not ideal for every patient. Moreover, the ability of CMR to differentiate muscle from thrombus, both by steady state free precession (SSFP) and DHE imaging, has been shown to be superior to transesophageal echocardiography (TEE). For example, during the course of late hyperenhancement imaging for viability, abnormal intraluminal processes, such as thrombus can be readily identified. In the setting of an apical mass in a post-MI patient, following late hyperenhancement imaging, the patient will have a bright endocardial signal with a very dark, generally homogeneous, signal surrounded by a bright chamber (see Fig. 15-8). Stated simply, there is a dark region sandwiched between bright regions. Since thrombus does not take up contrast well, confirmation of the presence of a thrombus can be made. At our institution, despite a very strong echocardiography program, it is not unusual for masses that have been labeled as apical thrombus, even in the setting of prior MI, to be identified by CMR to be aberrant papillary muscles or prominent apical trabeculations. If the left ventricle ejection fraction (EF) is <35%, the patient is considered for initiation of warfarin (Coumadin) anticoagulation therapy. However, in a setting of an EF >35%, where the thrombus is clearly visualized, conventional therapy would still be instituted, making this an important diagnosis by CMR. In patients considered for initiation of Coumadin therapy, despite a low EF, the unequivocal demonstration of an apical thrombus well serves the clinician and patient.

## CARDIOVASCULAR MAGNETIC RESONANCE AS A SCREENING TOOL

As described in Chapter 12, the ability of CMR to detect ischemic pathology provides the clinician with an unparalleled noninvasive tool. Employing a strategy of systematic evaluation with SSFP, double inversion

presentation (see Fig. 15-1). No pericardial effusion was seen and left ventricular function was normal. However, on delayed hyperenhancement imaging several areas of epicardial enhancement are seen (arrows) consistent with myocarditis. Note the distinct absence of an endocardial or midwall pattern, which can distinguish between a MI and myocarditis.

**Case Study 2.** After a viral prodrome lasting 2 weeks, a healthy 32-year-old man presents with angst and growing chest discomfort for which he can find no relief. While not typical for coronary artery disease (CAD), given his strong family history, he undergoes an uneventful cardiac catheterization, which reveals normal coronary arteries. His echocardiogram is normal, and he is referred for cardiovascular magnetic resonance (CMR) which reveals several areas of mid and epicardial enhancement (see Fig. 15-2, left panel). The patient returned 1 week later for further evaluation of the acute versus chronic nature of his presentation, to aid prognosis (right panel). No distinct change was noted, preliminarily suggesting that this process resulted in damage to the myocardium.

**Case Study 3.** 40-year-old man with insidious onset of progressive shortness of breath (SOB) and fatigue over a 3-week period. CAD is ruled out by catheterization. While the author was in service we performed a CMR to assess functional and structural details of the heart (see Fig. 15-3). CMR showed severe LV systolic dysfunction with following functional data:
Left ventricular end-diastolic volume index (LVEDVI) = 101.1 mL/m$^2$; left ventricular ejection fraction (LVEF) = 27.2%; right ventricular end-diastolic volume index (RVEDVI) = 86.6 mL/m$^2$; right ventricular ejection fraction (RVEF) = 23.3%; left ventricular end-systolic volume index (LVESVI) = 73.7 mL/m$^2$; left ventricular mass index (LVMI) = 78.8 g/m$^2$; and right ventricular end-systolic volume index (RVESVI) = 20.2 mL/m$^2$. CMR DHE images demonstrated widespread, extremely heterogeneous, dense and patchy areas of myocardial enhancement of left ventricles (LVs) and right ventricles (RVs). This is consistent with a severe inflammatory process. A diagnosis of giant cell myocarditis was made by CMR. One day later endomyocardial biopsy (EMB) confirmed the diagnosis of giant cell myocarditis.

**Case Study 4.** An 18-year-old male adolescent with progressive SOB and fatigue over 4 days before presentation. CAD is ruled out by catheterization. The patient had a paternal cousin who had similar presentation when he was 23-year-old and received heart transplant. CMR was performed to assess functional and structural details of the heart. CMR data is as follows (see Fig. 15-4):

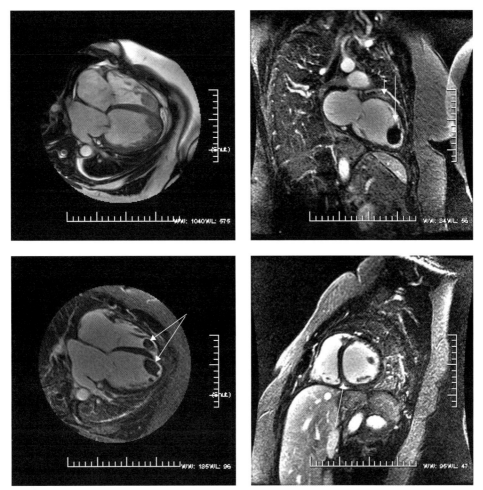

**FIGURE 15-8**  Steady state free precession (SSFP) images (left panel) demonstrating high resolution of biventricular dilation and biventricular apical densities that by the lack of delayed hyperenhancement (DHE) post–contrast enhancement (right panel), are morphology and by location diagnostic of biapical thrombus. Note the heterogeneous uptake in the DHE sequences of the hinge point enhancement suggestive of a dilated viral cardiomyopathy (*small arrows*). Images relate to case study 8.

recovery (DIR), triple inversion recovery (TIR), perfusion followed by DHE sequences allows discrimination between pathologies, thereby avoiding invasive strategies (see Fig. 15-9).

## UNUSUAL PRESENTATIONS OF CARDIAC PATHOLOGY

### Normal Variants

Unusual presentations of normal anatomy and abnormal pathology fall well into the purview of CMR's capabilities. In addition to its well defined use for standard clinical imaging, it is also well known as a "problem solver." Differentiating cysts from abnormal masses, interrogating LV myocardial structures such as diverticuli (see Fig. 15-10), aneurysms that masquerade in the form

$LVEDVI = 175.9 \text{ mL/m}^2$; $LVEF = 4.7\%$; $LVESVI = 167.5 \text{ mL/m}^2$; and $LVMI = 77.5 \text{ g/m}^2$. CMR functional images demonstrated markedly dilated LV and RV. The LV myocardium was thinned. On DHE sequence there was a midwall septal stripe of enhancement (arrows). To date this is considered as a sign of viral myocarditis (most commonly HHV-6); therefore a preliminary diagnosis of viral myocarditis was made. The patient underwent percutaneous EMB which showed hypertrophy of myocytes but no myocyte destruction or cellular inflammation (middle panel). Viral cytopathic effects were not identified and staining did not show fibrosis or amyloid deposition. He underwent cardiac transplantation and the explanted heart tissue was examined by staining and electron microscopy, which again did not show signs of viral myocarditis (right

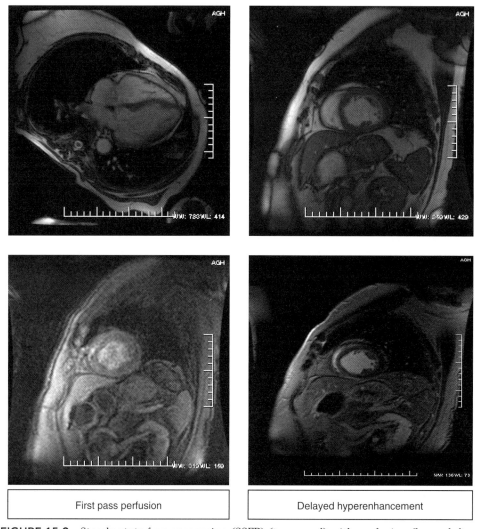

| First pass perfusion | Delayed hyperenhancement |

**FIGURE 15-9** Steady state free precession (SSFP) (top panel) with perfusion (lower left panel) and delayed hyperenhancement (DHE) (lower right panel) demonstrating integration of three sequences to determine the etiology of a patient presenting with an unknown cardiomyopathy without the use of cardiac catheterization. Images relate to case study 9.

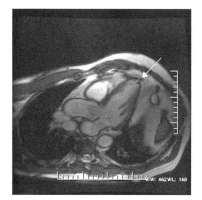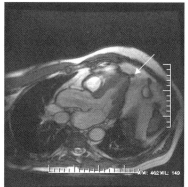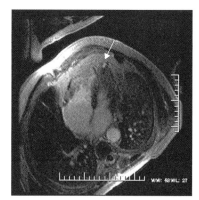

**FIGURE 15-10** Steady state free precession imaging (left and middle) with a delayed hyperenhancement (DHE) image revealing no evidence of enhancement in a very thinned left ventricular (LV) diverticulum. The wall thickness in this segment is 1.1 mm, therefore the ability to detect lack of enhancement at that resolution is a major advantage in cardiovascular magnetic resonance (CMR). Images relate to case study 10.

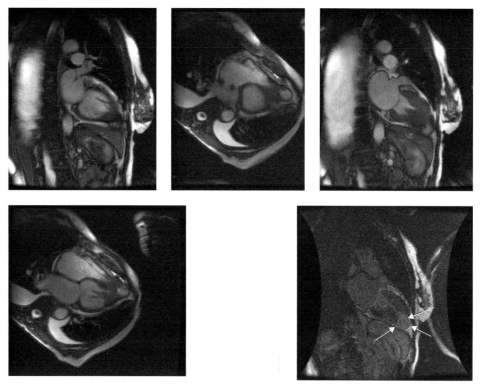

**FIGURE 15-11**    Steady state free precession (SSFP) in all images but the lower right (delayed hyperenhancement [DHE]) in a patient with a most peculiar left ventricular (LV) apical defect, initially thought to be a pseudoaneurysm or an LV diverticulum. The diagnosis was neither. Note the thin shell of endocardial enhancement and epicardial "viability" seen in this normal but high-resolution DHE acquisition, helping to narrow the differential diagnosis. Images relate to case study 11.

of hematomas (see Fig. 15-11) and intra- and extracardiac masses, are easily characterized by CMR. Other creative uses incorporating contrast are seen at the end of the chapter.

## INFILTRATIVE CARDIOMYOPATHIES

### Sarcoidosis

Infiltrative cardiomyopathies can be identified using CMR to determine the cardiac involvement in a patient with known extracardiac manifestations of sarcoidosis. In the patient population with known sarcoidosis, such as pulmonary sarcoidosis, the natural clinical question that follows is, "does the patient have evidence of infiltrative granulomatous disease within his myocardium." Heretofore, cardiac catheterization with biopsy of the right ventricular intraventricular septum would be performed to determine histopathologically whether the clinical suspicion was correct. However, importantly, the nature of the pathology of sarcoidosis is that of "skip" lesions with a very heterogeneous intermyocardial pattern. This leads to a moderate-to-high likelihood

panel). An inconclusive diagnosis of idiopathic dilated cardiomyopathy (DCM) was made based on the pathologic information. However, later his younger sister was screened by CMR for myocardial structure and function and was found to have biventricular dilatation with mild LV systolic dysfunction. On the basis of these findings, diagnosis of idiopathic DCM was reversed to familial DCM.

**Case Study 5.** A 45-year-old man presents with signs and symptoms consistent with congestive heart failure, and is demonstrated to have a DCM by echocardiography. Delayed hyperenhancement sequences demonstrate a striking midwall stripe tracking through the anterior septum and inferior septal territories without any other regions of hyperenhancement, consistent with viral cardiomyopathy (see Fig. 15-5). This has recently been reported to be nearly pathognomonic with a viral cardiomyopathy, suggesting that this is the etiology for this patient's presentation.

**Case Study 6.** 65-year-old white woman presents with SOB, fatigue, and left bundle branch block (LBBB)

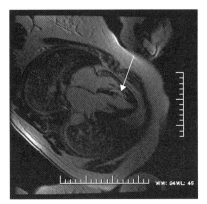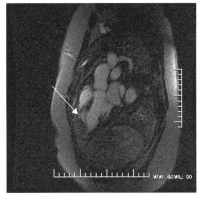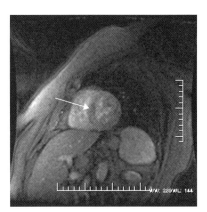

**FIGURE 15-12** Abnormal washout kinetics in the septum through delayed hyperenhancement (DHE) sequences are shown (left and middle panels, *arrow*) and matched reduced uptake in the perfusion sequence (right panel, *arrow*). The heterogeneous DHE pattern is atypical for infarct or myocarditis and in the correct clinical setting suggests an infiltrative process. DHE is highly sensitive for infarct patterns but has exceptional and expanding indications for noninfarct imaging such as in this patient with known pulmonary sarcoidosis. Images relate to case study 12.

of a negative study being a falsely negative study. Additionally, the naturally invasive technique is not without its own obligate morbidity and mortality. Therefore, a tool that could more completely evaluate cardiac myocardial tissue, would have a natural advantage if it could be shown to have high sensitivity and specificity. Late hyperenhancement, performed using the same sequence described for MI and myocarditis, depicts areas of interstitial changes and granulomatous formation due to the natural trapping of gadolinium within the lymphatic obstruction (see Fig. 15-12). In our experience, patients with moderate to high pretest probability of cardiac sarcoidosis, as well as more advanced extracardiac sarcoidosis, can be reliably screened by CMR without the need for biopsy. We have evaluated more than 20 patients with sarcoidosis, with biopsy confirmation in 12 patients, and 1 incorrectly diagnosed. In that patient, who presented early with no cardiac manifestation, the initial biopsy was read as negative, whereas 6 months later the patient underwent re-biopsy and had evidence of mild (early) cardiac sarcoidosis. Therefore, in our practice, when possible, patients with clinical suspicion for cardiac sarcoidosis either by electrocardiogram (ECG), clinical history, or Holter monitoring, undergo confirmation by CMR. In those patients with negative findings, if done early, no biopsy is needed. In those patients with negative findings and in whom good image quality is obtained, this author has high confidence in relating to the referring physician that the patient has no CMR evidence of sarcoidosis. Only in those cases in which there is a high clinical pretest probability biopsy is indicated. The diagnosis of cardiac sarcoidosis is critical for the optimization of therapy, including

pattern; what is the etiology (see Fig. 15-6)? There is no evidence of a subendocardial hyperenhancement pattern to suggest a MI. A specific linear dense DHE pattern is seen in the basal anteroseptum. In approximately 40% of patients who are ultimately defined to have viral cardiomyopathy, a similar linear DHE pattern is present within the midwall. In early reports, this pattern denotes an adverse cardiovascular prognostic finding.

**Case Study 7.** A 55-year-old man presents with a history of the viral prodrome that occurred approximately 1 year before his presentation for CMR (see Fig. 15-7). Delayed hyperenhancement imaging demonstrates a midwall stripe (arrows) supporting a diagnosis of a viral cardiomyopathy. Recent data suggest that the septal pattern, in addition to carrying a bad prognosis, may be due to the viral antigen HHV-6. This is in stark contrast to an infralateral or posterolateral pattern, which in many cases is of the antigen parvovirus, which carries a more favorable prognosis.

**Case Study 8.** A 67-year-old black woman presents with 2 years of fatigue, SOB, and weight gain and peculiar findings on echocardiography in which there were biapical intermediate echoic signals. A CMR was performed (see Fig. 15-8) demonstrating severe biventricular dysfunction with moderate (2+) mitral and tricuspid regurgitation. Delayed hyperenhancement was performed, which demonstrates the following: (a) no evidence of a typical infarction pattern, (b) bilateral apical densities that fail to enhance with hyperenhancement imaging, (c) subtle, but important midwall interior post–contrast enhancement, as well as right ventricular

pacemaker and/or alternate medical therapy, as well as intensification of ongoing medical therapy.

## Amyloidosis

Evaluation of cardiac amyloidosis by CMR is less well defined. However, utilizing the late hyperenhancement sequences, a number of patterns have been described, including a diffuse hypertensive pattern, as well as a more generalized septal homogeneous pattern. Unlike sarcoidosis, in which there is true infiltration, the amyloid proteins are generally more diffusely dispersed throughout the myocardium, therefore the late hyperenhancement signal is less well defined. The combination of visualizing interstitial septal thickening, atrial wall thickening, occasionally valve thickening, a generalize thickened myocardial wall with a restrictive filling pattern, and an abnormal late DHE signal is highly suspicious for cardiac amyloidosis. Amyloidosis, once diagnosed allows the physician and patient to understand the extent of the disease as well as permits intensification of medical therapy.

## Hypertrophic Cardiomyopathy

Hypertrophic cardiomyopathy is evaluated well using noncontrast CMR, which provides evaluation of left ventricular mass, left ventricular function, localization of hypertrophic process, coexisting mitral regurgitation and its mechanism, and the calculation of the left ventricular outflow tract (LVOT) gradient. However, to understand the tissue characteristics and the extent of collagen/abnormal hypertrophic process better, several investigators have added DHE imaging. Using standard DHE imaging, interrogation of areas of abnormal signal have been demonstrated to be beneficial in understanding the pathophysiology of hypertrophic cardiomyopathy (see Figs. 15-13 and 15-14). Specifically, areas that demonstrate increased contrast enhancement typically correspond to the area of greatest hypertrophy, greatest myofibrillar disarray, and areas of greatest collagen deposition in the extracellular matrix. Early evidence from several investigators has demonstrated that those presenting with a positive DHE signal within the myocardium possess an adverse cardiovascular prognostic indicator. These patients are at increased risk of syncope, sudden death, and subsequent pacemaker placement compared to a non-DHE matched cohort. DHE may be a particular egregious imaging marker for sudden death, and has prompted many centers, including ours, to believe that CMR is capable of dichotomizing patients who are believed to be at lower risk, into a low or high risk group depending on the absence or presence of a DHE signal, respectively. Those patients in whom high adverse clinical risk factors are present may also

septal insertion point hyperenhancement. This pattern is diagnostic for a viral cardiomyopathy with resultant severe biventricular dysfunction and biventricular apical thrombus formation assessed using only two CMR sequences.

**Case Study 9.** Evaluation of cardiomyopathy; part of an integrated approach. Using a combination of SSFP functional images, first pass perfusion, and delayed hyperenhancement, a myriad of cardiac pathology can be identified, allowing the clinician to determine with a high probability the etiology of the patient who presents with cardiomyopathy (see Fig. 15-9). An integrated imaging approach that is rapid, efficient, noninvasive, with no morbidity or mortality has clear advantage over current standard approaches which incorporate traditionally invasive cardiac catheterization and radionuclide imaging with or without biopsy. Such an approach that is also inexpensive has obvious, clinical translation, as well as socioeconomic implications.

**Case Study 10.** A routine cardiac CMR is performed in a middle-aged woman and an abnormality is seen in the very tip of the LV apex (see Fig. 15-10, arrows). Using SSFP images to demonstrate the contractile nature of the myocardium, with delayed hyperenhancement to demonstrate the lack of post–contrast enhancement, the abnormality is defined to be a benign LV diverticulum. No further therapy was needed. However, it is prudent to periodically follow this every one to 2 years to assure that no increase in size has occurred. Theoretically, if enlarged, this could be a favorable milieu for clot formation and therefore, warrant anticoagulation.

**Case Study 11.** A 54-year-old white woman presents with dyspnea on exertion, early exercise fatigue, and a peculiar mass seen on an echocardiogram. CMR demonstrates a hyperdynamic LV with 3D EF of 80% and a moderately sized circular thin walled apical mass with flow in it (see Fig. 15-11). The limited differential diagnosis is LV aneurysm, LV pseudoaneurysm, or LV diverticulum, or something rare. She had no history of an MI, making the first unlikely, but either of the first two as occult findings could be possible. However, there is a narrow neck, pointing toward either a pseudoaneurysm or an LV diverticulum. The radio frequency (RF) tissue tagging (not shown) demonstrates no contraction to the apical region, discounting these as the diagnosis. The DHE image is used to evaluate for the presence of occult infarction, which is clearly demonstrated, and shown in lower right panel (arrows) as a very thin, well delineated, nearly transmural DHE signal. From this we concluded this was a psuedoaneurysm both by

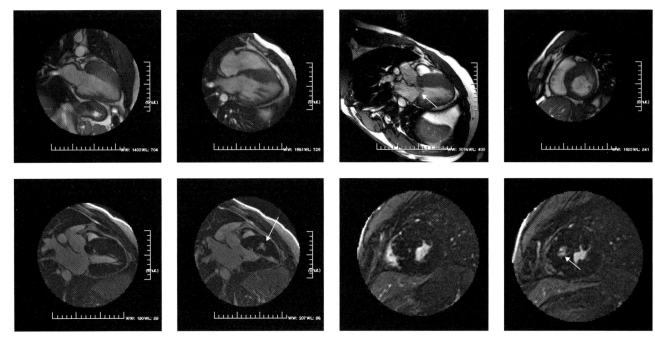

**FIGURE 15-13** Steady state free precession (SSFP) (top panel) in multiple views with delayed hyperenhancement (DHE) (lower panel) with several areas (*arrows*) of heterogeneous post–contrast enhancement, a pattern of important and independent adverse cardiovascular prognosis. Images relate to case study 13.

be further stratified by DHE examination. Additionally, in those patients who are referred for possible myomectomy, an exact description of the area for resection can be indicated to the surgeon. A roadmap can then be displayed in the operating room, giving dimensional information, aiding in septal resection. Upon completion of the surgery, a postoperative CMR can be obtained, which can also delineate the area of resection and the allow assessment of the completeness of the myomectomy. Similarly, in those patients in whom alcohol ablation might be considered, both the preoperative, as well as a postoperative DHE studies clearly delineate the area of abnormality preintervention, as well as display the area of infarct post alcohol injection.

## Takotsubo Cardiomyopathy

The presentation of this recently recognized cardiomyopathy is characterized as similar to that of an acute MI. Patients present with sudden onset of chest pain, ST elevation, and a ventricular function study demonstrating severe anteroapical and often inferior wall hypokinesis or akinesia, with paradoxical hyperdynamic basal function. On an x-ray angiogram examination, the coronary arteries conventionally show no or trivial disease, and the severely depressed ventricular function is markedly disproportionate to the nearly normal, if not completely normal, coronary arteriogram. In fact, on careful evaluation of the ventriculogram, echocardiogram, or CMR,

morphologic features of a narrow neck and by occult DHE. As the patient was extremely symptomatic, she underwent surgery for excision, under the premise that her hyperdynamic state was exaggerated (or caused) by this lesion, with high velocity "to and fro" flow seen in the apical mass. Surgical pathology however demonstrated that this was a hamartoma. Embryologically, a hamartoma is nearly identical to cardiac muscle. This is a case where DHE cannot differentiate cardiac muscle versus a muscle-like structure, leading to an erroneous, but logical CMR conclusion. Review of the histology did not completely negate the findings on CMR, because a layer of endocardial scar was clearly visible and hamartomas are *not* contractile. Apical resection, however, did not cure her problem.

**Case Study 12.** A 57-year-old woman presents which dyspnea on exertion and SOB with a known history of pulmonary sarcoidosis. CMR was performed to evaluate for the possibility of cardiac sarcoidosis—she did not want to undergo EMB (see Fig. 15-12). Using standard DHE sequence, an area of diffuse heterogeneous contrast uptake was seen within the septum. This pattern is atypical for MI, myocarditis, or amyloid, and in the setting where the pretest probability is high, the sensitivity and specificity for this being cardiac sarcoidosis is extremely high. The patient was diagnosed as having

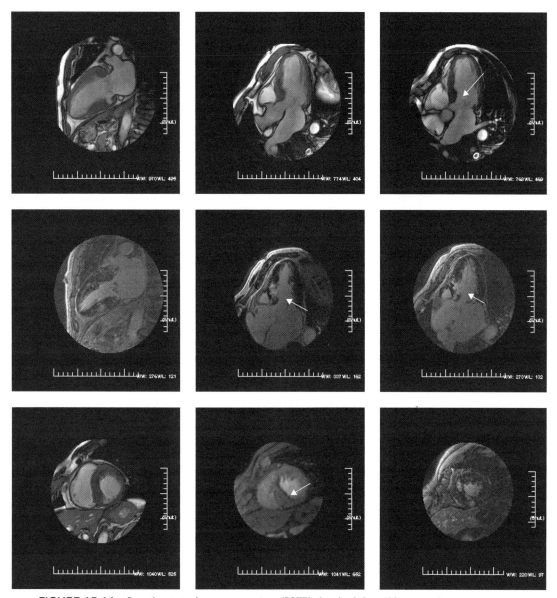

**FIGURE 15-14** Steady state free precession (SSFP) (top), delayed hyperenhancement (DHE) (middle), SSFP (lower right), perfusion (lower middle) and DHE (lower right) revealing multiple areas of irregular enhancement through the septum with matched hypoperfusion septal defects. Images relate to case study 14.

the left ventricular function is seen to be compartmentalized. Specifically, there is mid, distal, and apical hypokinesia to akinesia in a circumferential pattern with hyperdynamic basal circumferential function. This unusual pattern is under intense investigation, because the presenting symptoms are most often seen in middle-aged women who have had a dramatic recent experience. For instance, witnessing a traffic accident, seeing the death of their spouse, seeing their house burned down, or in a recent case in which the first anniversary of the sudden passing away of a lady's husband was the trigger (see Fig. 15-15). Prevailing theories suggest that this is a hyperadrenergic, catecholamine-driven

cardiac sarcoidosis and was treated with intensification of her medicines.

**Case Study 13.** A 25-year-old man with a family history of sudden cardiac death presents for evaluation with a "peculiar" ECG. A hypertrophic obstructive cardiomyopathy (HOCM) is demonstrated, with DHE signal in the area of greatest wall thickness (see Fig. 15-13). Note the top arrow pointing at the LVOT obstruction, measured by phase velocity mapping to be 41 mm Hg, likely greatly reduced owing to gradually dysfunctional anterior

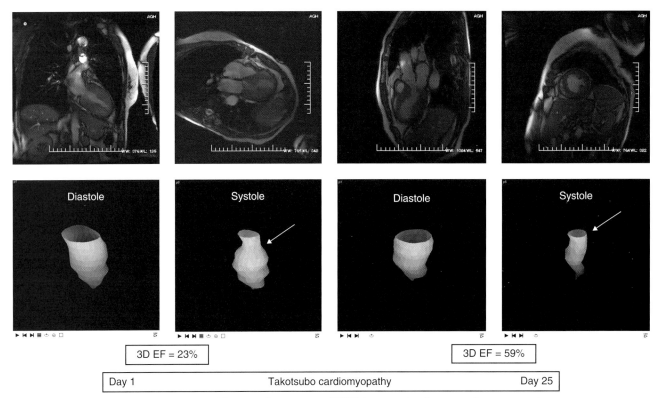

**FIGURE 15-15** Delayed hyperenhancement (DHE) images (top) suggesting an transient apical-ballooning syndrome with preserved hyperdynamic basal function and hypokinetic mid and apical segments (diastole to systole) compared at initial presentation and 25 days later. Lower row demonstrated 3D reconstructions of the preceding SSFP images, helping to define the physiologic perturbations of segmental hyperkinesia and lack of normalization nearly 1 month later in this patient with Takotsubo cardiomyopathy. Images relate to case study 15.

response. We and others have performed contrast perfusion imaging as well as late hyperenhancement imaging and have been unable to detect a clear hypoperfusion defect, nor a signal consistent with acute or subacute infarct. This helps to very clearly distinguish this pattern from an acute infarct with spontaneous lysis because there is no residual perfusion deficit, nor matched area of infarct by DHE imaging. As this diagnosis has only recently been considered, but probably more frequently seen and unrecognized, the additive value of CMR in confirming this diagnosis is clearly obvious.

An interesting pattern that helps in confirming the diagnosis is the remarkable ventricular recovery capable by the myocardium in relatively short order following simple supportive care. As no specific therapy is known to ameliorate the disease process, standard pharmacologic strategies such as ACE-inhibitor, β-blocker, and aspirin appear warranted. Yet, even in the absence of standard therapy, repeat CMR almost universally depicts complete resolution of the dysfunctional segments. Indeed, we have mathematically segmented the

septal mechanics and paradoxical reduction in his gradient as the hypertrophic process progresses.

**Case Study 14.** A 51-year-old white man developed syncope while watching a hockey game. CMR (see Fig. 15-14) shows a "moth-eaten" anterior septum (top panel), delayed enhancement in anterior septum (middle panel), and abnormal LV septal perfusion (lower middle panel). Despite the appearance, the patient denied prior septal modification procedures in the setting of a hypertrophic cardiomyopathy (not the obstructive subtype-likely due to autoinfarction of his septum).

**Case Study 15.** An elderly woman presents in acute extremis with sudden onset of chest pain and ST elevations across her precordium for which she is immediately taken to the cardiac catheterization suite, fully expecting to have a left anterior descending artery occlusion. Surprisingly, her coronary arteries are entirely patent. Yet there is striking, mid and distal left ventricular wall dysfunction with near

ventricular function into the basal and nonbasal my-ocardium at the time of CMR and analyzed these patients at baseline and at 4 to 6 weeks following their initial presentation. An interesting finding is that, despite normalization of the myocardial segments over time, the hyperdynamic basal function remains. This suggests that hyperadrenergic tone may not completely explain the pathophysiology. Logically, if elevated catecholamine states induced the event, upon normalization, one would expect to see a return of the basal myocardial function towards normal, which is not the pattern we have observed. Considerable work remains to be done in this patient population, but CMR appears to be very helpful in understanding and diagnosing this disease process, as well as reinforcing its important clinical recognition in what is otherwise a most vexing disorder.

## Arrhythmogenic Right Ventricular Dysplasia

As discussed earlier, arrhythmogenic right ventricular dysplasia (ARVD) is defined by meeting a group of characteristic major and minor criteria, and CMR evaluation can raise or lower probability for the disease. CMR is especially useful in the evaluation of right ventricular function, and can evaluate focal areas of right ventricular wall thinning, sacular aneurysms, crenulations, and colocalize fatty–fibrotic transformation. Recently, investigators from two universities have demonstrated that addition of contrast to patients with a high pretest probability for ARVD, can further increase the specificity for this otherwise difficult diagnostic evaluation. The finding of a bright DHE signal within areas of right ventricular free wall confirms that there is a fibrotic pathology present. This observation has helped to establish a variant of ARVD known as the *fatty–fibro subclass*. Particularly, if the hyperenhancement pattern is seen within the epicardium and extends into the endocardium, the specificity of this diagnosis is further increased.

## EXPERIMENTAL USES OF CONTRAST

### Pulmonary Vein Identification

Identification of the pulmonary veins is increasing in importance because of the observation that, especially in young patients presenting with atrial fibrillation, the *os* of the veins has atrial muscular tissue that can serve as the focus for the arrhythmia. Several investigators have described atrialized pulmonary veins that can extend up to several centimeters into the veins, each capable of sustaining ectopic foci. More recently, the age of the patients in whom this has been observed has crept up, such that it is now reasonable to see foci initiating the arrythmogenic circuit in patients

akinesis. An echocardiogram confirms the severe LV dysfunction, occupying the entire mid and apical LV. The patient is sent for a CMR (see Fig. 15-15). The LV dysfunction is confirmed, but is noted to be a segmental pattern with hyperdynamic basal function with a kinetic mid and distal function. Both perfusion and hyperenhancement (not shown) are strikingly normal. More in-depth conversation with her reveals that the scan day is close to the anniversary of her husband's sudden death. The constellation of presentation, electrocardiographic, angiographic perfusion and delayed hyperenhancement pattern denote a diagnosis of Takotsubo cardiomyopathy. As this is essentially a diagnosis of exclusion, follow-up CMR was performed 25 days later, revealing remarkable improvement in the segmental dysfunction. Indeed, based on CMR an alternate hypothesis to the hyperadrenergic explanation was considered. Because the basal systolic function in a 3D segmental analysis remained unchanged over time, and the improvement occurred only in the mid and apical zones, a pure catecholamine-driven pathology that resolved over time would have more likely shown incremental decrease in basal systolic function. Yet this was not observed, suggesting an alternative, nonadrenergic explanation. The patient returned at 1 year with no change in either global or segmental systolic function or evidence of a perfusion/DHE abnormality.

**Case Study 16.** An elderly man older than 80 years presents for echocardiogram following a motor vehicle accident in which he sustained chest wall trauma. While the technologist and the physician were watching a "strange feature" on the echocardiogram the patient experienced sudden death. He was resuscitated, and an hour later was sent for CMR (see Fig. 15-16). SSFP imaging demonstrates an abnormality outside the right ventricular free wall. Perfusion imaging demonstrates a contrast that appears outside the ventricular free wall, which is caught in a spectacular manner on an intentionally planned early DHE sequence. The patient fortunately had undergone a coronary artery bypass graft (CABG) 15 years earlier which formed the basis of an unlikely salvation for his otherwise complete RV perforation. Most certainly, the decade of scar and fibrosis prevented complete right ventricular free wall rupture and sudden death.

**Case Study 17.** A patient sent for CMR before routine pulmonary vein isolation for atrial fibrillation (see Fig. 15-17). magnetic resonance angiography (MRA) was performed, which identified seven isolated pulmonary veins. This information is critically important to the electrophysiologist, who after having ablated

older than 70 years. The varied anatomy both in location and number of veins affected, although long known to the anatomists, has only been more recently recognized by imagers. CMR provides a roadmap for the electrophysiologist, interventionalist, or cardiothoracic surgeon when atrial vein modification procedures, such as pulmonary vein isolation, Maze, Mini-Maze, or focal ablation, are contemplated. The frequency with which atypical location of pulmonary veins, *not* equal to four, occurs is in our practice more than 50% of the time, helping to permit plastic corrective strategies *before* the procedure, thereby limiting morbidity and mortality (see Figs. 15-15–15-16).

## Valvular Enhancement: Does it Account for Progressive Mitral Regurgitation?

Multiple explanations exist for the etiology of left ventricular annular dilation that begets mitral regurgitation. The current assumptions suggest an active process, reflecting remodeling of adjacent and remote myocardium. However, nongeometric, passive mechanisms have not been considered, and are potentially important. CMR late hyperenhancement postcontrast techniques describe a myriad of left ventricular histopathology in addition to infarct, including infiltration and inflammatory perturbations within the LV myocardium, and may also be sensitive to nonmyocardial pathology. We had an opportunity at our center to look at occult annular and/or mitral enhancement in patients with postmyocardial infarction (see Case Study 20): 82 subjects underwent evaluation by CMR, 49 were post-MI patients whereas 33 patients formed the control group. The presence or absence of a DHE pattern in the mitral valve apparatus was visually assessed

the usual four pulmonary veins would have naturally thought that he had incomplete transmural burn when the atrial fibrillation returned. It is clear that as more experience is gained, the normal variant anatomy of the pulmonary veins requires understanding before the current practice of ablating only four veins. CMR can provide the necessary anatomic detail for the electrophysiologist.

**Case Study 18.** An 82-year-old healthy man presents for routine follow-up status post an MI more than 10 years ago (see Fig. 15-18). Note, the evidence of prior large inferior and posterolateral infarct, but more interestingly, on SSFP imaging, the dark thin rim along the subendocardium, which appears to be a highly calcified subendocardium. This is an unusual postinfarct remodeling pattern that, on rare occasion, can be seen. Delayed hyperenhancement imaging demonstrated no uptake in that region.

**Case Study 19.** A 67-year-old white man presents routinely status post a 12-year-old large anterior wall MI. Standard SSFP imaging was performed (see Fig. 15-19), revealing a bright signal within the endocardium and midwall. Using a series of DIR, TIR sequence, perfusion, and delayed hyperenhancement, systematic evaluation of the underlying tissue characteristics was performed. Since the tissue in question was bright on DIR, dark on TIR, hypoperfused on first pass imaging, but modestly enhanced with late DHE, we concluded that this was evidence of fat within the myocardium. Because the patient had colocalization of both fat and infarct in this region, his infarct was more than 12 years ago, his

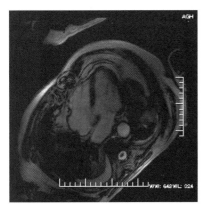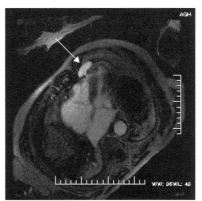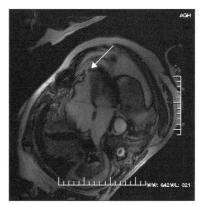

**FIGURE 15-16** Steady state free precession (SSFP) four-chamber sequences (left and right panels) with an abnormal extracardiac signal (*arrow*). The middle panel is 2 minutes post–contrast enhancement demonstrating a mushroom-shaped extracardiac collection (*arrow*) in this elderly patient, hours following a motor vehicle accident. By SSFP imaging, the pericardial and extrapericardial collection is a fibrotic postsurgical finding and likely a life-saving pathologic process. Images relate to case study 16.

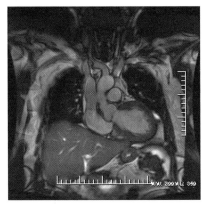 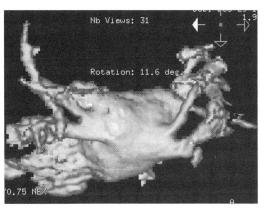

**FIGURE 15-17**   Steady state free precession (SSFP) (left panel) with 3D reconstruction of the left atrium (LA) and pulmonary veins (right panel) demonstrating more than four pulmonary veins. The timing was made from the main pulmonary artery using a manual 3-mL gadolinium pre-scan with surface rendering performed in less than 60 seconds. Images relate to case study 17.

binarily: (a) notation of presence or absence of a DHE pattern involving the mitral annulus and/or valve was made, (b) patients were specifically excluded if the MI pattern involved basal myocardium to avoid confounding signal etiology. We found that all post-MI patients demonstrated an area of infarct by functional analysis, as expected. In the post-MI group at >6 weeks, the DHE signal was observed in the mitral valve in 31 of 36 (86%) patients, and the mitral annulus was enhanced in 19 in 36 (53%). Only 1 of 13 (8%) patients at <6 weeks post-MI had a positive DHE signal. In the post-MI patients, the region of infarction was confirmed by functional analysis and DHE. In the control group, only 2 of 33 (6%) of the patients showed mitral valve/annular enhancement. The specificity of this finding was 94%. Cases of valvular enhancement occurred in one case of hypertrophic cardiomyopathy, and in one of three patients with dilated cardiomyopathy (DCM). Importantly, despite a prominent systemic inflammatory pattern in patients with sarcoidosis, myocarditis, and a resected hematoma and lupus, no cases of valvular or mitral annular enhancement occurred. The size of the infarct pattern appears to have no impact on the presence of valvular or annular enhancement. Indeed, only one infarction pattern before 6 weeks demonstrated any significant degree of enhancement, and in that case the patient had an infarct size >40% of their myocardium with extensive microvascular occlusion and necrosis. The mechanism for this observation is currently unknown, but we postulate that it may be due to an inflammatory process, triggered by the MI. This response may be initiated by the hypoxic effect that causes apoptosis and cell death. The elution of several cytokines known to be present postinfarction may also have an effect such as that of IL-6, IL-1, tumor necrosis factor (TNF),

ECG showed "Q" waves in the anterior and anteroseptal leads when the underlying tissue characteristics were incorporated, the most likely explanation was a rare observation of fatty transformation of the myocardium post-MI. The composite figure demonstrates the considerable utility that CMR grants to the imager; multiple sequences, each with its own ability to identify tissue characteristics, providing an answer to a particular clinical (or research) question.

**Case Study 20.** CMR DHE depicts a focal annular and/or valvar enhancement in a large number of post-MI patients, suggesting a specific, as yet unknown reactive process that may contribute to annular dilation and/or mitral leaflet pathology (see Fig. 15-20). This passive phenomenon was not suspected as a contributor to the post-MI phenotype, but may portend primary or secondary mitral regurgitation. Rarely is it associated with other systemic or local cardiac entity.

IL-25, or C-reactive protein (cRP). Further support that this observation is related to an inflammatory mechanism is derived from concordant visualization of the hyperenhancement phenomenon within the aortic, tricuspid, and pulmonic valve, the aortic and atrial walls, hepatic capsule, and in the pulmonary artery in these patients with both MI and hyperenhancement of the mitral valve. This passive phenomenon is currently not a suspected contributor to the post-MI phenotype, but may predict late left ventricular dilation and either primary or secondary mitral regurgitation. Importantly, does valvular/annular DHE portend late emergence of mitral regurgitation through a

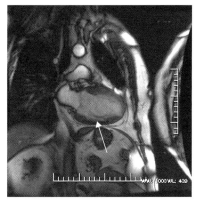 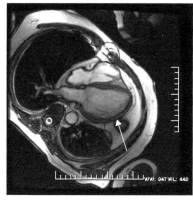 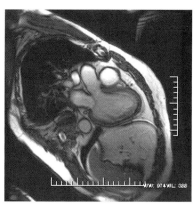

**FIGURE 15-18** Steady state free precession (SSFP) images demonstrating an unusual hypointense subendocardial rim that failed to enhance following contrast (not shown). This T1/T2 signal is most consistent with myocardial calcification, an uncommon finding, but occasionally observed >10 years following a myocardial infarction. Images relate to case study 18.

**FIGURE 15-19** Postinfarct myocardial transformation to fat can also occur. A series of steady state free precession (SSFP), double inversion recovery (DIR), TIR, perfusion, and delayed hyperenhancement (DHE) imaging delineate this rarely seen pathology integrating four common sequences. The abnormalities seen on the DHE sequence mostly depict the bright fat signal. Note the near circumferential hyopointense signal in the same location as the fat in the middle right panel. Images relate to case study 19.

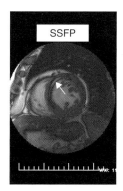 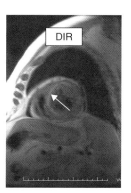 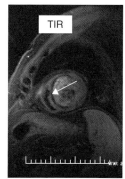

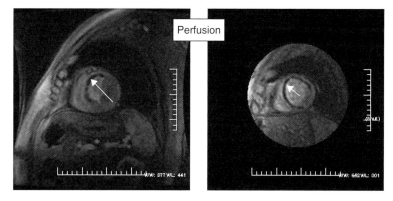

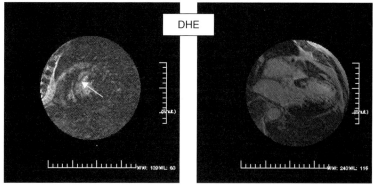

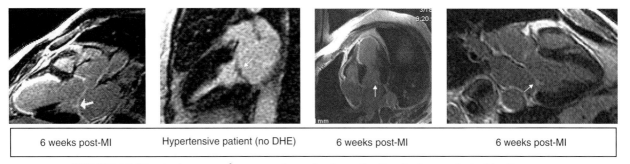

| 6 weeks post-MI | Hypertensive patient (no DHE) | 6 weeks post-MI | 6 weeks post-MI |

**FIGURE 15-20** A phenomenon currently under investigation is demonstrated by the contrast uptake observed in the valve structure through delayed hyperenhancement (DHE) imaging in patients with myocardial infarction, but rarely seen in those without infarction. *Arrows* point to the unquestionable increased signal in the mitral valve, but also other valves, not always in the left ventricle (note, the tricuspid valve (TV) in the third panel from the left). The mechanism of uptake is currently unknown, but speculation suggests that there is increased neovascularization in the endothelium of the valvular tissue. Images relate to case study 20.

*passive* component? Until now, the process of mitral regurgitation has been thought to be *active*: (a) active destruction of the mitral valve leading to loss of structural integrity, and (b) weakening of the fibroannular skeleton leading to active annular dilation. To our knowledge, this is the first formal identification of this phenomenon. Further efforts aimed at determining whether this, in fact, does predict a greater degree of mitral regurgitation is an area of active research.

# CHAPTER 16

# Miscellaneous Uses of Cardiovascular Magnetic Resonance Imaging

Robert W. W. Biederman

Perhaps the most interesting aspect of cardiovascular magnetic resonance (CMR) involves the myriad number of novel applications to which it can be applied. Given the multitude of CMR sequences, combined with the plasticity with which they can be utilized, one might feel that we are only limited by our imagination. Innovative uses for CMR can be obtained by using standard sequences, but applied in a nonstandard manner. This aspect is distinctly different as compared to other modalities that have limited body applications, as well as limited physical characteristics, which prevent their widespread application. It is for this reason that great creativity can be brought to bear by the imaging physician and technologists. Listed in the following text are a few of the more interesting and imaginative application areas.

## CONSTRICTIVE PERICARDITIS

Evaluation of constrictive pericarditis in conventional modalities requires high-quality imaging of the pericardium. Echocardiography has a well-defined limited ability to delineate the anatomic features of the pericardium. Although the posterior wall is often seen to be thick, it is due to a far-field artifact, generating a hyperechoic signal, often mimicking a thickened, highly calcified pericardium. Pulse-wave Doppler techniques demonstrating evidence of a restrictive pattern, as well as an abnormal tissue Doppler signal with an exaggerated "e" and blunted "a" wave are helpful in the evaluating the presence of constricted physiology. When a respirometer is available, the perturbed physiology can be evaluated more accurately, whereupon inspiration and expiration produce a characteristic Doppler pattern that can aid in diagnosis. In the catheterization suite, reliance on a morphologic "square root sign" is the cardinal feature. When fluid boluses are given, the specificity is increased, but still is far from diagnostic in many cases. A technique that has received some popularity in the catheterization suite is using the concept of "ventricular interdependence" in which during inspiration and expiration there is a characteristic separation in contraction of right and left atrial pressures. This can be a cumbersome technique, and requires invasive instrumentation to make this diagnosis, but in expert hands has high accuracy. Because physical examination, although helpful, has very limited sensitivity and specificity and is chiefly detected by a most subtle pericardial knock, is often not present until middle stages of disease, requiring an astute clinician and high clinical suspicion, there exists a great need for a technique that is both noninvasive, easy-to-use, and near foolproof. It is important to note that the ability to accurately detect constricted pericarditis has tremendous upside and downside potential (see Fig. 16-1). In these patients, who often present late, with months to years of vague progressive indolent symptoms that culminate in severe right heart failure, the accurate diagnosis leads to median sternotomy and pericardial stripping with dramatic improvement in the patient's symptomatology (see Fig. 16-2). However, in the same setting, with the patient *in extremis*, an incorrect diagnosis can lead to needless open-heart surgery. Consider the following hypothetical conversation with the cardiothoracic surgeon, in whom you have misdiagnosed constriction in a patient, "Would you please come down to the operating room to show me where *you* think I should cut the pericardium. By the way, would you mind telling the patient why I needlessly opened this patient up?" When stated in this graphic manner, it is clear that a versatile technique, such as CMR, would be advantageous (see Fig. 16-3).

The technique of radiofrequency tissue tagging, in which saturated lines of magnetization are placed in

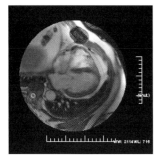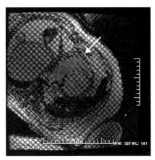

**FIGURE 16-1**   Steady state free precession (SSFP) in a four-chamber view (left) demonstrating a normal thickness pericardium and a sternal wire artifact. On the right is a radiofrequency tissue tagging image with the arrow pointing at the visceral–parietal interface. Note the distortion of the tagging pattern, indicating adherence between the two layers. By observing normals, an understanding of the typical interaction between the visceral and parietal layers can be appreciated while permitting a better understanding of the range of abnormal possible. The radiofrequency tissue tagging sequence is a standard option on all vendor protocols. Images relate to case study 1.

either a radial or gridlike pattern across the myocardium noninvasively, is useful in assessing pericardial disease. Typically, radiofrequency tagging is used to determine myocardial contraction patterns, and has been well described by us and others to provide knowledge of segmental myocardial deformation and measurement of strain in a transmural manner across the myocardium. This has been used to evaluate the post–myocardial infarction (MI) remodeling process and assess the effects of myocardial performance before and after surgical intervention. Measurement of circumferential, longitudinal, and radial strain patterns in one, two, and three dimensions has been performed, detailing high-fidelity physiologic patterns of normal and deranged

## CASE STUDIES

**Case Study 1.** A 64-year-old man status post CABG presents with mild chest pain (CP) for which echocardiography revealed an abnormal right ventricular (RV) free wall motion. CMR demonstrates a normal pericardial signal throughout the entire left ventricular (LV) with the exception of the most anterobasal RV free wall, whereby the signal is no longer homogeneous (see Fig. 16-1, left). Tissue tagging (right panel) demonstrates focal adherence, denoted by deformation of the basal RV free wall, indicative of focal lack of slippage between the visceral and parietal pericardial layers (*arrow*) with normal slippage otherwise noted. Because this is the only abnormal region, this is regarded as a normal finding, and not as evidence of constrictive anatomy. The perfusion sequence (not shown) reveals a dense inferior septal hypoperfusion defect that becomes nearly circumferential toward the apex. Ten years following emergency bypass, all three saphenous vein grafts (SVGs) showed evidence of moderate occlusion, for which he underwent rebypass, following confirmation of the lack of constrictive pericarditis.

**Case Study 2.** Adherence between the visceral and parietal RV pericardium in a 76-year-old status post CABG 2 years ago (see Fig. 16-2). Note, the normal thickness of the pericardium (best seen in middle panel) and deformation of the radiofrequency tissue tagging stripes. These signs are indicative of an adherence between the two pericardial layers (visceral and parietal). Upon surgical pericardiotomy, the noninvasive diagnosis was confirmed. We use this technique preferentially to volume loading in the catheterization suite or to ventricular interdependence in the echocardiography laboratory. To date, we have not been proved incorrect: if there is slippage seen between the two pericardial layers, the

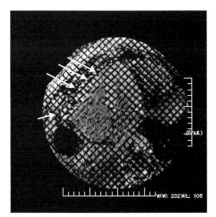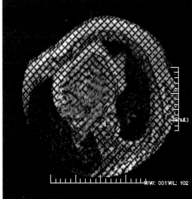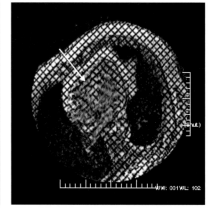

**FIGURE 16-2**   Radiofrequency tissue images taken of a patient with surgical proven constriction (right and middle) and a normal for comparison (left). This pattern is best seen in the enclosed DVD. Images relate to case study 2.

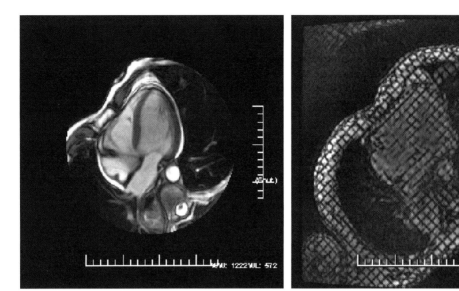

**FIGURE 16-3** A steady state free precession (SSFP) four-chamber view demonstrated a small pericardial effusion (left) with a radiofrequency tissue tagging image (right) demonstrating normal pericardial slippage as expected between the two clearly separate pericardial layers. Images relate to case study 3.

physiology. However, the clinical applicability is only now becoming recognized for quantitation of myocardial mechanics using this technique. An offshoot of this technology has been applied to evaluation of constrictive pericarditis in which tissue tagging has proved to be a robust and clinically applicable technique. The grid pattern is placed over the entire field of view (FOV), which includes the myocardium and pericardium by definition, and allows separation of pericardial signal from myocardial signal. Except for bulk translation, the pericardial signal is fixed in healthy individuals; therefore the epicardial signal should "slide" past the pericardial surface during systolic contraction and diastolic relaxation. Therefore, the visceral surface of the pericardium (epicardium) should migrate past the stationary parietal pericardium. Failure to see slippage between the visceral and parietal pericardium, evidenced by lack of relative motion, is diagnostic of adherence between the two layers. The observation of a fixed or grid pattern, without slippage, demonstrates that there is fibrosis, scarring, or union between the parietal and visceral pleura. This observation is the *sine qua non* of constrictive pericarditis (see Fig. 16-4). In our practice, in which we see sliding between the two pericardial layers, despite evidence by echocardiography or catheterization suite of constriction, we are confident in assuring the surgeon that there is no reason to take the patient to surgery. On the other hand, despite absence of constriction by other imaging modalities including the presence of a thin pericardium on computed tomography (CT), if there is no slippage in the major portion of the pericardium by CMR, we can assure the surgeon

diagnosis of constrictive pericarditis (constriction) is excluded. The left panel demonstrates normal slippage for comparison (well seen along the RV).

**Case Study 3.** A 50-year-old white woman with CP was sent for CMR evaluation (see Fig. 16-3). A very small pericardial effusion (bright) is present, which by use of radiofrequency tissue tagging, reveals no evidence of constriction (there is no adherence between the visceral and the parietal pericardium and there is a clean slippage plane). There is no evidence of tamponade physiology due to lack of right ventricular (RV) compression, lack of septal bounce, and no RA inversion.

**Case Study 4.** A 65-year-old white woman with recurrent pericardial effusions (see Fig. 16-4). CMR demonstrates no effusion, but limited excursion between the visceral and parietal pericardium is seen focally in the lower left along the right ventricular outflow tract (RVOT) and anterior RV free wall (note the clean slippage plane through systole) best seen in right panel.

**Case Study 5.** Standard double inversion recovery sequences obtained in a 54-year-old, demonstrating in axial and parasagittal images, a widely patent left main, proximal, and middle left anterior descending and proximal left circumflex vessels (see Fig. 16-5).

**Case Study 6.** SSFP imaging performed in a 59-year-old, referred for evaluation of the coronary arteries (see Fig. 16-6). The patient refused invasive cardiac

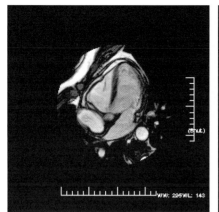
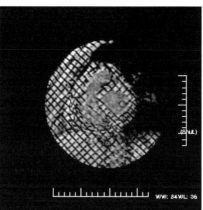
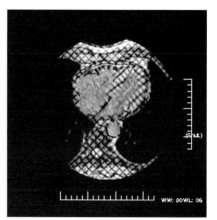

FIGURE 16-4 A steady state free precession (SSFP) (left) modified four-chamber view demonstrating a trace pericardial effusion, around the distal right ventricular free wall and left ventricular (LV) apex. Radiofrequency tissue tagging images in the short axis (middle) and four-chamber view (right) depict limited slippage between the visceral and parietal pericardium. Images relate to case study 4.

that they will find an adherence pattern consistent with constrictive pericarditis upon opening the chest. In our series of more than 50 patients, we have never been incorrect.

With reference to diagnostic strategies, it is worth commenting on the change in natural history of constricted pericarditis, which leads to ambiguity in detecting this elusive disease. Over the last 20 years, the natural history of constricted pericarditis has changed from the classic effusive-constrictive pattern of tuberculosis, which was the leading cause of constriction. In the late 1990s, with the advent of better

catheterization. The vessels were shown to be widely patent.

**Case Study 7.** Two-dimensional (see Fig. 16-7A) right coronary artery (RCA) and 3D surface rendered imaging of the same vessel in a 54-year-old man with ST depression in the inferior leads suggestive of RCA ischemia.

**Case Study 8.** A 67-year-old man, 1-month status post CABG presents with CP. Typically, a cardiac catheterization would be considered. However, the referring

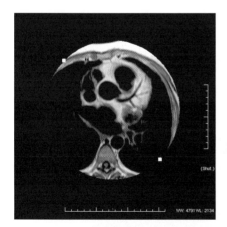
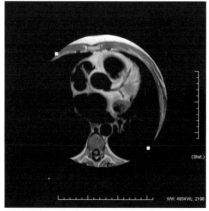
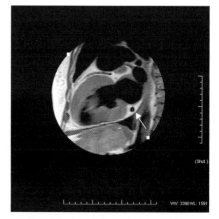

FIGURE 16-5 Breath-hold double inversion recovery sequence are obtained in the multislice axial (left and middle) and standard two-chamber (right) acquisition. The left main and the bifurcation into the left anterior descending (LAD) and left circumflex in this black blood sequence are easily seen as well as small diagonals emerging from the LAD. This sequence with this quality is enough to assure the referring physician that the left main and proximal/middle left coronary system is widely patent. The more distal aspects of the left courses are not visualized in this sequence. Note the coronary sinus seen in the right panel (*arrow*). Images relate to case study 5.

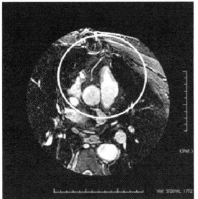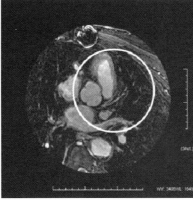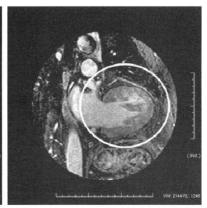

FIGURE 16-6   Three-dimensional (3D) steady state free precession (SSFP) images without contrast obtained in multiple projections delineating the conus branch (left), and left anterior descending (middle and right panel). In the right panel, the distal LAD is visualized. Images relate to case study 6.

surveillance and aggressive therapeutic strategies, the pattern has changed to one in which either unknown causes or, more likely iatrogenic constrictive pericarditis has become the norm. Unlike effusive-constrictive pericarditis, where the pericardium is thickened, forming an often-calcified rind that is unmistakable, the constrictive pericardium is very frequently of normal thickness (<3.5 mm) making standard techniques virtually ineffective when based solely on anatomic evaluation of the pericardium (i.e. CT Scans). In our practice, more than 50% of patients who were sent to surgery have normal thickness of their pericardium, but marked abnormalities in visceral–parietal slippage patterns.

cardiologist felt the CMR breath-hold angiogram might be sufficient (see Fig. 16-8). Shown are of the 3D reconstructed images of a 22-second acquisition, demonstrating three widely patent saphenous vein grafts.

**Case Study 9.** The double inversion recovery images in a 38-year-old man who presented with atypical CP (see Fig. 16-9). Cardiac catheterization revealed an anomalous origin of the RCA. Although unusual for the RCA to travel in the intra-arterial course when originating from the left coronary cusp, imaging was performed

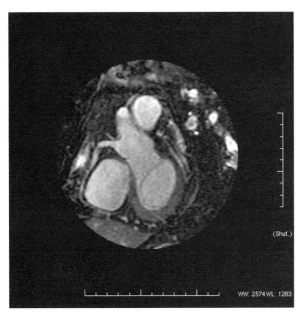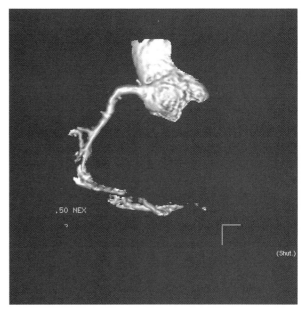

FIGURE 16-7   Two-dimensional (2D) (left panel) right coronary artery and 3D surface rendered imaging (right panel) of the same vessel. The right panel was a contrast-injected acquisition with manual surface rendering. Images relate to case study 7.

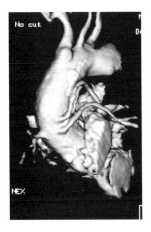
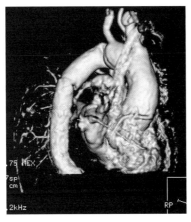

**FIGURE 16-8** Magnetic resonance angiography (MRA) performed in 22 seconds manually timed from the proximal ascending aorta, depicting the proximal mid and distal coronary artery bypass grafts, and their widely patent status. On the left is the saphenous vein graft (SVG) to D1 and SVG to OM1 (top graft) whereas the SVG to posterior descending artery (PDA) graft is seen on the right. Images relate to case study 8.

## CORONARY ARTERY IMAGING

Practitioners of CMR have long held the notion that the coronary arteries could be imaged noninvasively. Historically, perhaps the most long-awaited advance for noninvasive imaging by CMR has been the accurate and practical visualization of the coronary tree structure. A tremendous amount of effort has been applied, and many advances have been made, over the last two decades. We have now reached a point where image quality and scan speed have provided an early ability for CMR to delineate atherosclerotic disease within the coronaries. A caveat is necessary; the current techniques that are available when used in the ideal patient and ideal circumstances offer a reasonably suitable alternative to the current "gold standard" of cardiac catheterization. Many single study–single vendor studies have been performed and, when matched with a very small, but growing, number of multicenter trials, give credence to the concept that practical coronary imaging, although not as fast and easy to perform as CT, is possible.

demonstrating the posterior course of the RCA, which finally emerged and travel in the usual trajectory along the atrioventricular (AV) groove.

**Case Study 10.** A cardiac catheterization was performed on a 41-year-old man who presented with shortness of breath and an enlarged right heart by echocardiogram. The catheterization revealed an unusual directed anteriorly vessel, arising directly, and running superiorly from, the left anterior descending artery (LAD). The mid and distal course of the vessel was unknown, prompting CMR for further valuation (see Fig. 16-10). Seen in these SSFP sequences is a vessel traveling superiorly to, and anteriorly around the RVOT to empty into the supravalvular pulmonary artery. The course of this vessel is circuitous, taking a very serpentine pathway as it finally drains into the pulmonary artery. This prominent pulmonary artery fistula was quantified by Phase velocity mapping (PVM) to have a Qp:Qs of 1.3:1, which is a very small left-to-right shunt. Incorporating short-axis imaging of the right

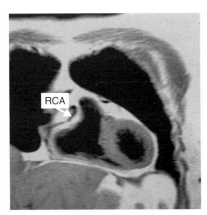
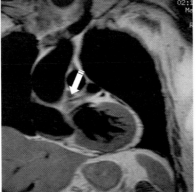
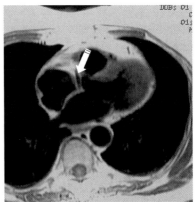

**FIGURE 16-9** Double inversion recovery sequences in multiple projections delineating the course of the anomalous left circumflex vessel, as well as its proximal and mid patency. Images relate to case study 9.

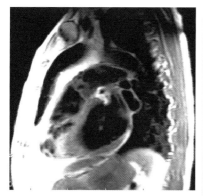 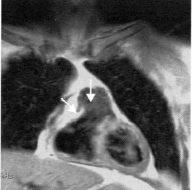 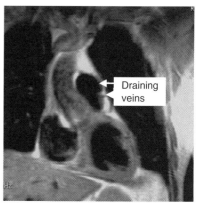

**FIGURE 16-10** Double inversion recovery sequences in the sagittal (left panel) and coronal projections (middle and right panels) demonstrating multiple left anterior descending (LAD) pulmonary artery fistulae. Not shown is the ability to utilize phase velocity mapping to quantitate the extent of the intracardiac shunt. Images relate to case study 10.

## NATIVE CORONARY ARTERY IMAGING

Traditionally, standard double inversion recovery sequences were used to delineate the coronary arteries (see Fig. 16-5). Now, several options are available, including rapid breath-hold two-dimensional (2D) segmented gradient recalled echo, steady state free precession (SSFP) imaging (see Fig. 16-6), magnetic resonance angiography (MRA) (see Figs. 16-7 and 16-8), and 3D noncontrast breath-hold imaging. With this wide variety of approaches, the field of CMR coronary artery imaging has seen an increase in popularity. Interestingly, contrast infusion techniques have been relegated to techniques of last resort and do not constitute the workhorse strategy for coronary imaging.

Clinical applications of existing coronary CMR techniques include the following:

1. Determining the patency and direction of flow in native coronary arteries
2. Evaluating the patency of native vessels following coronary stent placement
3. Evaluating congenital and acquired coronary anomalies
4. Screening and evaluation of patients with ischemic heart disease
5. Routinely delineating the ostial, proximal, and mid portions of the major coronary arteries and visualization of some coronary artery branches
6. Evaluating the patency of coronary artery bypass grafts (CABGs)

Currently, limitations for coronary imaging strategies by CMR still exist, including the inability to visualize the more distal segments and their respective branches, and that generally the scan time is in the order of 10 minutes. Because the distal vessels are generally not

and left ventricles, the shunt was confirmed to be small. However, the RV was at the top of normal size. He was offered prophylactic coiling of the coronary fistula but the patient decided against any intervention.

**Case Study 11.** A 32-year-old man presents with typical CP prompting a cardiac catheterization. The angiogram reveals a common ostium for all three of the coronary vessels. Clarification of the etiology, as well as determination of the trajectory of the anomalous vessels is performed by CMR (see Fig. 16-11). No single view reveals the common ostia of all three vessels, but through triangulation, it is clear that there is either a large ostia, or an adjacent, but near contiguous large ostia for all three vessels. In the left panel, the RCA is visualized whereas the mid and right panel depicts the left circumflex artery. The mid panel reveals the large common ostia for both the LAD and circumflex arteries traveling in separate directions. The LAD is seen in the right panel, derived from the common ostia (*right arrow*) whereas the *left arrow* signifies the RCA. This is an extremely rare congenital anomaly, whereby essentially all three vessels are derived from one common ostia, which is the right coronary cusp.

**Case Study 12.** A 62-year-old white man with transient ischemic attacks (TIA) presented for transesophageal echocardiography (TEE) unable to be intubated. Subsequently, he was found to have esophageal strictures that were not amenable to Hagar dilation. Because he was not in normal sinus rhythm (NSR), exonerating his left atrial appendage (LAA) as the cardiac source of embolus was important; therefore a CMR was ordered (see Fig. 16-12). The LAA is seen in the SSFP with the pectinate muscles shown, despite a respiratory artifact

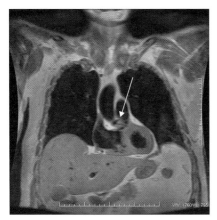 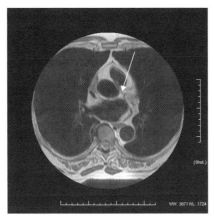 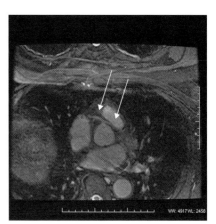

**FIGURE 16-11**    Selected double inversion recovery sequences for the evaluation of anomalous coronary arteries (left and middle panel) with a dedicated fast spoiled gradient recalled echo (FSPGR) sequence (right). Images relate to case study 11.

regions for major interventional strategies (including CABG and angioplasty/stent placement) this is not a major limitation, yet may still be a source of angina for the patient. With stated ability of the CMR to define with high-resolution cardiac structure, function, valves, perfusion and viability, the missing ingredient for complete interrogation of the frequent and the occasional cardiac perturbations remains only the complete portrayal of the coronary bed.

Several vendors have utilized a 3D noncontrast volume block acquisition in which depiction of the entire coronary tree can be performed in as little as one long breath-hold. Others employ a 3D non-breath hold navigator technique. The striking 3D depictions of the coronary arteries leads one to speculate that the era of 2D reconstructions is likely soon over. Support for this notion comes from the encouraging 3D CT coronary imaging that is now routinely being performed. It is our belief that when CMR coronary imaging is recognized as relatively inexpensive, noninvasive, and not requiring of either iodinated contrast, high-dose x-ray, or β-blockade administration for heart rate modulation that, when

from his inability to breath-hold. A 2 NEX scan with a 196 × 196 matrix was employed. PVM demonstrated a transappendageal emptying velocity of 50 cm per second supporting the lack of visible thrombus or a favorable milieu for its subsequent formation. The patient was not placed on Coumadin.

**Case Study 13.** A 73-year-old woman presents with a CVA as an esophageal stricture not amenable to intervention. A para-axial (see Fig. 16-13, left panel) as well as a two-chamber view (right) demonstrate a normal size for the LAA with normal contraction. The left panel reveals small pectinate muscles without any evidence of thrombus.

**Case Study 14.** A 43-year-old black man who presents with atypical CP, negative workup for coronary artery disease including negative CKMB and troponin-I. Knowing the potential for detecting subclinical disease, the accepting physician referred him for CMR (see Fig. 16-14). The *arrows* delineate small focal regions of myocarditis

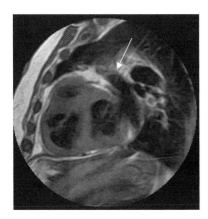 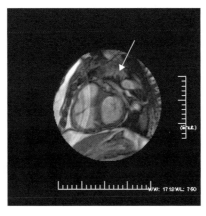

**FIGURE 16-12**    The left atrial appendage (LAA) is seen in the steady state free precession (SSFP) (right) with the pectinate muscles shown, despite a respiratory artifact from his inability to breath-hold. A 2 NEX scan with a 196 × 196 matrix was employed. Phase velocity mapping (PVM) demonstrated a transappendageal emptying velocity of 50 cm per second supporting the lack of visible thrombus or a favorable milieu for its subsequent formation. Double inversion recovery sequences in the two-chamber projection is seen in the left panel. Images relate to case study 12.

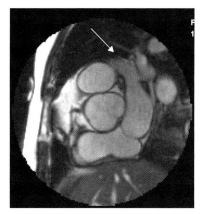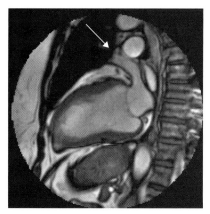

**FIGURE 16-13**    Steady state free precession (SSFP) images taken in the para-axial (left) and the two-chamber view (right) depicting the left atrial appendage (LAA) (*arrows*) and the lack of thrombus formation. Phase velocity mapping can be performed by measuring the transappendageal velocities. Placing a slice perpendicular to the long axis of the LAA (at the LAA os) and setting the velocity encoding gradient to 1 m per second permits measurement of both systolic, and end-diastolic filling velocities. While this sequence is sensitive to low velocities, it is highly sensitive to motion and noise. Emptying velocities in excess of 50 cm per second are considered normal and at low risk for thrombus presence or is subsequent formation whereas velocities between 40 and 50 cm are indeterminate, velocities <40 suggest a favorable milieu for thrombus formation. Images relate to case study 13.

added to the "one-stop shop" philosophy, it will become the definitive, decisive, and indefatigable technique of choice.

## ANOMALOUS CORONARY ARTERIES

For the last 10 years, CMR has become the gold standard for delineation of anomalous coronary arteries. This stems from the ability of CMR to depict multiple vascular structures and their interrelationship, which is a product of the large FOV that is possible (see Fig. 16-9). Therefore, when an x-ray angiographer identifies an apparent origin for a coronary artery, the ability to detect the trajectory of the vessel often remains equivocal. The ability to detect not only the origin, but to track the direction and plot through which vascular structures the vessel traverse is the major contribution of CMR to coronary artery imaging (see Fig. 16-10). It provides a roadmap for the coronary bed in the context of its anatomic relationship to other cardiovascular structures. Despite substantial strategies that provide a mechanistic approach to systematically delineate the path of the anomalous coronary such as the "i" or "dot" sign, considerable pragmatic limitations exist and this approach, in our experience, has fallen out of practice. This may be related as much to the local imaging capabilities that are available, making the absolute need to unequivocally identify the aberrant course less critical if a good CMR program is nearby (see Fig. 16-11).

in the absence of either wall motion irregularities or effusion. Note the nonendocardial distribution of the DHE pattern as distinctly different from that of an MI pattern.

**Case Study 15.** A 37-year-old white man with periodic syncope, especially when dehydrated from playing softball. Three successive SSFP images demonstrating the hyperdynamic systolic function, anatomic LVOT obstruction with minimal leaflet SAM (see Fig. 16-15), eccentric posteriorly directed moderately severe (3+) mitral regurgitation, as well as turbulence radiating off the aortic leaflets (three different levels for systolic murmurs; left panel, best seen in the DVD). Note the very narrow LVOT at exactly the area where the systolic turbulence starts (*arrow*). Also present are pleural effusions in the more axial acquisitions, but not seen in the pure coronal view.

**Case Study 16.** A 69-year-old white man with muscular sclerosis and dyspnea on exertion with positional desaturation. TEE examination demonstrated "bizarre anatomy," with suspicion of an anomalous pulmonary vein. Further investigation showed that the only anomaly was a distorted *cardia* due to RA compression from an unknown source (see Fig. 16-16). CMR clearly shows on SSFP coronal imaging a narrow slit with relatively high velocities due to compression from the liver and elevated right hemidiaphragm. In middle panel, real-time

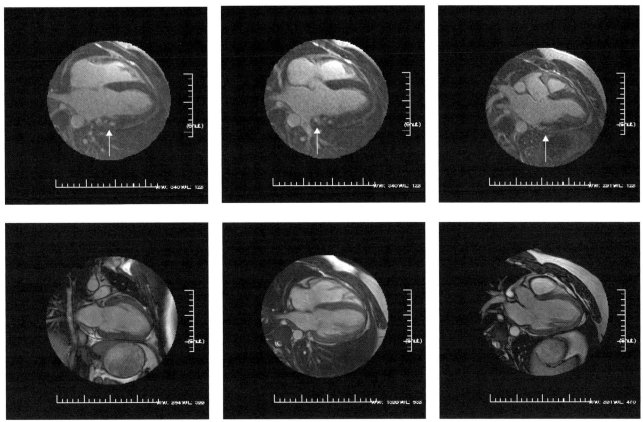

**FIGURE 16-14**  Delayed hyperenhancement images taken in multiple projections with the *arrows* pointing to several small punctate hyperenhancement zones in the midwall of the basal lateral wall corresponding steady state free precession (SSFP) images are shown. Imaging was acquired at 2 to 3 minutes after contrast enhancement for maximum sensitivity. Images relate to case study 14.

We and other investigators have demonstrated the continued utility of accurate delineation and confirmation of anomalous coronary arteries by CMR, with independent confirmation in those cases referred to the surgical suite. At our institution, given the accuracy of CMR for assessing anomalous coronary arteries, a young person presenting with typical chest pain (CP), will undergo noninvasive CMR coronary imaging, under the presumption that the risk of an invasive approach is neither warranted, ideal, or accurate enough to justify the risks of the diagnostic procedure.

Recently, several investigators have described use of CMR coronary artery imaging for evaluation of Kawasaki disease. By definition, limiting the use of invasive techniques and contrast administration in the pediatric patient population, for which this disease has its highest prevalence, would be a major advantage. Therefore, in centers where CMR is available, patients presenting with initial diagnosis of, or in follow up for, Kawasaki disease, CMR is preferred.

We and others have described the use of CMR for the delineation of the emptying chamber for coronary artery

imaging was employed on the suspicion that it was a paralyzed right hemidiaphragm, owing to the demyelenating disorder, affecting thoracic nerves 3, 4, and 5 (the phrenic nerve). Analogous to fluoroscopy, CMR in the coronal plane clearly demonstrated a paralyzed right hemidiaphragm, confirming the diagnosis. Interestingly, upon showing the patient that, although he had no congenital heart disease he did have a paralyzed diaphragm, he responded, "Oh I've had that since I was a small boy when my brother was removed from my right chest injuring my lung." Conjecture suggests that large teratoma was resected with surgical phrenic nerve damage. He subsequently went for percutaneous patent foramen ovale closure, which was very positional and with extensive right to left shunting, only when he lay down on his left side as he did for the TEE. No CMR shunting was noted (QP:QS was 0.99:1.0 by PVM).

**Case Study 17.** A pregnant 34-year-old presents with gradual weight gain for 6 to 7 months, now urinary

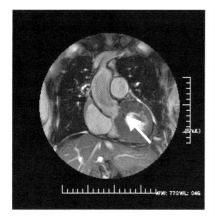
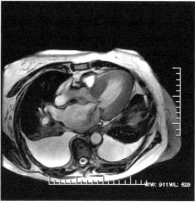
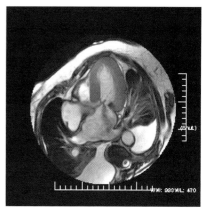

**FIGURE 16-15**   Steady state free precession (SSFP) images taken in the coronal (left panel), high three chamber (middle), and low three chamber (right) illustrating systolic anterior mitral motion (SAM) and subsequently the centric posteriorly directed moderately severe (3+) mitral regurgitation due to an left ventricular outflow tract (LVOT) obstruction. In this situation, the SSFP images portray the high spatial and temporal resolution necessary to detect the Venturi effect due to the low pressure along the anterior septal wall and subsequent invagination the anterior mitral leaflet creating the LVOT obstruction. This is exceptionally well depicted in the DVD. Note also the moderate bilateral pleural effusions best seen in the middle and right panels, helping to confirm the severity of this patient's condition. Images relate to case study 15.

fistulae. In the cardiac catheterization suite, often the origination of the coronary system is easily visualized. The definitive description of where the vessel empties into is often much more equivocal. In addition, through the use of phase velocity mapping (PVM), quantitation of flow volume can be performed and described in terms of Qp:Qs.

## LEFT ATRIAL APPENDAGE

The reference standard for the evaluation of patients with either transient ischemic attacks (TIA) or cerebrovascular accident (CVA) is transesophageal echocardiography (TEE). However, it is not infrequent that for

hesitancy and bloating, and a report of an extracardiac mass by ultrasonography. She was sent for CMR evaluation after a fetal echocardiogram failed to define the anatomy suggestive of tetrology of Fallot (see Fig. 16-17). A CMR was performed, demonstrating the ventricular septal defect (VSD) with a narrowed infundibulum. Most importantly, the main pulmonary artery and its respective small branches were seen (middle panel) permitting definitive surgical correction to be performed at 3 months post delivery, not emergently upon birth, favoring long-term outcome and depicting a unique and new use of CMR. The child is now nearly 1 year old and was recently introduced to the author as a healthy baby boy.

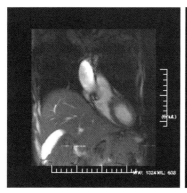
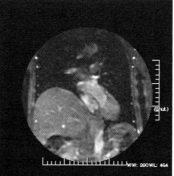
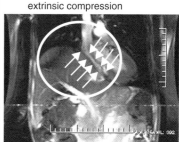

Marked hemiparesis of right hemidiaphragm resulting in RA extrinsic compression

**FIGURE 16-16**   Selective coronal steady state free precession (SSFP) images (left and right panels) with a real-time image (middle panel) depicting the dynamic compression of the inferior vena cava (IVC) from the right diaphragmatic hemiparesis. The real-time sequence is best seen in the enclosed DVD. Images relate to case study 16. RA, right atrium.

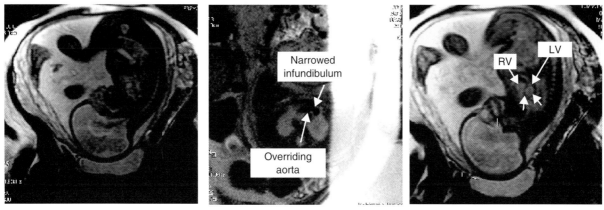

**FIGURE 16-17** *In utero* imaging was performed with the baby's heart rate of 140 beats per minute. As such, no direct cardiac gating was possible. Therefore, reliance on the less sensitive sequence such as the DIR was used for the bulk of imaging. When the baby is resting quietly, reasonably high-quality information can be obtained. However, because the mother, not the baby, can be insulated from the gradient switching noise, after a short while, our experience has shown that the baby awakes, hindering continued scanning and subsequent degradation in quality. Often, more can be gained with less, that is, pulling the mother out and letting her rest, permits the baby to fall sleep, affording another scanning opportunity. Images relate to case study 17. RV, right ventricle; LV, left ventricle.

any number of reasons, the patient is unable to be intubated or is not a candidate for TEE. Formally, transesophageal echocardiography was the only option. CMR can also be used to evaluate this population, with the main sequence being SSFP imaging, used to visualize the left atrial appendage (LAA) (see Fig. 16-12). Using serial SSFP images oriented parallel to the LAA it is typically well visualized (see Fig. 16-13). When decreasing the FOV and increasing the NEX and matrix, identification of the presence or absence of left atrial thrombus is often possible. Identification of normal anatomy, such as the pectinate muscles, is often quite easily performed, and at a minimum, can raise or lower the threshold for atrial thrombus detection. The delineation of slow flow is also helpful, analogous to the detection of spontaneous echo contrast or "smoke". Using PVM, a plane placed 1 cm into, and perpendicular to, the LAA os allows quantification of emptying velocities. If the velocity is >50 cm per second, then the milieu favorable for the formation of thrombus is not present. Therefore, if no thrombus is seen, no slow flow pattern is observed, and velocities are normal or above, our center defines the LAA to be free of clot and its likelihood for its formation to be low. Variants of the above raises suspicion for increased likelihood for appendageal clot formation. When added to the ability of CMR to detect ventricular thrombus (described in Chapter 15), CMR has the ability to evaluate for cardiac sources of emboli in this patient population. An important limitation exists in patients who present with atrial fibrillation. In the absence of a reasonably regular heart rhythm, images

**Case Study 18.** A 65-year-old man status post CABG ×3, and mitral valve replacement with equivocal transthoracic echocardiogram, TEE, and cardiac catheterization after volume loading is referred for CMR (see Fig. 16-18). An equivocal "square root sign" is present. However, he is hypotensive, intubated, and in great *extremis*. Understandably the cardiothoracic surgeons want a more definitive diagnosis before considering surgery. He is referred for high pretest probability constrictive pericarditis but has a pacemaker. Although extremely controversial, under very careful circumstances in which the pretest probability is high (as in this case), judicious use of CMR is potentially life saving. The implanted pacemaker is seen in most of the images, especially the right upper region as a black paramagnetic artifact. The thickened pericardium that extends throughout the right ventricular free wall and into the right atrial wall is easily seen. In various images, the failure for slippage is appreciated. Physiologic assessment of the importance is also obtained through the abnormal septal motion ("septal bounce") that is highly supportive of this diagnosis (left panel). Marked pericardial/diaphragmatic adherence was also present. There was complete failure of slippage between the parietal and visceral pericardium and although the examination took <7 minutes to complete, it was extraordinarily conclusive that constrictive pericarditis was the unifying diagnosis. However, because only CMR supported this diagnosis, it was with great reticence that the chair of cardiothoracic surgery looked at me and asked, "How certain are

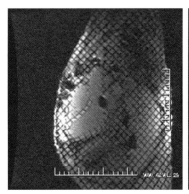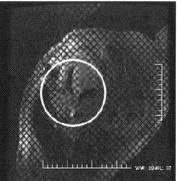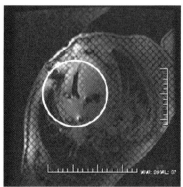

**FIGURE 16-18** Selective radiofrequency tissue tagging of a patient with a pacemaker. Note the circled dark artifact of the pacemaker. Also note the prosthetic mitral valve field defect noted in the panel on the left. An appreciation for the abnormal septal motion that was present in this patient was obtained with radiofrequency tissue tagging, with constricted pericarditis seen in the left panel. Note the marked visceral–parietal pericardial adherence pattern involving, not only the right ventricular free wall, but the right atrial wall. The DVD demonstrates the abnormal respiratory-phasic changes that were present in this surgically confirmed constricted pericarditis. Placing the pacer in V00 mode, using a sequence with a very low specific absorption ratio (SAR) such as the gradient recalled echo (GRE) sequence (SAR <0.15) will minimize heat and conductivity, minimizing the time in the scanner and centering the pacemaker (not the patient) in the bore of the scanner are some of the techniques that one can implement to minimize, but not eliminate the pacemaker risk. Images relate to case study 18.

are often suboptimal. However, because this population is generally in need of anticoagulation, independent of the diagnosis, coumadinization therapy should be considered.

## MYOCARDITIS

As described in Chapter 15, myocarditis evaluation has become an important part of the evaluation of patients who have CP of unknown etiology. Briefly, using the delayed hyperenhancement sequence, the complete interrogation of myocardial tissue characteristics can be performed, such that evaluation for acute, subacute, or chronic MI, infiltrative or inflammatory processes can be detected. Typically MI patterns, as described earlier, are distinctly endocardial in origin, migrating toward the epicardium as the infarct pattern becomes larger. However, the appearance of a distinct midwall and/or epicardial processes allows clinical distinction of these two entities to be made (see Fig. 16-14).

## VALVULAR HEART DISEASE

Although covered extensively in Chapter 9, the high temporal and spatial resolution necessary to capture dynamically induced valvular heart disease is a feature that is underappreciated, but, on occasion, critically important. Figure 16-15 demonstrates a patient with a

you?" He became even more surprised by my response, "100%!" The patient was taken to surgery that evening, and I heard the surgeon reply, "This is not only constrictive pericarditis but the worse case I've ever seen." The patient survived the surgery only to succumb 2 months later.

several-day history of the severe gastrointestinal virus and subsequent severe shortness of breath. On examination, she had decreased breath sounds at the lung bases and was presumed to have had pneumonia. However, a dynamic systolic ejection murmur was present, worsening with squat and Valsalva maneuvers. A CMR was performed demonstrating a slightly redundant anterior mitral leaflet and hyperdynamic (near-cavity obliteration) left ventricular systolic function. Marked systolic anterior mitral motion (SAM) involving the posterior leaflet (P3 scallop) and the anterior-medial papillary muscle, all contributed to substantial left ventricular outflow tract (LVOT) obstruction. The investigation of the anterior mitral leaflet toward the anterior septum created a very eccentric moderately severe jet of posteriorly directed mitral regurgitation. The treatment of choice for her was aggressive fluid resuscitation to relieve the relative hypovolemic state. Within 1 hour of the 3 L fluid infusion, the murmur of mitral regurgitation, as well as the LVOT murmur had mostly disappeared. This example highlights the spatial and temporal resolution possible by CMR, the cardinal role of incorporating a solid understanding of pathophysiology, auscultation, and CMR imaging to aid in accurate diagnoses. Integration of this diagnostic armamentarium prevented needless ancillary studies, rapidly facilitated her appropriate therapy and, most importantly, prevented potential invasive strategies that might have culminated in mitral valve repair or replacement.

## CONGENITAL HEART DISEASE: DIAGNOSIS *IN UTERO*

A few attempts have been made worldwide to image an infant's heart *in utero* using CMR. We have had some recent success either diagnosing or confirming congenital abnormalities. Because CMR is a noninvasive imaging modality it is considered a safe procedure for pregnant women after the teratogenic period. It should be noted that, after decades of CMR use, and many systematic retrospective and prospective investigations in both human and nonhuman studies, there have never been any definitive studies that indicate that high field magnets have an adverse impact on fetal growth and development. In generations of animal models, namely mice, there is no increased rate of fetal demise or abnormal fetal development. Nevertheless, the recommendation for magnetic resonance imaging (MRI) is that no female patient is imaged before 12 weeks, unless the risk of nondetection is inordinately high to the mother. However, at any time during the pregnancy, we as a matter of policy, obtain written consent from the patient after a careful explanation detailing what is known and not known about CMR imaging. This imaging is far from a matter of routine in that gating algorithms are well established for the mother, but currently, the ability to gate to the fetal heart rate is beyond most centers' capabilities. Therefore, reliance on double inversion recovery (DIR) is the workhorse all of our sequences. Limited SSFP sequences are possible, but require cooperation of mother and baby, the latter being more difficult to train! Indeed, the fetus has an impeccable ability to know just when the key sequences are being performed, choosing the most inopportune moment to move. Orientation within the body is not standard such that a few added minutes of triangulation and reorientation of the baby in a more standard imaging coordinate system is needed. As expected, as soon as that is accomplished it is time for the baby to reposition itself. Additionally, we have used real-time imaging with some success to derive limited functional information about the left ventricle and right ventricle (RV). When the mother, baby, and sequence are all optimally aligned, impressive image quality can be obtained, permitting for a noninvasive diagnosis (see Fig. 16-16). This allows

for either reassurance of the family and physician or for optimally timing peridelivery surgical correction.

## REAL-TIME IMAGING

In certain situations, the application of real-time imaging, available on most scanners, adds another element of clinical utility (see Fig. 16-17). Initially designed for more rapid scouting and identifying standard prescriptions, more creative uses have been recently employed. Investigators have used real-time imaging to evaluate for a patent foramen ovalis (PFO) disease using the four-chamber view, and careful synchronization of gadolinium injection and watching it cross from the right atrium (RA) to the left atrium when either a Valsalva or a cough was performed. It should be noted that the sensitivity for TEE is higher, but given intrinsically higher temporal resolution of the TEE, the ability to see a bubble crossing through the limbus of the PFO is likely lower. We have used real-time imaging for evaluation of diaphragmatic palsy associated with neuromuscular disorders, evaluation of swallowing in a patient presenting with *dysphagia Lusoria* in this setting of aberrant subclavian artery, congenital heart disease *in utero*, and other applications, recognizing that it adds another tool to the imager's armamentarium when complex imaging is considered.

## CARDIOVASCULAR MAGNETIC RESONANCE AND PACEMAKERS

Pacemaker use in CMR has traditionally been thought to be an absolute contraindication. The risks of sudden death due to the induction of heart rates equivalent to the RF frequency, the potential for magnetic field causing displacement of the can or lead(s), heating of the tip, causing either coagulation of blood or necrosis of the myocardial/tip interface, among others have paralyzed the field in recent years into near unanimity that the potential for disaster is too high to warrant the potential benefit. Over the recent 3 or 4 years however, intrepid investigators have carefully performed CMR in selected patients with compelling results. Careful selection of sequences that reduce the specific absorption rate (SAR), limiting exposure to imaging sequences, positioning the pacemaker/lead in the center of the bore, switching the magnet to a nonpaced mode (V00), and imaging only non–pacemaker-dependent patients are among some of the techniques recommended by proponents of imaging in this population. These measures minimize, but cannot absolutely eliminate, the potential for tragedy. Above all, a "heart-to-heart" discussion with both the patient and especially the relatives is mandatory. At our center, we will not image anybody in this situation unless the CMR physician has personally reviewed all prior diagnostic tests to ascertain that all other strategies have been exhausted, and that the potential to benefit the patient with the knowledge gained is high. As a clinical cardiologist with training in CMR, this balance is a delicate one. Our ability to determine the clinical need for further investigation beyond what has been done adds another advantage by having such personnel either in charge or actively involved in this decision making (see Fig. 16-18). Ultimately, however, the decision for proceeding rests on the director of the CMR center, who must assume full responsibility for either the resultant success or failure. To date, we have imaged only four patients and have done so without complications. However, demonstrating that the patient survived the scan is *not* our definition of success, and we judge that answering the clinical question at the conclusion of the study, with no change in pacemaker lead impedance compared with the preimpedance check, and no evidence of intracurrent complications, is the true measure of success. The clinical indications for which we have performed imaging in patients with pacemakers have been as follows: (i) constrictive pericarditis, (ii) aborted pacemaker lead implantation (accurate determination of LV function), (iii) evaluation of cardiac sarcoidosis using delayed hyperenhancement (DHE) in a patient with known pulmonary sarcoidosis under the premise that we were not only reducing the risk of a biopsy, but given the known skip-lesion pathology of sarcoidosis, potentially avoiding a false-negative biopsy result, and (iv) extracardiac mass encroaching on the myocardium/pericardium. It should also be stated that we are not cavalier in our approach, having turned down three times as many for unfounded clinical reasons.

# PART III

# Advanced Training

# CHAPTER 17

# Gradient Echo

Mark Doyle

## OVERVIEW

Gradient echo imaging is one of the fundamental imaging sequences used in cardiovascular applications. This is mainly because it lends itself easily to cine imaging, and is therefore used in applications that assess cardiovascular function, such as the following:

- Velocity
- Perfusion
- Delayed enhancement viability imaging

These application areas may either directly use classical gradient echo imaging or some variant on the basic sequence. Important variants on gradient echo imaging and specialized applications are discussed in more detail in separate chapters. Here, the basics of the technique are introduced, together with a brief outline of how gradient echo imaging is applied to assess myocardial function, blood flow, and perfusion.

## GRADIENT ECHO IMAGING—BASIC PRINCIPLES

Spatial information is encoded by application of magnetic gradients to the spin system. The local magnetic field experienced by each spin, $\mathbf{B_0}$, results in the spin precessing at a fixed angular frequency, $\omega$, which is characteristic of the gyromagnetic ratio, $\gamma$, of the nuclear species. The relationship linking these three qualities is termed the *Lamor equation*:

$$\omega = \gamma \times \mathbf{B_0}$$

Therefore, if the local magnetic field varies in a linear manner, from a low field at one position in the body to a high field at another position (a magnetic gradient), the nuclear spins will experience a linear range of frequencies. Therefore, signal acquired in a magnetic gradient directly relates spin frequency to spatial

position in the one-dimensional (1D) case. However, the body is 3D. After performing slice selection, the problem of imaging reduces to a 2D situation. However, this may present a conceptual problem, that is, if a linear gradient relates only to one dimension, then how is the second dimension encoded? To address this, we quickly introduce the conceptual framework of k-space: which can be regarded as a signal space in which frequency information is encoded along the two dimensions. Other chapters give a fuller description of k-space, but here the important features to be aware of are that the 2D gradient echo signals are arranged to fill k-space directly. Once the k-space data set has been compiled, application of a single Fourier transform operation is sufficient to generate an image. Therefore, k-space forms the signal domain and the Fourier transform, which is a signal processing operation, is applied to form an image. In 2D magnetic resonance imaging (MRI), the k-space signal is arranged in a 2D matrix and is commonly represented as a series of parallel lines. Most MRI sequences populate k-space one line at a time. To encode each k-space line requires application of two separate gradients:

Frequency encoding gradient, for example, X

Phase encoding gradient, for example, Y

Note in Fig. 17-1, illustrating the acquisition of two lines of k-space, that the frequency encoding gradient is applied identically for each line. However, the phase encoding gradient is required to ensure that successive lines are stepped through to cover the second dimension of k-space. Also note that the phase encoding gradient is applied before signal detection, which occurs at the frequency encoding stage.

## SIGNAL PREPARATION

The phase encoding gradient is applied before the signal read out because the spin system has to be prepared.

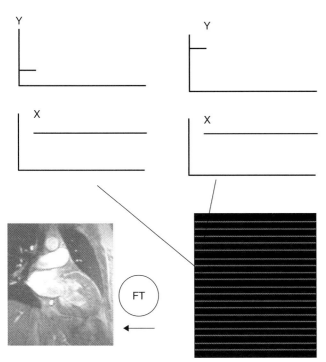

**FIGURE 17-1** K-space encoding is illustrated. Each line of the k-space matrix (*series of lines*) are encoded by applying an X gradient in a uniform manner as indicated. Each line of k-space is distinguished from other lines by the Y gradient applied. The Y gradient is applied in the stepped manner indicated in the top panel. Therefore, to acquire the complete k-space matrix requires successive application of the sequence: the Y gradient applied in a stepped manner, and the X gradient applied in a uniform manner. When the k-space matrix is complete, application of the image-processing step of the Fourier transformation (FT) is all that is required to form an image. Note that there is a time delay between application of the X and Y gradients.

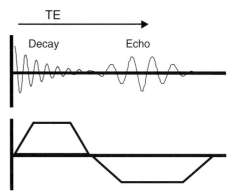

**FIGURE 17-2** The time delay between application of the phase encoding and frequency encoding gradients is accomplished by generation of a gradient echo. First, a positive gradient is applied, which causes the signal to decay rapidly, because spins at multiple spatial locations become dephased with respect to each other. This gradient is followed by a negative gradient that refocuses spins. When the spins come into phase, they form an echo peak. After the echo peak is attained, the signal dephases, and again decays. The echo formed by this means is symmetric. The time from spin excitation to the echo peak is termed the *echo time* (TE).

Therefore, we require the signal to be delayed from its inception at slice selection to the time of detection. This small delay is accomplished by the maneuver of forming a signal echo. Here, we will consider the gradient echo variant of forming a signal echo.

## GRADIENT ECHO

By applying a positive gradient for a time period, and following it by a negative gradient, we can appreciate that the spins initially advance in phase in the positive gradient and reverse in phase in the negative gradient (see Fig. 17-2). Since spins at physically different locations along the gradient direction experience a range of rotation frequencies, when the positive gradient is applied, the signal is observed to decay as spins progressively lose phase coherence with respect to each

other. Conversely, application of the negative gradient results in signal regrowth, as spins progressively come back into phase, forming an echo peak. Because the negative gradient continues to be applied following the echo peak, the spins progressively lose phase, and signal decay is again observed. Therefore, the positive gradient followed by a negative gradient results in a signal echo, characterized by a signal buildup to a peak, which then decays to zero in a time-symmetric manner. The echo time (TE) is defined as the time from signal origination at slice selection to the echo peak.

## GRADIENT-RECALLED ECHO PULSE SEQUENCE

The gradient-recalled echo (GRE) sequence is composed of the following steps:

- Slice selection
- Phase encoding gradient
- Gradient echo formation, which also forms the frequency encoding or measurement gradient

We note that each application of the phase gradient only generates data for one k-space line, and consequently, multiple applications of the basic imaging sequence are required to compile a complete k-space matrix (see Fig. 17-3). Further, to form a cardiac cine image series, multiple k-space matrices are required, that is, one complete matrix for each point in the cardiac

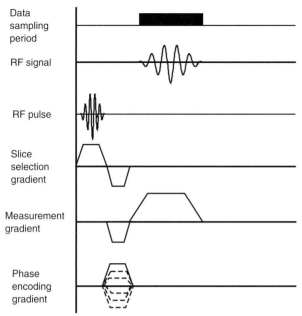

Data
sampling
period

RF signal

RF pulse

Slice
selection
gradient

Measurement
gradient

Phase
encoding
gradient

**FIGURE 17-3** The gradient echo pulse sequence is shown. Each line represents an activity, such as application of a gradient, an RF pulse, or performing signal detection. The first RF pulse is applied by the system in conjunction with the slice selection gradient, and is the combination that is responsible for accomplishing slice selection. The gradient echo forms the frequency encoding gradient, and data is sampled as the echo is formed. The phase encoding gradient is applied in successive steps as indicated. RF, radio frequency.

cycle where an image is needed (see Fig. 17-4). Because each k-space matrix is compiled one line at a time, data must be acquired over multiple cardiac cycles to build up the set of k-space matrices required to generate temporally resolved images. This is achieved by synchronizing the acquisition with the cardiac cycle to form a cine image series.

## GRADIENT ECHO TERMINOLOGY

Some of the terminology associated with gradient echo imaging is as follows:

- TE; echo time
- TR; repetition time of the basic "pulse sequence"
- Pulse sequence; the imaging procedure, gradient-recalled echo
- Relaxation times; spin–lattice relaxation, T1; spin–spin relaxation, T2

Typical values for gradient echo imaging parameters are as follows:

- TR; low, 4 to 10 milliseconds
- TE; short, 1 to 6 milliseconds

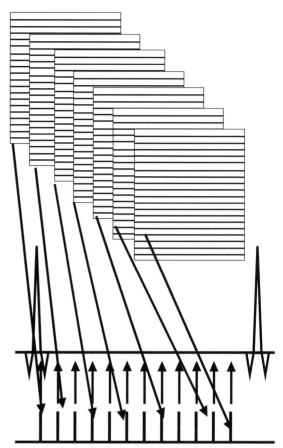

**FIGURE 17-4** To acquire a series of images over the cardiac cycle, a series of k-space matrices are required, each matrix corresponding to a point in the cardiac cycle. Multiple cardiac cycles are required to acquire the time-resolved cardiac image series.

- Blood signal; bright, owing to flow refreshment
- Fat signal; bright, owing to short T1
- Myocardium signal; intermediate intensity

## FREQUENCY AND PHASE ENCODING GRADIENTS

To encode each k-space line requires application of the following two separate gradients:

- Frequency encoding
- Phase encoding

For a transverse image of the body, that is, an image in the X-Y plane, the frequency encoding gradient could be assigned to the X gradient, or equivalently it could be assigned to the Y gradient. Is there a preference in the selection of each gradient direction? To examine this question, consider what happens when the frequency encoding gradient is applied to sample a line of k-space data. We note that the digital sampling rate determines the highest frequency that can be sampled. Further, the outer limits of the body in the imaging plane experience the highest magnetic field due to the gradient. Therefore, to correctly sample data to describe the outer extremities of the body requires a high data-sampling rate. This allows signal from spins at the extreme edges to be correctly sampled and represented in the image. Technically, the feature of the data described by the sampling rate is the bandwidth (BW). The BW of the measured signal is given by the equation:

$$BW = No. \text{ of samples}/T_{sample}$$

where $T_{sample}$ is the sampling interval between individual sample points. Wide BWs are required for signals with high frequency components, which corresponds to a high number of sampled points. In the frequency encoding direction, there is no penalty for sampling at a high temporal rate (corresponding to a wide signal BW), and full representation of this information is typically easily accommodated. Similarly, the BW in the phase encoding direction is determined by how many lines are acquired to sample that dimension of k-space. In the phase encoding direction there is a very large penalty for sampling at a higher rate, because each sample *point* along the *phase encoding direction* requires application of a separate gradient echo sequence, which necessarily leads to an increased scan time. Because acquiring data to map out the phase encoding gradient dimension is time consuming, it is always set at the smallest possible value consistent with the imaging dimensions of the body (see Fig. 17-5). When imaging the body in a section where one dimension is lower than the other (e.g., for an elliptical cross-section of the body), it is common to use a rectangular field of view, matching the long and short dimensions to the long and short axes of the ellipse. When using a rectangular field of view, two numbers represent the scan matrix, the first is the frequency encoding and the second the phase encoding resolution, for example, $256 \times 196$. From the arguments discussed in the preceding text, we can appreciate that the periphery of the body is problematic for the phase encoding direction, because sampling at a high rate (i.e., more lines of k-space) is required to correctly represent these outer regions. For this reason, the field of view is often set slightly smaller than the dimensions of the body, which will result in signal fold-over, that is, the edges of the body are "folded" over other image features, partially obscuring them. A small amount of fold-over is generally acceptable (see Fig. 17-6).

## FLIP ANGLE

There is a relationship between the radiofrequency (RF) flip angle used and the signal strength of the

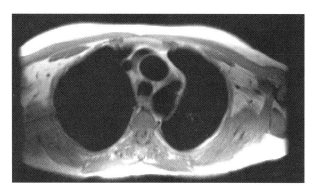

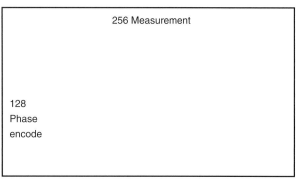

256 Measurement

128
Phase
encode

**FIGURE 17-5** Because there is a high time penalty to acquire each k-space phase encoded line, rectangular fields of view are typically employed to reduce the number of lines. The short dimension of the body is aligned with the shorter phase encoding direction, whereas the longer dimension of the body is aligned with the frequency encoding direction.

gradient echo image. For each RF pulse applied at a certain flip angle, we only see the component of spins that are in the transverse plane. Initially, a large flip angle generates a large transverse component (see Fig. 17-7). When considering the spin system as being resolved into a "vertical," longitudinal component, and a "horizontal" transverse component, we can appreciate that increasing the horizontal component of the spins by applying a large RF pulse flip angle proportionately diminishes the longitudinal component. However, more than one RF pulse is required to generate an image. If the time interval (TI) between application of successive RF pulses is short relative to the tissue's T1, then the longitudinal magnetization will not have recovered sufficiently to contribute a high signal as the train of RF pulses progresses. Therefore, under conditions of a high flip angle and a short TR, the longitudinal signal quickly diminishes to zero, and consequently the steady state transverse signal also diminishes to zero. Richard Ernst calculated the optimal angle for a given TR and T1 to maximize the signal:

- Ernst angle = EA
- $Cos(EA) = exp\ (-TR/T1)$

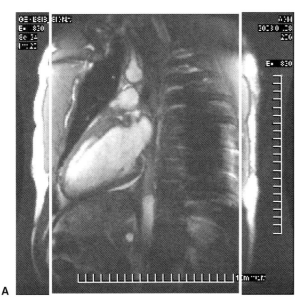 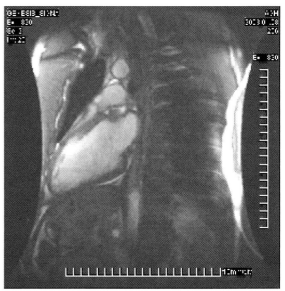

A                                                                                                          B

**FIGURE 17-6** For a full field of view image, the image is well represented up to the edges of the body. To reduce the scan time, the field of view may be selected within the boundaries of the body. When this occurs in the phase encoding direction, the resulting image will experience a folding over of the boundaries of the body beyond the field of view. This is the so-called aliasing artifact.

At this angle, transverse magnetization quickly attains a sustainable steady state value, because spin relaxation occurs at a sufficient rate to replenish the longitudinal magnetization. As a rule of thumb for cardiac imaging, short TRs are generally used, and under these conditions the Ernst angle approximately equals the TR. However, what we generally require is optimal contrast not optimal signal. Typically, a higher flip angle than the Ernst angle is used to optimize contrast between myocardium and blood.

## PHASE VELOCITY IMAGING

It is possible to quantify blood flow velocity using a modification of the GRE imaging sequence. Consider that spins are really vector quantities, and that they have the properties of magnitude and phase. These vector properties can be used to encode velocity (see Fig. 17-8). A spin moving along a magnetic field gradient experiences a progressively increasing precessional frequency. Compared to static spins, moving spins will not completely refocus in a gradient echo sequence due to the velocity dependence of the precessional frequency. In terms of the spin system then, motion results in the spin vector attaining a different phase angle compared to the static spins. We can arrange for the phase difference between a static spin and a moving spin to be linearly proportional to the moving spin's velocity:

- Phase = Velocity × constant

Addition of a bipolar gradient pair will encode velocity in the signal phase in a predictable manner (see Fig. 17-9). A set of bipolar gradients can be added to any imaging axis

- X
- Y
- Z

When separately applied to an imaging axis, bipolar gradients encode velocity along that axis. However, k-space data are imperfectly acquired owing to a number of equipment features, including lack of truly linear gradients and inhomogeneities in the main magnetic field. Consequently, the phase information in the velocity image is rarely flat in regions of static tissue, and the velocity information is therefore distorted. To correct for these phase distortions, a reference image is acquired. The reference image is typically flow compensated, such that static and moving spins each possess nominally zero phase. This is compared with the flow-encoded image, in which, nominally, only static spins have zero phase. The imperfections in phase are arranged to be common to both images, and upon subtraction, the true, undistorted, velocity data can be extracted.

## FLOW VISUALIZATION

Because through-plane velocity can be either positive or negative, and because display systems can only

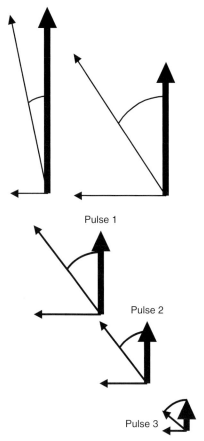

**FIGURE 17-7** The effects of RF pulse angle are illustrated. In the upper panel, the thin arrows indicate the $M_0$ magnetization vector position following application of low and high angle RF pulses. In the case of the high RF flip angle, the transverse component of the $M_0$ vector is the larger. In the lower panel, the effects of applying successive RF pulses with a relatively high flip angle are seen. Following each pulse, the longitudinal component of magnetization diminishes, such that as successive pulses are applied at the same angle, the transverse signal rapidly diminishes.

represent positive intensities, through-plane velocity is typically represented using a gray-scale convention:

• Gray—static
• Dark—negative velocity
• Bright—positive velocity

The conventional magnitude images are generated as a by-product along with the velocity images. The most common problem in velocity imaging is "aliasing". Aliasing is caused when the velocity encoding limits are set too low, and the phase exceeds 360 degrees. The cure for aliasing is to repeat the scan, typically with the velocity sensitivity limit increased appropriately. When in-plane flow is encoded, two velocity directions are separately acquired. However, visualization of in-plane velocity is more involved than that of through-plane

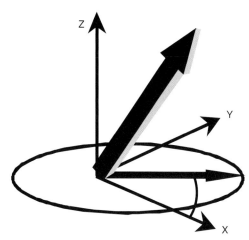

**FIGURE 17-8** The vector properties of the magnetization $M_0$ are illustrated. Relative to a fixed reference frame (e.g., the X-axis) the transverse component of $M_0$ has a phase angle. This phase angle can be used to directly encode velocity information.

flow. Here, there is no standard visualization approach. Each component of velocity can be viewed using the gray-scale approach explained in the preceding text. However, this requires the viewer to integrate the information mentally. Alternatively, arrow plots can be used, where in each frame the instantaneous length and direction of each arrow relates to the velocity at that pixel. Other schemes are possible using color displays.

## INVERSION RECOVERY

Inversion recovery (IR), is a contrast mechanism that is typically used to distinguish tissues based on their T1 properties. Typically, IR is used in conjunction with contrast agent imaging. In equilibrium, spins are aligned with the main magnetic field. Following inversion by applying a 180-degree RF pulse, spins relax back to realignment over time (see Fig. 17-10). However, no signal is seen in the basic IR operation. In order to see a signal, a second RF pulse is required. Following the initial inversion and partial recovery of the spin system, application of a second 90-degree RF pulse flips the spins into the transverse plane. Following the 90-degree pulse, signal is seen from the net magnetization vector in the transverse plane.

## INVERSION RECOVERY CONTRAST

Consider inversion and partial recovery for two spins, each with distinctly different T1 values:

• Short T1
• Long T1

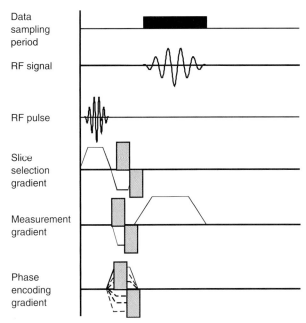

FIGURE 17-9 By adding bipolar gradients to individual axes, shown in gray shading, the velocity of moving spins can be encoded separately along the slice select, frequency encoding (or measurement) and phase encoding directions. Consider that the bipolar gradient initially dephases static spins and then refocuses them, resulting in a net zero phase accumulation. However, moving spins will not fully refocus, and will be left with a velocity-dependant phase angle. Note that the bipolar gradients are applied to only one axis at a time. RF, radiofrequency.

After a suitable IR delay, when the spins are partially recovered, applying a 90-degree RF allows detection of the spin signal. Since the recovery rates are different for the two spins, the net signals will also be different. The origin of the IR signal contrast is when the positive and negative longitudinal spin component tends to cancel for spins with one T1 value and are either mostly positive or mostly negative for spins with another T1 value. In this way, cancellation of signals leads to low or zero signal for spins with one T1 value, whereas the spins with a distinctly different T1 value are seen with relatively high signal. By selecting a long IR TI, both long and short T1 components will be seen, whereas selecting a short TI preferentially suppresses short T1 components, such as fat. Because two pulses are required to view the IR signal, one feature of IR is that moving blood, which does not experience both pulses, is well suppressed. Therefore, the process of IR offers an additional way of suppressing moving blood signal. As the blood velocity approaches zero, this mechanism is less effective. However, it is possible to apply two or even three IR pulses before signal read out to allow increased blood signal suppression.

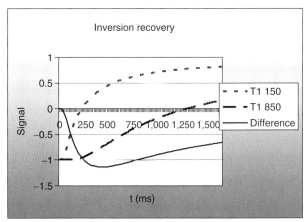

FIGURE 17-10 The basis of the inversion recovery contrast is graphed for spins with two distinct T1 values: 150 milliseconds and 850 milliseconds. Upon inversion of the spin system, both spins have a value of −1, and therefore provide no net contrast. As the lower T1 spins relax back to +1 faster than the longer T1 spins, the contrast between them initially grows. As time goes on, the lower T1 spins have almost fully relaxed and the longer T1 spins will approach full relaxation, leading to reduction of contrast.

## INVERSION RECOVERY AND MYOCARDIAL PERFUSION AND VIABILITY IMAGING

By introducing a gadolinium contrast agent intravenously, the T1 of myocardium is shortened, but only during passage of the agent. Therefore, contrast agent administered as a bolus, accompanied by rapid imaging using an IR contrast pulse, allows identification of myocardium that is perfused by the agent. In myocardial perfusion imaging, multiple slices are imaged as the contrast agent passes through the cardiovascular system, first its arrival is observed in the right ventricle, then the left, and lastly as it perfuses the myocardium. Therefore, it can be appreciated that myocardial perfusion imaging is accomplished during passage of a single administration of a contrast agent. Typically, this requires compromises to be made concerning selection of the TI and image resolution parameters. For this reason, perfusion contrast is not high, and perfusion images typically require careful evaluation to detect perfusion defects, and can benefit from quantitative analysis. After 5 to 10 minutes following administration of gadolinium, the agent accumulates in regions of infarct. In this case, static, as opposed to dynamic imaging can be used employing the IR contrast and consequently close to optimal contrast is obtained. The presence of a bright delayed enhancement signal indicates lack of viable tissue, and can typically be seen with high spatial resolution and excellent contrast.

## SUMMARY

Gradient echo imaging forms images by recalling the signal as an echo when applying two gradients of opposite polarity. Gradient echo images typically employ a short TR, and incorporation of cardiac gating is typically employed to produce cine images. The spin phase information can be used to encode velocity, and IR contrast can be used to assess myocardial perfusion and viability.

# CHAPTER 18

# Cardiac Triggering

Mark Doyle

## MOTIVATION

It has been said "In CMR, triggering is everything." Although there is always the promise that one day real-time imaging will invalidate that statement, that era is yet to dawn. Given this situation, the following three important prerequisites for cardiac magnetic resonance (CMR) remain:

- Triggering
- Triggering
- Triggering

In short, there is no cardiac image without triggering.

## ESTABLISH A CLEAN ELECTROCARDIOGRAM SIGNAL

First, to establish a strong electrocardiogram (ECG) signal, good contact between the skin and the ECG electrodes is required (see Fig. 18-1). To accomplish this, certain precautions and procedures should be followed:

- If body hair intrudes, it should be shaved off.
- The skin should be abraded to allow effective electrical contact.
- A gel should be used.
- Electrodes of the highest quality should consistently be used.
- The patient should be mandated to wear loose clothing to prevent buildup of sweat, which destroys electrical contact as the study progresses. This is a particularly troubling problem, because to remedy it the patient must be withdrawn, the leads repositioned, and scout scans repeated.
- The airflow in the scanner should be adjusted to keep the patient at a comfortable temperature.

## TIPS AND TRICKS: ELECTROCARDIOGRAM

To ensure good scan quality, it is advisable to spend time up front to obtain a good ECG signal. If signal is weak or otherwise poor, consider the following hierarchy of solutions:

- Change the reference lead at the scanner console.
- Reposition the leads.
- If not contraindicated by the scanner manufacturer, consider positioning the leads on the patient's back (over the heart region).

If the patient has a known myocardial infarction (MI), the triggering signal may be weaker than for a normally functioning heart. Be cognizant that the lead positions may not be the exact configuration required for a patient without an MI. If the location of MI is known, consider positioning the leads toward the side of the heart with the most function. If, after these precautions, the signal is still too weak, only spend a minimal of time changing the signal leads because the solution likely requires repositioning of the leads on the patient. It is therefore advisable to put a few extra pads on in anticipation of this, to allow easier repositioning.

## POSITION ELECTRODES FOR SAFETY

Formally, electrodes could be positioned at widely separated sites on the chest. This effectively formed a wide conductance loop, but the high performance gradients and radiofrequency (RF) of modern scanners can induce currents sufficient to burn the patient. Currently, a tight configuration of electrodes is generally required for safety (see Fig. 18-1).

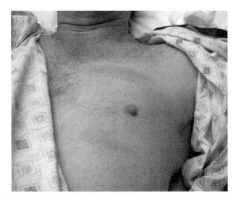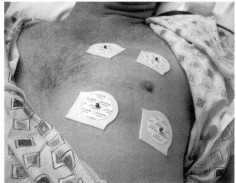

FIGURE 18-1    Patient preparation is shown, whereby hair is shaved and skin abraded in preparation for placement of electrocardiogram (ECG) pads (left panel). The configuration of the ECG pads is shown in the right panel. Note the relatively tight configuration centered on the heart.

## ESTABLISH SIGNAL

After observing normal screening precautions, position the patient on the scanner table, typically feet first. Connect the ECG leads, respiratory gating device, and blood pressure cuff for full monitoring capability. Before positioning any receiver coils, check the adequacy of the signal at the console.

## MANY WORDS ONE PHENOMENON

In the same manner that Eskimos are reputed to have more than 20 words to describe snow, magnetic resonance imaging (MRI) personnel have a wide vocabulary to describe the condition of the ECG signal:

- Normal (a highly nuanced term)
- Weak
- Distorted
- Respiratory breakthrough
- Inverted
- "We can live with it"

## Normal Electrocardiogram Signals

Even the "normal" ECG signal has a grossly distorted "T" wave (see Fig. 18-2). The "T" wave corresponds to a period in the cardiac cycle when blood is rapidly ejected from the heart to the vascular system. Blood, which is a conducting fluid moving in a magnetic field, will generate an electrical signal of its own. This electrical signal adds to the natural "T" wave, essentially broadening and elevating it.

## Weak Electrocardiogram Signals

A weak ECG signal often suffers from "respiratory motion breakthrough" (see Fig. 18-3). In this situation,

the whole ECG drifts up and down with the respiratory cycle, usually resulting in a very erratic triggering capability. To remedy this, consider repositioning leads or reattaching the leads at the same position. Changing the signal lead at the scanner console rarely remedies this problem, and only a minimum amount of time should be spent trying this approach.

## Distorted Electrocardiogram Signals

Distortions take many forms, and surprisingly it is often possible to trigger with grossly distorted waveforms (see Fig. 18-4). The key features to look for in an ECG signal is that the "r" wave is higher and sharper than any other wave feature. If the scanner software detects the trigger point based on signal amplitude, a higher signal is required for successful and consistent triggering. However, in some scanners, the trigger point is sensitive to the maximum rate of change of the signal,

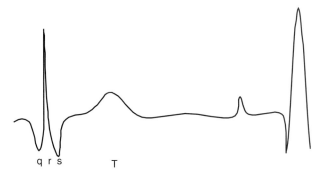

FIGURE 18-2    A normal electrocardiogram (ECG) signal, typical of that obtained in the MRI system featuring the "qrs" complex and the "T" wave. Note that the "T" wave appears elevated compared to a conventional ECG signal due to the electrohemodynamic effect associated with blood moving through a magnetic field and generating its own electrical signal.

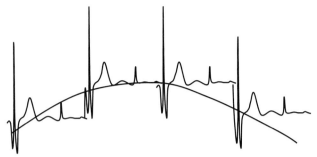

**FIGURE 18-3** A weak ECG signal is susceptible to respiratory breakthrough, whereby the whole of the ECG signal rides up and down with the respiratory cycle.

and therefore a sharply increasing signal is required for consistent triggering.

### Inverted Electrocardiogram Signals

Normally, the "r" wave should be upright. Occasionally the "q" wave will be higher than the "r" wave (see Fig. 18-5). If triggering off the "q" or "s" waves, owing to an inverted "r" wave, the first phase may not reliably correspond to end-diastole. A possible solution is to invert the signal at the console. Alternatively, change the lead positions at the patient.

## PATIENT SCANNING

Once on the scanner table and a strong ECG signal is established, "center" the patient on the midline of the chest, approximately 3 in. above the zyphoid notch.

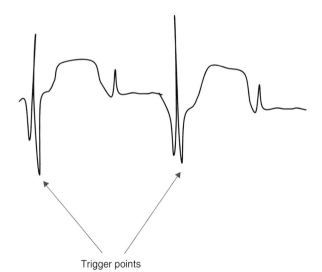

Trigger points

**FIGURE 18-4** A severely distorted ECG signal is shown. In this case, triggering would likely be successful because of the sharp and high waveform features indicated as triggering the scan.

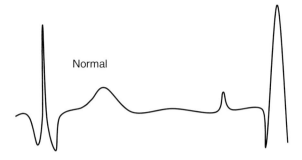

Normal

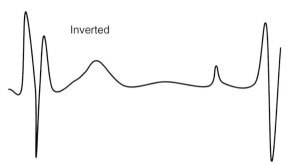

Inverted

**FIGURE 18-5** A normal and an inverted ECG signal are shown. The inverted "r" wave may cause unreliable triggering, and depending on whether the "q" or the "s" waves formed the trigger point, the first phase may be either early or late relative to end-diastole, respectively.

After performing appropriate scout scanning, plan the standard views, such as:

- Vertical long axis, two-chamber view
- Horizontal long axis, four-chamber view
- Short axis views

Each of these views will typically be acquired in a cardiac triggered mode, and it is essential that the cardiac cine data be acquired throughout the full cycle. On some scanners, internal algorithms automatically set cardiac triggering requirements, whereas other scanners may require manual calculations to be performed. In either situation, it is beneficial to know what considerations enter into these calculations.

## IMPORTANCE OF CARDIAC TRIGGERING

For imaging sequences that are triggered to the cardiac cycle we note that individual excitations contribute to a specific k-space map, assigned to that particular part of the cycle (see Fig. 18-6). The nature of MRI requires that each image is generated from a complete k-space matrix. At each point in the cardiac cycle, a complete k-space matrix is built up, line by line. Therefore, to acquire enough k-space lines to form an image at each point in the cycle, data generally have to be acquired

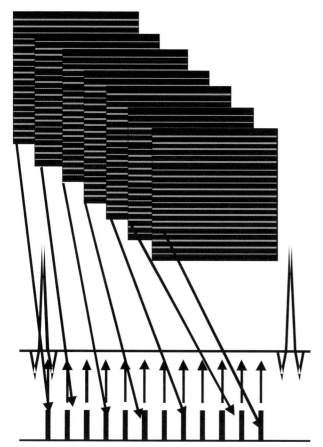

**FIGURE 18-6** At each point in the cardiac cycle where an image is required, a k-space matrix is needed. The requirements of cardiac triggering are to synchronize the acquisition of k-space lines to specific points in the cardiac cycle. Because each k-space map cannot generally be compiled within a single cardiac cycle, it has to be compiled over several cardiac cycles.

over several cardiac cycles. For this reason, reliable cardiac triggering is required.

## SEGMENTED SCANNING

Segmentation is employed to reduce the number of cardiac cycles over which k-space data are obtained. The scan time is reduced in direct proportion to the segmentation factor (see Fig. 18-7). To illustrate how segmentation reduces scan time, consider the following example:

- Basic repetition time (TR) = 4 milliseconds
- Number of views per segment (VPS) = 12
- Segmentation duration = $12 \times 4$ milliseconds = 48 milliseconds
- For a $256 \times 256$ matrix, the scan time is reduced to $256/12 = 21$ heartbeats, allowing it to be performed within a typical breath-hold time

## MAXIMUM NUMBER OF CARDIAC PHASES

The maximum number of cardiac phases that are allowed in segmented scanning can be calculated from knowledge of a few basic parameters:

- RR interval = 60,000/heart rate
- Segmentation duration = VPS × TR
- Maximum number of cardiac phases = RR interval/segmentation duration

  For example:

- TR = 5 milliseconds
- VPS = 10
- Segmentation duration = 50 milliseconds
- Heart rate = 60 beats per minute (BPM)
- RR interval = 1,000 milliseconds
- Maximum number of cardiac phases = 1,000/50 = 20

Depending on the cardiac triggering mode available on your scanner, you may have to set the number of cardiac phases to be less than the maximum allowed to avoid missing detection of the next ''r'' wave (see Fig. 18-8). In this case, it is convenient to make a chart of the maximum number of cardiac phases that can be acquired for a range of heart rates and scan parameters. As we have seen, there are two key variables that determine the maximum number of cardiac phases:

- RR interval
- Segmentation duration

However, it may be more convenient to express these in terms of scanner related variables, such as VPS, TR, and so on.

## VIEW SHARING

Some scanners have ''view-sharing'' options whereby intermediate cardiac phases are generated and inserted in between each of the directly acquired phases (see Fig. 18-9). For example, consider that 15 cardiac phases are specified, then 29 (i.e., $2 \times n - 1$) phases may be generated by a basic view-sharing algorithm. Alternatively, view sharing may be implemented such that the number of phases output is independent of such simple algebraic relationships, that is, these approaches allow freedom of choice of the represented number of cardiac phases, and is independent of the acquired number of cardiac phases. In general, it may be best to consistently select view sharing, because it generally provides increased temporal resolution relative to the acquired phases, and further provides a consistent number of phases, which may streamline additional processing. You will have to determine for your scanner,

**FIGURE 18-7** To speed up the acquisition of each k-space matrix, data segmentation is used. In this example, at each nominal cardiac phase point, three successive lines of k-space are acquired and assigned to the k-space matrix for that cardiac phase. This process is repeated for each nominal cardiac phase, and the k-space acquisition is achieved in one third of the conventional time.

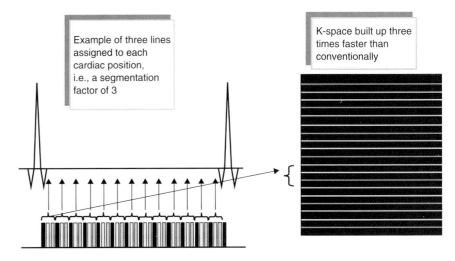

whether you set the number of cardiac phases based on the view-sharing formula or on the basic formula for the maximum number of phases.

## BENEFICIAL VIEW SHARING

It is important to set the segmentation parameter so as to realize a practical benefit. There are two incorrect ways to set the segmentation and view-sharing options:

- Setting the segmentation duration too high will result in motion-related blurring. In general, 50 milliseconds is considered to be the upper limit to obtain sharp cardiac features.
- Setting the segmentation value too low may result in the loss of data due to the appearance of temporal "gaps" that appear between the represented phases in the cardiac cycle.

Consider the following example, where the basic TR is 4 milliseconds, and a segmentation value of 8

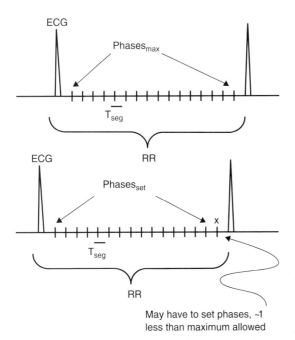

**FIGURE 18-8** A major requirement for cardiac cine imaging is to obtain images over the whole of the cardiac cycle. The maximum number of cardiac phases ($Phases_{max}$) is determined by the time duration of each segment ($T_{seg}$). In the lower panel, the situation is illustrated where one less than the maximum phases is prescribed. This allows the scanner time to detect the next r wave. Some scanners do not have this requirement and can scan up to the last available segment slot.

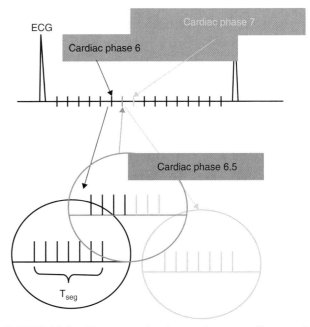

**FIGURE 18-9** The principle of view sharing is illustrated, whereby data from cardiac frames 6 and 7 are combined to form an intermediate cardiac phase (6.5). Ideally, the data from cardiac phases 6 and 7 should be exactly adjacent to each other without any additional time gap between them.

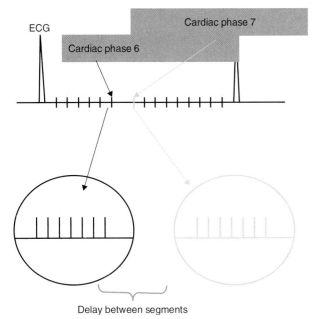

**FIGURE 18-10** Incorrect parameters for view sharing are illustrated. In this example, there is a time delay between cardiac phases 6 and 7. This delay essentially corresponds to loss of data (i.e., dead time when no data are acquired). The segmentation duration and the number of cardiac phases to be acquired should be adjusted to eliminate such gaps.

is chosen, then the segmentation duration is 32 milliseconds. If the RR interval is 1,000 milliseconds and

20 phases are requested, then each represented phase is separated by 50 milliseconds, which in this case results in a gap of 18 milliseconds between each segment. In effect, this is equivalent to throwing away data (see Fig. 18-10). Ideally, the segmentation value should be set high enough such that there is an overlap between the acquired phases and the phases generated by view sharing. For example, if the RR interval is 1,000 milliseconds and the segmentation duration is 50 milliseconds, then the maximum number of acquired phases is 20 (1,000/50). In this case, selecting a number of phases >20, for example, 30 to 40, will allow the view-sharing algorithm to function correctly.

## SUMMARY

"In CMR, triggering is everything."

The three important prerequisites for CMR are:

- Triggering
- Triggering
- Triggering

There is no cardiac image without triggering. Great care should be taken to establish a strong ECG signal upfront and select scan parameters to benefit from the various acquisition and reconstruction options available on your scanner.

# CHAPTER 19

# Inflow Refreshment Angiography

Mark Doyle

## OVERVIEW

Inflow refreshment is a means of achieving bright blood signal, especially for angiographic purposes. The basic mechanism relies on the physical displacement of blood, which quite literally introduces fresh blood signal between slice selective radiofrequency (RF) pulses. The means of applying this in two-dimensional (2D) and 3D imaging will be discussed.

## INFLOW REFRESHMENT MECHANISM

In standard imaging, the signal of interest is usually not the signal produced by an isolated RF pulse, but the signal resulting from a train of RF pulses, that is, under conditions of dynamic equilibrium. Following each RF excitation, the magnetization vector, $\mathbf{M_0}$, relaxes back to alignment with $\mathbf{B_0}$ by the T1 relaxation process. The strength of the transverse signal following a train of RF pulses depends on the imaging parameters and the intrinsic properties of the body:

- TR
- RF pulse angle
- Tissue T1

The optimum equilibrium signal for static tissue is achieved when the Ernst angle is applied. Using a larger flip angle results in a lower equilibrium signal, that is, a degree of signal suppression is achieved. This feature is exploited in 2D time of flight (TOF) or inflow refreshment imaging, to preferentially suppress static tissue.

## FLOW REFRESHMENT

Flowing blood that continuously refreshes the imaging plane does not achieve the equilibrium signal reached by the static tissue, and therefore appears as a relatively bright signal (see Fig. 19-1). This is the basis of the inflow refreshment phenomenon:

- Suppression of static tissue, by means of a high RF flip angle and short TR
- Enhancement of blood signal by virtue of it refreshing the imaging plane

This so-called TOF mechanism relies on blood spins physically refreshing the imaging plane and exiting the plane rapidly, and thereby avoids becoming suppressed in the manner of static tissue signal.

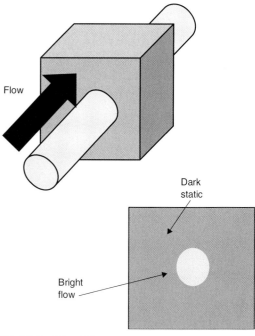

**FIGURE 19-1** Blood flow that traverses the imaging slice at a faster rate than the imaging repetition time (TR) results in fresh blood being excited for each application of the basic imaging sequence. Consequently, flow appears bright, because it essentially contributes a fresh signal for each RF pulse experienced. Conversely, static tissue within the slice, after experiencing a train of RF pulses, will become partially saturated, and suffer loss of signal. This is the basis of the inflow refreshment phenomenon.

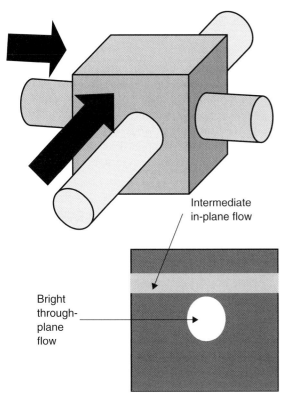

**FIGURE 19-2**   Blood flow that travels predominantly within the imaging plane (*short arrow*), fails to completely refresh the plane during each repetition time (TR) interval, and consequently experiences multiple radiofrequency (RF) pulses before exiting the imaging plane. The signal from this blood flow is therefore lower in intensity compared to the more rapid through-plane flow, and may become isointense with the static tissue signal.

## IN-PLANE FLOW SIGNAL

Flow refreshment is incomplete if the flowing blood has a long residency time in the imaged slice. This occurs primarily under the following three conditions:

- A large in-plane flow component is present
- Slow flow conditions dominate
- Flow which reverses in direction and retraverses the image plane

Under these conditions blood clears the plane slowly, and therefore experiences multiple RF pulses, serving to reduce the signal contribution from flow.

## TIME OF FLIGHT ACQUISITION

In the 2D TOF acquisition, each slice is fully acquired before advancing to the next slice location. In this way, extended coverage of the body is achieved by performing multiple slices, sufficient to cover the region

of interest. In general, the slices are oriented orthogonal to the major direction of flow. Rapid through-plane flow generally appears bright, whereas in-plane flow or slow through-plane flow appears darker or even isointense with the static tissue (see Fig. 19-2). Signal saturation is particularly problematic for the following:

- Tortuous vessels
- Thick slab 3D imaging
- Slow flow near boundary walls

In-plane signal loss is known to be problematic for certain body regions, such as the carotid arteries where they undergo an excursion perpendicular to the main axis of the neck. However, for regions where blood flow is sufficient to refresh each slice, contrast can be very good (see Fig. 19-3). In the abdomen, respiration and peristaltic motion can result in some residual "static" tissue signal, which may obscure arteries when vessel rendering on the basis of signal brightness is used.

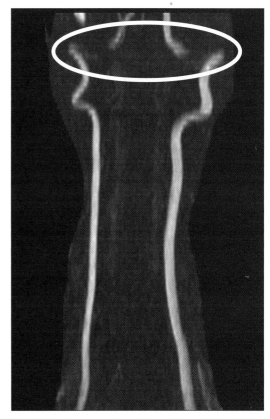

**FIGURE 19-3**   An example of signal loss attributable to the blood vessel path presenting a higher in-plane competent relative to the imaging slice. In this example of the carotid arteries, most vessels are bright, exhibiting high contrast where flow is perpendicular to the imaging slice, but contrast is diminished (*circle*) where the vessels become parallel to the imaging slice.

## TURBULENT FLOW SIGNAL LOSS

Signal loss in gradient echo imaging also occurs in regions of turbulence or high velocity gradients. Signal loss is attributable to the T2* signal loss mechanism. Effectively, T2* increases with turbulence and with high velocity gradients. Under normal arterial flow conditions, the lumen appears bright across its entire diameter on a TOF image. At a region with plaque, signal loss is commonly experienced because of the turbulence. Downstream from the plaque site, as the vessel returns to its normal diameter, the blood flow may experience jet flow. Therefore, in this downstream region, signal loss may be experienced in TOF images. Additionally, high flow gradients that occur within a voxel result in spin dephasing and contribute to signal loss. Therefore, it is common for TOF images to exhibit signal loss over a region larger than the physical extent of the vascular plaque (see Fig. 19-4).

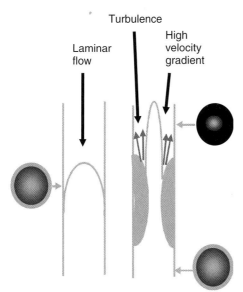

**FIGURE 19-4** Comparison of normal and stenotic vessel flow. On the left, a parabolic flow profile through an unobstructed vessel segment is indicated (*laminar flow*). The corresponding appearance in the TOF image is that of a bright circle, representing the true cross-sectional view of the vessel at that position. On the right, a stenotic vessel is represented with laminar flow before the stenotic region, and jet and turbulent flow in the immediate poststenotic region. Before the stenosis, the TOF appearance of the vessel cross-section correctly corresponds to the true vessel section, but after stenosis the bright signal region is restricted to the central region of the jet flow, whereas the surrounding region of turbulent flow is represented as a region of signal loss. In this way, the region of signal loss may artifactually extend beyond the region of plaque.

## VENOUS SUPPRESSION

To suppress venous flow, a saturation slab can be applied before slice selection, suppressing all inflowing spins from one direction. This approach relies on the predominant direction of arterial and venous flow being opposite each other (see Fig. 19-5). By applying the saturation slab on the venous inflow side of the slice, the venous flow, which is relatively slow, typically experiences several RF saturation pulses before reaching the imaging slice.

## TIME OF FLIGHT IMAGING SEQUENCE

The TOF approach is based on the gradient-recalled echo (GRE) imaging sequence and comprises the following:

- Slab selection
- Slice selection
- Frequency encoding gradient
- Phase encoding gradient
- Signal sampling period

Before slice selection, the slab selection procedure, involving application of an RF pulse and gradient, is applied (see Fig. 19-6). Following slab selection, the remainder of the sequence is identical to a conventional GRE.

## SLICE PROFILE

Ideally, the slice profile is described by a square function with sharp edges. In reality, it is rarely this sharply

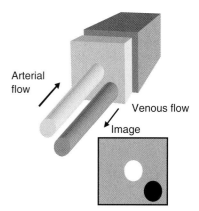

**FIGURE 19-5** The preferential suppression of venous flow is achieved by preceding the slice selective imaging sequence with a suppression slab, positioned on the "downstream" side relative to arterial flow. The suppression slab consists of a selective RF pulse employing a high flip angle. As the venous flow travels through the wide suppression slab, it becomes well suppressed by the time it reaches the imaging plane.

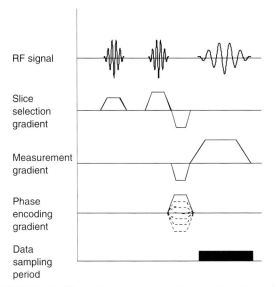

RF signal

Slice
selection
gradient

Measurement
gradient

Phase
encoding
gradient

Data
sampling
period

**FIGURE 19-6** The pulse sequence diagram for time of flight (TOF) imaging is shown. The sequence is similar to the conventional gradient-recalled echo sequence, with the addition of the venous suppression slab selection segment, consisting of the radiofrequency (RF) and the slab selection gradient (*preceeding the main sequence*).

defined, because of the compromises made in selecting a short RF pulse (see Fig. 19-7). The slice profile is more likely tapered at each edge. Owing to the tapered shape of the slice, after application of several RF pulses, the edges of the slice tend to become exaggerated relative to the center. Similar reasoning also applies to the slab

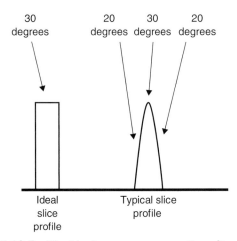

30
degrees

20          30          20
degrees  degrees  degrees

Ideal
slice
profile

Typical slice
profile

**FIGURE 19-7** The ideal square cross-section slice profile (left) is compared against the profile that is more realistically achieved. Ideally, a radiofrequency (RF) flip angle of 30 degrees is to be applied across the slice thickness. In reality, because of the compromises made in the excitation time, the true flip angle may only be realized in the center of the slice, with lower angles being achieved toward the edge of the slice.

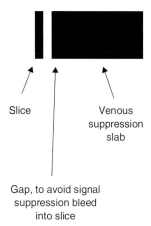

Slice               Venous
                 suppression
                      slab

Gap, to avoid signal
suppression bleed
into slice

**FIGURE 19-8** Owing to imperfections in the imaging slice and venous suppression slab excitations, a gap of several millimeters is left between the slice and suppression slab to avoid cross contamination. Venous flow is not suppressed in the gap, but this is not generally problematic for typical venous flow velocities and sequence repetition times.

selection pulse. Thus, owing to these imperfections, it is usual to allow a gap of approximately 2 to 5 mm between the imaged slice and the venous suppression slab, thereby avoid contamination of the imaging slice due to nonideal slice profiles (see Fig. 19-8).

## TRIGGERED TIME OF FLIGHT

Blood flow is maximal during systole in most of the arterial system, and therefore triggering the acquisition to this part of the cycle increases signal in TOF images (see Fig. 19-9). In a triggered TOF acquisition, two parameters generally control the acquisition window relative to the cardiac cycle:

- Trigger delay from R wave
- Width in milliseconds of the data sampling window

In triggered TOF images, blood vessels are seen with good contrast against a low static tissue signal. Another advantage of triggering the acquisition is that pulsatile flow artifacts are generally low. However, there may be some residual breathing artifacts present. Cardiac triggering does not necessarily avoid respiratory displacement related artifacts that manifest as sudden displacements of the vessels from one slice to another.

## THREE-DIMENSIONAL TIME OF FLIGHT

When imaging body regions supplied by small, tortuous vessels, a 3D approach generally produces better results. The 3D TOF acquisition is applied in the same

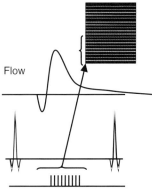

Flow

Data sampling

**FIGURE 19-9** The triggered time of flight sequence is shown. The timing and manner of arterial flow are illustrated in the flow graph. The imaging sequence is triggered to only acquire data during the period when substantial forward arterial flow is present. During this time, several lines of k-space are acquired. When data are not being actively taken, the sequence may perform "dummy acquisitions", whereby the radiofrequency (RF) and gradients are applied, but no data are taken. This maintains the steady state conditions necessary for the sequence to suppress static tissue.

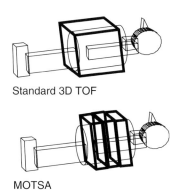

Standard 3D TOF

MOTSA

**FIGURE 19-10** Standard and multiple overlapping slab three-dimensional (3D) approaches are illustrated. In the standard approach, a single 3D slab is excited and directly acquired. To accommodate slower flow, thinner slabs may be acquired, each requiring a proportionately lower number of slice encoding steps. Because the edges of each 3D slab are not generally well defined, a couple of slices are typically discarded at each end. For this reason, overlapping slabs are required to maintain contiguous coverage of the body region. The approach shown here is termed *Multiple Overlapping Slabs For TOF Angiography* (MOTSA). TOF, time of flight.

manner as 2D TOF, with the exception of using a lower flip angle to avoid flow saturation in the wider slab. The wider slab results in a longer transit time for moving spins. Further, the lower flip angle also means that there is lower suppression of static tissue signal. By comparison with 2D TOF, where the slice thickness is typically 4 to 8 mm, 3D encoded slices of thickness of 2 mm are common. Since thinner slices require stronger gradients, in 2D acquisitions they result in long echo times (TEs). One advantage of 3D TOF is that the wide slab can be excited with a weak gradient, and therefore shorter TEs are realizable. Shorter TEs give increased sensitivity to moving blood. However, a major disadvantage of 3D imaging is that flowing blood has a longer residency time in the slab compared to the 2D approach, resulting in increased flow signal saturation. To avoid flow signal saturation, especially toward the

exit plane of the 3D slab, multiple thin slabs can be used, with each slab arranged to overlap the other slabs by a small amount. This approach is termed *Multiple Overlapping Slabs For TOF Angiography* (MOTSA) (see Fig. 19-10). In general, in 3D TOF data a smaller "slice" dimension of the voxel is allowed, because it is encoded rather than excited.

## SUMMARY

TOF angiography relies on physical motion of blood to achieve the desired contrast. Both 2D and 3D approaches are possible, with 3D being used when vessels with a high degree of tortuosity are imaged, because 3D approaches permit smaller voxels. In each case, a TR sufficiently long to allow blood to at least partially refresh the imaging volume is required.

# CHAPTER 20

# Three Dimensional Contrast Angiography

Mark Doyle

## OVERVIEW

Contrast angiography relies on administering a contrast agent that is imaged in a three-dimensional (3D) manner. Here we discuss the acquisition and contrast mechanism, and examine the issues associated with timing the sequence to maximize contrast. Lastly, approaches to rendering the 3D data sets will be discussed.

## BASIC PRINCIPLES

The conventional 2D angiographic approach provides limited coverage because each acquisition is restricted to one slice, although multiple acquisitions can be combined. However, when using an exogenous contrast agent, it is impractical to apply multiple 2D acquisitions, because each requires its own administration of contrast. To extend coverage, a 3D acquisition is used to image a contiguous volume during a single acquisition. Just as two dimensions of k-space are required to represent a 2D spatial slice, similarly three dimensions of k-space are required to represent a 3D volume (see Fig. 20-1). The 3D gradient-recalled echo (GRE) pulse sequence comprises a slab selection pulse (as opposed to a slice selection pulse), a frequency encoding gradient (which is formed by the gradient echo maneuver), a phase encoding gradient, and a slice encoding gradient that is not present in 2D imaging (see Fig. 20-2). The nature of phase encoding gradients is that they are applied multiple times to encode each dimension of k-space. Therefore, because the 3D acquisition requires two separate phase encoding gradients, the acquisition time is inherently long. Consider a 3D acquisition with the following parameters:

- Repetition time (TR) 8 milliseconds
- 256 Frequency encoding points

- 128 Phase encoding points
- 64 Slice encoding points
- Scan time = 8 × 128 × 64 = 66 seconds

## CONTRAST MECHANISM

To perform body angiography, a contrast agent is administered through an intravenous line as a bolus, and is followed by a saline flush to ensure that the agent enters the vasculature. The contrast agent reduces the T1 of the blood as it comes in contact with it. When using a short TR imaging sequence with a relatively high radiofrequency (RF) flip angle, the images become T1 weighted. Under these conditions, tissues that have short T1 relaxation times contribute the highest signals, which in this case would be blood. To obtain optimal contrast, it is important to image the contrast agent during its arterial phase. By waiting too long, venous contamination will occur, obscuring the arterial system. However, because contrast transfers from the arterial to the venous system in 15 to 20 seconds, it is imperative to reduce the 3D acquisition time <1 minute (see Fig. 20-3). This can be partially accomplished by the use of a reduce scan matrix. Consider the following modified 3D acquisition parameters:

- TR 8 milliseconds
- 256 frequency encoding points
- 128 phase encoding points
- 32 slice encoding points
- Scan time = 8 × 128 × 32 = 33 seconds

Another approach to reduce the 3D scan time is to perform centric coding. In this scheme, instead of sampling a full k-space matrix, only the central region is sampled, typically in the shape of an ellipse (see Fig. 20-4). However, this may lead to further reduction in resolution.

**FIGURE 20-1** A two-dimensional (2D) image only provides limited information concerning a thin slice of the body, whereas the vasculature is inherently a 3D structure. The right panel shows the corresponding k-space matrices, that is, a 2D image is formed from a 2D k-space matrix, and a 3D image is formed from a 3D k-space matrix.

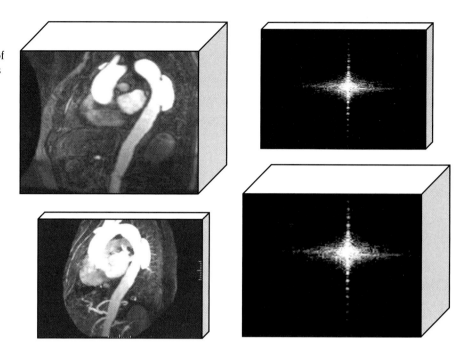

## BOLUS INJECTION

A bolus of gadolinium contrast agent is rapidly introduced using a power injector, which employs a dual syringe system. Because optimal contrast is reliant on precisely timing (to within a second or two) the arrival of the contrast bolus with the imaging sequence, bolus administration is under programmable control from the operator's console. Optimal contrast is also reliant on correct dosage of the agent, which is calculated on the basis of several factors: the extent of the body region to be imaged, the particular contrast agent used, and the imaging purpose. Formulas are used to calculate half dosage (for perfusion), single dosage (for 3D angiography of one region) and double dosage (for 3D angiography of two or more regions).

## IMAGE CONTRAST AND K-SPACE

Image contrast is largely determined by the contrast conditions that pertain for lines acquired near the center of k-space. In contrast angiography, we arrange for the central k-space lines to be acquired during the time interval corresponding to peak contrast conditions as the agent traverses the vascular system. Because there is a fairly wide (~30 seconds) passage time for the contrast agent, it is important to know when the center of k-space is being acquired during this extended acquisition time (see Fig. 20-5). There is varying scanner terminology to indicate when the center of k-space is scheduled to be sampled, for example:

- Centric—the k-space center is sampled at the start of the acquisition
- Reverse-centric—the k-space center is sampled at the end of the acquisition

Additionally, to determine when to start the acquisition relative to the bolus injection, a "timing sequence" is used:

- Inject a small amount of contrast agent.
- Continuously image using a rapid 2D approach.
- Determine (by counting frames) how many seconds after injection it takes for the contrast to arrive in the vasculature of interest.

Usually, the 2D timing bolus scan allows the arrival time of contrast to be easily calculated. However, if there is any doubt about the exact time to initiate the 3D acquisition, it is usually safer to "err on the side of being a little late as opposed to being too early."

## BOLUS FOLLOWING

To obtain a 3D view of the vasculature from several body regions, for example, (1) abdomen, (2) legs, and (3) feet, the patient must be physically moved to image each successive section (see Fig. 20-6). This is referred to as *bolus following*. Typically, up to three "stations" are imaged. The first two stations generally have good contrast, whereas the third station has lower contrast due to venous and tissue contamination.

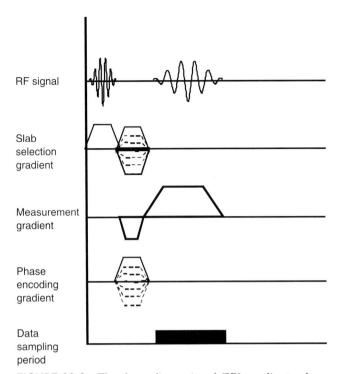

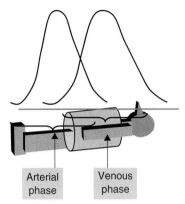

**FIGURE 20-3**  Illustrated here is the timing of the arterial phase of the contrast agent, following a bolus injection, relative to the venous phase. Depending on the length of the bolus injection, the two phases will overlap to some extent. The 3D acquisition has to be accomplished mainly during the arterial phase, and has therefore to be accomplished within 30 seconds.

**FIGURE 20-2**  The three-dimensional (3D) gradient echo imaging sequence is shown. Most features are common to 2D gradient echo imaging, with the exception that instead of slice selection, a slab is selected (however, this is accomplished in exactly the same manner as slice selection), and that an additional phase encoding gradient is applied along the slab selection direction, as indicated by the multiple phase encoding gradients in the slab selection direction. The 3D acquisition is inherently longer than the 2D acquisition because two phase encoding gradients have to be cycled through. RF, radiofrequency.

## TIME-RESOLVED ANGIOGRAPHY

Sometimes, there is no correct timing for the 3D acquisition. This may be due to the physiology of the vascular lesion, which results in differences in opacification times for multiple vessel segments. The best solution to such difficult timing problems in 3D angiography is to obtain the 3D data in a time-resolved manner. However, because the 3D acquisition is a fairly long sequence, this is not normally possible. Fortunately, additional acquisition strategies have been developed specifically for time-resolved protocols. Note that successive frames in a time-resolved angiographic sequence have a high degree of similarity. This high degree of temporal correlation can be exploited to allow k-space sampling in a sparse manner (thereby reducing the scan time) and filling in the unsampled data with interpolated data at the post-processing stage (see Fig. 20-7). By careful consideration of which lines of k-space are to be sampled and at which rate to sample them, the temporally interpolated data can be almost

indistinguishable from fully acquired data (if it were indeed possible to acquire the data fully). One such technique is termed TRICKS: Time Resolved Intensity Contrast KineticS.

Using the time-resolved approach, vessels that are either fast or slow to fill can be better seen. For instance, the late filling due to collateral flow is better appreciated, and superior venous and arterial differentiation can be achieved on a regional basis. However, there are some conditions where time-resolved approaches may fail. When dynamic changes are present that are not accounted for in the interpolation scheme, then artifact will result. Common sources of artifact include the following:

- Respiratory motion
- Peristaltic motion
- Bulk patient motion

## IMAGE RENDERING

3D data is inherently difficult to examine and measure because most of our tools are 2D. For instance, the viewing screen is 2D and it is easier to image and measure distances and areas, as opposed to volumes and depth. A number of 3D data viewing tools have been developed which invariably rely on rapidly viewing a series of successive views to appreciate the 3D nature of the data. In this sense, time has replaced the third spatial dimension. Common 3D viewing options include the following:

- Viewing 2D source images as a movie series
- Maximum intensity projection (MIP)
- Surface rendering

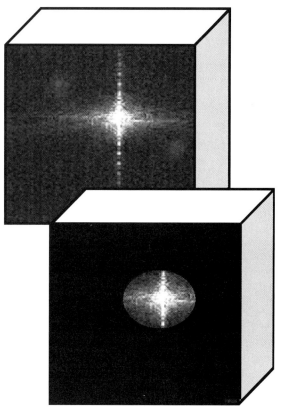

**FIGURE 20-4** In the top panel the full 3D k-space matrix is represented. To encode this fully necessarily requires a long scan time. It is observed that contrast is dominated by the center of k-space, and to speed up the acquisition, some 3D scans, optimized for contrast angiography, will only acquire the central region of k-space. This is termed *centric coding* (lower panel).

- Volume rendering
- Virtual reality

## Source Images

Source images can be viewed as a series of contiguous slices, and these "primary data" views allow measurements to be easily performed. Although these images are generally free of processing artifact, they rely on the user mentally relating each 2D view into a 3D set.

## Maximum Intensity Projection

In MIPs, the brightest (i.e., maximum) intensity value of the volume are projected on to the flat surface corresponding to the viewing direction (see Fig. 20-8). Because MIPs are sensitive to the highest signal, as opposed to the presence of contrast, either uniform signal reception is required or the extraneous high intensity signals have to be edited out. In the editing operation, features that are removed will not contribute to the final image. Projection images have the disadvantage

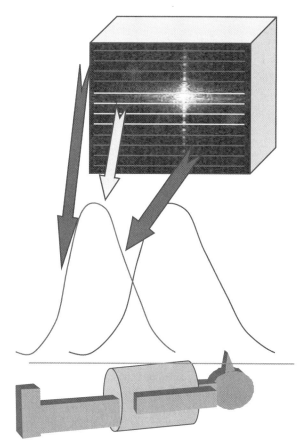

**FIGURE 20-5** A variant of the 3D acquisition designed to ensure capture of contrast during the arterial phase of the agent encodes the central lines of k-space at the time of peak contrast. The outer regions of k-space can in principle be imaged either before or following peak contrast; however, this requires being able to predict when maximal contrast will occur. An alternative is to start imaging when peak contrast is achieved, and in this case start by imaging the central lines of k-space, and then proceed to image the outer lines. This is termed *centric-out coding*.

that bright regions, such as fat around the periphery, may mask the edges of the vessel lumen, obscuring the vessel or making them appear narrower than they really are. Commonly encountered image features that can obscure arterial vascular features include the following:

- Fat signal
- Bright surface features
- Venous structures
- Motion artifacts

Nevertheless, MIPs often provide a quick and convenient way of viewing the vascular extent in the 3D volume (see Fig. 20-9). To enhance the 3D nature of the vasculature, the MIPS are often viewed in a rotating cine mode. Wide fields of views (FOVs) are obtainable for a

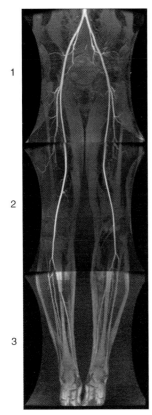

**FIGURE 20-6**   To image an extended region of the body, the concept of bolus following is used. The first station imaged is the region where the contrast arrives first (1). Following this, the body is rapidly advanced to allow imaging of the next station (2), and then advanced a third time to image the lower extremities (3). Notice that in these images, contrast is optimal for stations 1 and 2, but station 3 displays some highlighting of the musculature, because the contrast agent has entered the tissue phase.

single region, whereas lower FOVs are typically used if more than one station is to be imaged.

## Surface Rendering

When the surface of a vessel lumen can be identified by a combination of intensity thresholding and editing, then it is possible to "surface render" the vasculature. The high contrast of 3D angiography often makes surfaces easy to identify. Surface rendering has the following characteristics:

- It requires human interaction to identify vessels segments from a series of images and therefore relevant features may be erroneously excluded:
  - Branch vessels excluded
  - Stenosis missed because of defining generous vessel borders
- Solid surface mode
- Transparent surface mode

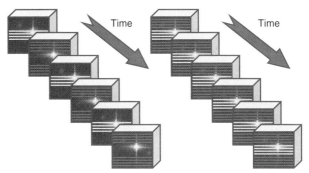

**FIGURE 20-7**   To dynamically image the contrast agent during passage of the contrast agent, a sparse sampling rapid imaging variant is shown. In the sequence illustrated here, only partial regions of k-space are imaged at each time point. The regions sampled are alternated over time (left panel). In the right panel, the completed k-space matrix is illustrated, composed of some regions that are directly sampled (left panel) and some regions that are filled in by mathematical processing. After the series of complete k-space matrices are generated, the passage of the contrast agent can be seen dynamically in 3D.

## Volume Rendering

Volume rendering is a hybrid of the surface rendering and MIP presentation modes. In volume rendering, both depth and brightness affect the image presentation, and a 3D rotation of the rendered image can be used to appreciate the depth and relative position of internal image features. Volume rendering has the following characteristics:

- Surfaces and internal detail can be appreciated.
- Little to no human interaction is required.

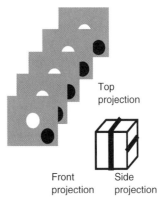

**FIGURE 20-8**   The principle of maximum intensity projection (MIP) rendering is illustrated. The left panel indicates the series of images (from the 3D volume) with vessels highlighted by the contrast agent. The right panel indicates projecting the maximum intensity onto various surfaces from the series of source images. When viewed in projection mode, the images resemble conventional x-ray angiograms.

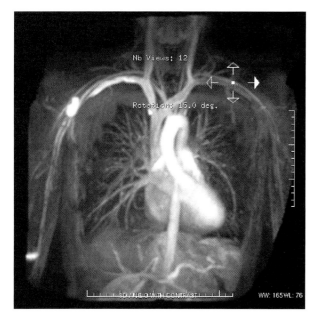

**FIGURE 20-9**    A maximum intensity projection (MIP) image (coronal projection) showing the thoracic vasculature.

- Features can be obscured by bright regions.
- 3D rotation is required.

## Virtual Reality

A view from within the vessel can be obtained using a virtual reality "fly through" (see Fig. 20-10). The vessel is opacified by image processing and the path is manually selected by user interaction. Different branches of vessels must be viewed by successively chosen paths through the vasculature. The closest paradigm for this type of viewing is intravascular ultrasound (IVUS).

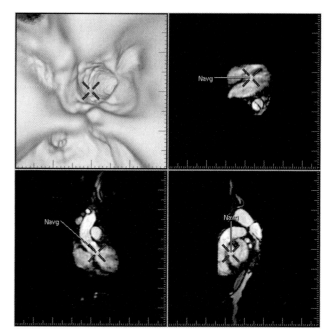

**FIGURE 20-10**    Virtual intravascular view. The top left panel shows the view of the vessel from the inside. The other three views are used to determine, in three dimensions, where the view is relative to the source images.

## SUMMARY

Contrast 3D angiography requires a rapid 3D acquisition, a timed bolus injection of contrast agent and special viewing software to measure and render the 3D angiographic data.

# CHAPTER 21

# Imaging Parameters

Mark Doyle

## OVERVIEW

A common starting point for many topic areas in magnetic resonance imaging (MRI) is the phenomenon of k-space. K-space is essentially the "raw material" from which magnetic resonance (MR) images are derived, that is, it is the signal space. There are a number of important options in the scanner interface that directly affect the manner in which k-space is acquired. These features or options can have a dramatic impact on imaging time, quality, and contrast. Here we will discuss scanner interface features in terms of k-space.

## K-SPACE PROPERTIES

To produce a cardiac image series, we have to balance spatial and temporal resolution features. These can be distributed in a variety of ways, each affecting a different aspect of image quality. Each k-space property has a direct impact on multiple aspects of image quality.

### Dimensions of k-Space

When considering a k-space matrix, "conventional" MRI acquisition methods essentially compile k-space one line at a time. The image is produced by performing the Fourier transform operation on the completed k-space data. Often, the Fourier transform is referred to as the *fast Fourier transform* (FFT), in reference to a particularly efficient mathematical algorithm that is used to perform the operation. One relationship linking the k-space data and the image data is that the dimensions of k-space are the same as the image, for example, a square k-space data set with $128 \times 128$ data points generates an image that is square, also with $128 \times 128$, picture elements, or pixels. In this respect there is a one-to-one correspondence between the number of k-space points and the number of image points.

## Temporal Blur

In cardiac imaging, each image at each cardiac phase is formed from a k-space data set, typically generated as a series of lines, (see Fig. 21-1). For breath-hold approaches, cine images are typically acquired in a "segmented" or "turbo" manner such that each cardiac view is rapidly compiled by acquiring a group of lines or views per segment (VPS), during successive cardiac cycles, (see Fig. 21-2). In a segmented scan, data for each cardiac phase are acquired by a short "string" of acquisitions (e.g., eight views). Each element of the segment has a duration, $T_d$, and thereby the duration of each segment, $T_{seg}$, is given by $T_d$ multiplied by the number of segments (in this example, $T_{seg} = 7 \times T_d$). It is apparent that for a cardiac image series, one of the determinants of scan time is the VPS factor that is used. For example, consider a matrix of $256 \times 256$ being acquired at a rate of one line per cardiac cycle. At this rate, the scan time required extends over 256 heartbeats (~4 minutes, depending on heart rate). By increasing the VPS beyond 1, the scan time is reduced in a linear manner:

- Matrix $256 \times 256$, VPS = 8 scan time = 256/8 = 32 heartbeats
- Matrix $256 \times 256$, VPS = 16 scan time = 256/16 = 16 heartbeats
- Matrix $256 \times 256$, VPS = 20 scan time = 256/20 = 12 heartbeats

The advantage of using a high VPS factor is that scan time is dramatically reduced. However, one disadvantage of selecting too high a VPS value is that temporal blur may result within the cardiac cycle. Consider the example where the repetition time (TR) is 4 milliseconds; the resulting segmentation time (Tseg) increases with increasing VPS values:

- TR = 4 milliseconds, VPS = 8, segment time = 32 milliseconds

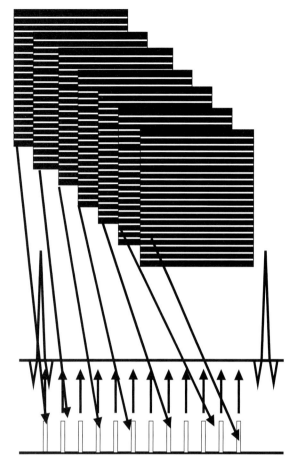

**FIGURE 21-1** In cardiovascular magnetic resonance imaging (MRI), a separate k-space matrix is compiled at each point in the cardiac cycle, that is, during each cardiac cycle, a number of k-space matrices are compiled, and this is necessarily a time-consuming process.

- TR = 4 milliseconds, VPS = 16, segment time = 64 milliseconds
- TR = 4 milliseconds, VPS = 20, segment time = 80 milliseconds

Therefore, as the VPS increases, the degree of temporal blur associated with each cardiac view also increases. Further, when employing data segmentation, the number of cardiac phases that can be fitted into each cardiac cycle is reduced in direct proportion to the VPS value. For example, consider a patient with a heartbeat interval of 1,000 milliseconds. As the VPS value increases, the number of intervals in which data can be acquired decreases:

- VPS = 8, segment time = 32 milliseconds, number of cardiac phases = 1,000/32 = 31
- VPS = 16, segment time = 64 milliseconds, number of cardiac phases = 1,000/64 = 15
- VPS = 20, segment time = 80 milliseconds, number of cardiac phases = 1,000/80 = 12

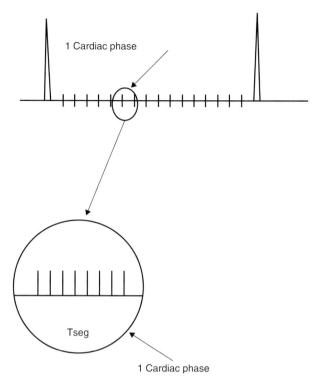

**FIGURE 21-2** In cardiovascular magnetic resonance (CMR), scan time is reduced by employing segmentation. In a segmented scan, each cardiac phase is acquired by a short "string" of acquisitions (eight views in this example). The scan time is reduced by a factor equal to the segmentation factor.

## View Sharing

A processing option that confounds the simple calculations in the preceding text is "view sharing". View sharing can be used to increase the temporal resolution within the cardiac cycle, irrespective of the VPS value selected! Essentially, the view sharing option allows generation of images at intermediate cardiac phases, that is, images are generated in between each directly acquired segmented data set (see Fig. 21-3). In view sharing, k-space data from two directly acquired adjacent cardiac phases are combined to construct an intermediate k-space data set, for example, in the VPS 7 example, the last four views of the cardiac phase number 5 are combined with the first three views of data from cardiac phase number 6 to form cardiac phase 5.5, and so on. In this example, the number of cardiac phases that are represented is almost doubled. For example, if 15 phases are directly acquired, 29 (i.e., $2 \times n - 1$) phases may be generated by view-sharing data. On some scanners, the number of views represented in the final cardiac series can be set almost arbitrarily when more general data interpolation and k-space combination approaches are used. Therefore, caution should be exercised when

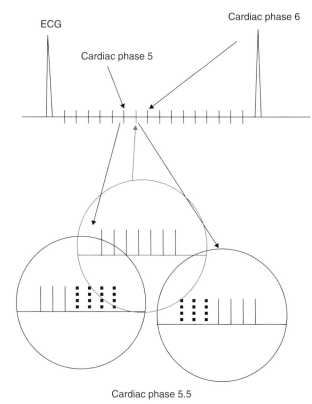

**FIGURE 21-3**    View sharing is a means to create intermediate cardiac phases, that is, between each directly acquired cardiac phase, when segmentation is employed. In view sharing, k-space lines are shared between adjacent cardiac phases, whereby the last few lines of the earlier cardiac phase data are combined with the first few lines of the later phase data (indicated by dashed lines). This process is performed for all phases across the cycle, effectively increasing the number of cardiac phases in the time series. ECG, electrocardiography.

using view sharing, because the statements in the preceding text concerning temporal blurring are still applicable, that is, when using view sharing, although an increased number of cardiac phases are available for inspection, the temporal blur present in each cardiac phase is ultimately determined by the segmentation duration. There are some guidelines in selecting the VPS, as follows:

- An acquisition time of 50 milliseconds per cardiac frame is generally regarded as adequate for imaging myocardial motion, and the selection of VPS should reflect this.
- When imaging faster moving features such as the valve leaflets, 25 milliseconds per frame is recommended, indicating that lower VPS values be used.

## Resolution

Although there are no limits to the extent of k-space, there are limits to the extent to which we sample it.

The extent to which k-space is sampled along any one axis determines the spatial resolution in the image along the corresponding axis. Therefore, to achieve increased resolution, k-space has to be sampled to a wider extent, which for a given field of view (FOV) is reflected in the k-space dimensions. Typical k-space dimensions are as follows:

- $384 \times 384$
- $256 \times 256$
- $256 \times 128$

For a given FOV, increasing the k-space dimensions corresponds to increasing the extent to which k-space is sampled (see Fig. 21-4). The center of reference for measuring distance in k-space is the "origin" of k-space, which corresponds to the center of the data set. The center of k-space is the brightest point, and corresponds to the point where all spins are in phase with each other. Of note, in the preceding examples of k-space dimensions, a matrix of $256 \times 128$ was used instead of a matrix of $128 \times 128$. This is due to the fact that time to obtain a $128 \times 128$ data set would be virtually identical to a $256 \times 128$ data set. This is due to the scan "overhead" required to set up each "measurement" gradient. For example, the TR for a line of resolution 256 could be 4.5 milliseconds, whereas the TR for a line of resolution 128 could be 4 milliseconds. Hence, it is usually more worthwhile to obtain the line that covers more of k-space (i.e., 256 vs. 128) compared to the slight time benefit of obtaining a line of half the extent, and consequently of half the resolution (see Fig. 21-5).

## K-Space Symmetry

K-space has the property of complex conjugate symmetry through the center (see Fig. 21-6). This means that relative to the center of k-space features demonstrate symmetry: consider a feature in k-space, when drawing a line from that feature that passes through the center of k-space, a similar feature will be seen at the same distance along the line on the other side of the origin. Given the observation that k-space is symmetric in this manner, it follows that it is only necessary to acquire one half of k-space, and the other half can be generated at the post-processing stage. In this scenario, the acquisition time should be halved compared to a full k-space scan, and the resolution should be retained, being governed by the extent of k-space sampled. What is affected in this reduced acquisition is the signal-to-noise ratio (SNR), which is reduced by a factor of the square root of 2 in this case. There is a practical caveat to the use of this symmetry feature, in that in reality, imperfections in the scanner system (e.g., gradient eddy currents) introduce distortions that disrupt the expected symmetry. However, by sampling a few percent of k-space

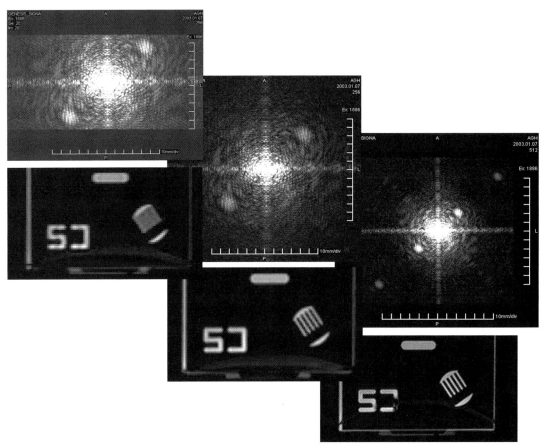

**FIGURE 21-4** Three examples of k-space sampling grids are shown: $256 \times 128$, $256 \times 256$, $384 \times 384$. By sampling k-space to a wider extent in each direction, the resolution is increased. The corresponding images are shown, revealing the increased resolution.

lines symmetrically about the origin, the nature of the distortions can be documented and corrected at the post-processing stage. On the scanner, the parameter that activates the asymmetric sampling of k-space may have terminology such as the following:

• Partial NEX (number of excitations)
• Partial FOV imaging
• Asymmetric k-space sampling

Typically, the parameter indicates the percentage or fraction of k-space that is sampled: for example, a value of 0.5 indicates that only one half of k-space is acquired (see Fig. 21-7). In practice, due to the requirement to sample a few lines symmetrically, even a 0.5 value only reduces the scan time by approximately 40%. A good practical compromise is to accept a lesser reduction in scan time, such as 0.75, which retains the regions of k-space that typically contain high signal. Using a value of 0.75 reduces the scan time by 25%, but only minimally reduces the SNR. In the partial k-space scanning approach, resolution is preserved compared to a full scan, the scan time is reduced, and the SNR is diminished.

## Field of View

Irrespective of the extent to which k-space is sampled, the sampling density, that is, the number of lines per unit k-space distance can be set separately. The density of sampling of k-space determines the FOV that can be imaged without being affected by aliasing artifacts. For example, if the heart were physically isolated in the center of the scanner, then to image it with high resolution would only require a low resolution k-space set, for example, $64 \times 64$ with the FOV set proportionally low at 10 cm (pixel resolution in this case is 1.6 mm$^2$). However, the heart is typically surrounded by the body, and therefore it is necessary to set the FOV accordingly, for example, at 40 cm, and appropriately increase the k-space sampling dimensions, for example, to $256 \times 256$ to maintain the pixel resolution of 1.6 mm$^2$. In this scenario, the resolution achieved in each image was equivalent, that is, 1.6 mm$^2$. Therefore, by the arguments developed so far, the extent of k-space must be identical in each case. Yet in the first example, k-space was fully represented by 64 lines whereas in the second case 256 lines were required. The feature that changed between

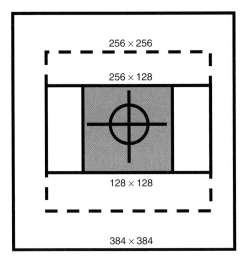

**FIGURE 21-5** For four different k-space matrices, the extent and relative position of each acquisition is shown: Each k-space matrix is "centered" on the center of k-space (defined as the point where all spins are in phase); the 384 × 384 matrix is represented by the large solid square, the 256 × 256 matrix is represented by the dashed square, the 256 × 128 matrix is represented by the solid rectangle and the 128 × 128 matrix is represented by the small shaded square.

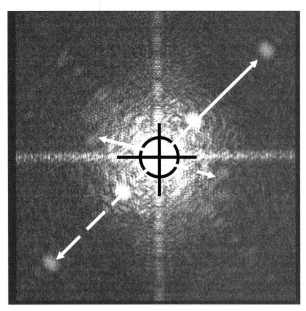

**FIGURE 21-6** K-space has a special type of symmetry: whereby the center acts as a mirror point, such that a line drawn from any k-space feature through the center and continued past the center to the equidistant point on the other side of k-space will show the same feature.

the two cases was the density with which k-space was sampled. Therefore, density of sampling k-space relates to the FOV that can be unambiguously represented: that is, when the extent of k-space sampling is fixed, doubling the number of k-space lines (i.e., number of lines representing k-space) will double the FOV, and similarly quadrupling the number of lines (e.g., from 64 to 256) similarly quadruples the FOV (e.g., from 10 to 40 cm). Conversely, if the imaged object extends beyond the selected FOV, the signal from it will not be correctly dealt with and the extra extent of the object will fold over into the image, that is, the so-called signal aliasing or fold-over artifact (see Fig. 21-8). One way to appreciate the signal aliasing artifact is to consider a one-dimensional (1D) signal sampling problem: a sinusoidal waveform is digitally sampled such that a maximum of 64 Hz can be detected. When a 10 Hz sinusoidal waveform is digitally sampled at the fixed sampling rate (i.e., sampling density), the Fourier transform of the signal correctly indicates that the resonant frequency present is at 10 Hz, indicated by a corresponding peak at the 10 Hz position. Similarly, when a sinusoidal waveform of frequency 50 Hz is sampled, and the signal Fourier transformed, the peak in the Fourier coefficient domain is positioned at 50 Hz. However, when a 100 Hz sinusoid is digitally sampled at the same fixed rate, in this instance the Fourier transformed signal indicates that the peak is positioned at 36 Hz. This is because 100 Hz is approximately 36 Hz higher than the maximum

frequency that could be represented by that sampling rate, that is, the signal has aliased because of using too low a sampling density. To prevent signal from aliasing, the waveform should be sampled at a higher rate. If this were performed, the total sample interval would remain the same whereas the sampling density would increase (i.e., the number of points describing the waveform would be increased). One practical outcome of this is related to the observation that in certain orientations and cross-sections, the body may have substantially lower physical dimensions in one direction compared with the other primary direction. In such cases it is advantageous to scan with a rectangular matrix, that is, a rectangular FOV. Under conditions that the matrix and FOV are both rectangular, the pixel resolution is preserved (i.e., pixels are square, e.g., 1 × 1 mm). A rectangular matrix can be initiated using a parameter such as "phase FOV" or "rectangular FOV", with a value selected <1.0, for example, 0.75. In this example, if the full k-space data set was 256 × 256, a rectangular FOV value of 0.75 will produce a k-space matrix of 256 × 192. Therefore, a partial, or rectangular phase FOV can be used to reduce the scan time while preserving resolution. The features that are diminished in a rectangular FOV image are the FOV in 1D and the SNR (see Fig. 21-9). It is possible to combine rectangular phase FOV and partial k-space sampling. However, the law of diminishing returns dictates that the time benefit becomes progressively less as multiple acceleration factors are compounded.

**FIGURE 21-7** Owing to the symmetry of k-space, it is possible to acquire as little as 50%, and by knowledge of the symmetric nature, generate the missing k-space data at the post-processing stage. Shown here is a close to 50% acquisition of k-space, which generates an image that is comparable to a fully acquired image.

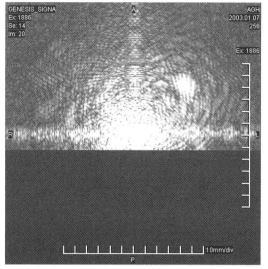
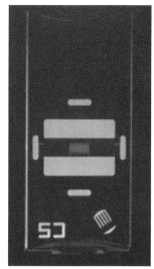
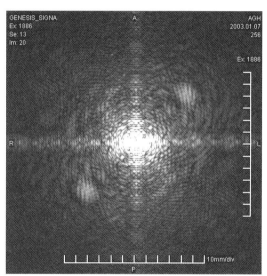
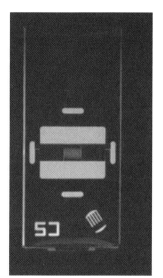

**FIGURE 21-8** To illustrate signal aliasing, compare an image of a fully-sampled k-space matrix, with an image of a k-space matrix sampled at half the density of lines. In this case, the signal aliases by 50%, but note that where image features are seen unobstructed, the resolution is identical in each case.

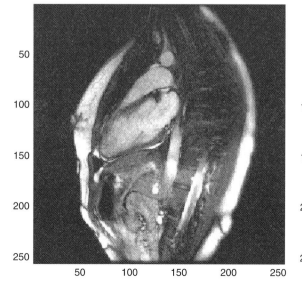
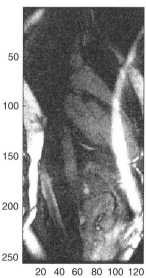

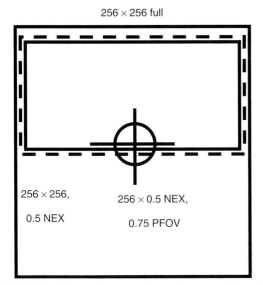

256 × 256 full

256 × 256, 0.5 NEX

256 × 0.5 NEX, 0.75 PFOV

**FIGURE 21-9**   Shown here are the relative position of k-space coverage for a full 256 × 256 scan (large square); a 50% partial matrix acquisition (solid rectangle); and a 50% partial matrix acquisition combined with a 75% rectangular field of view (dashed rectangle). Note that the dashed and solid rectangles are coincident, the feature that is different between them is the sampling density with which k-space is covered. NEX, number of excitations; PFOV, partial field of view.

## No Fold-Over Feature

We have seen that when sampling at too low a density (low compared to the FOV and resolution), aliasing will result. Some scanners may have a parameter to prevent signal aliasing. Without this parameter set, a conventional image will exhibit fold over when the FOV is set too small. In the conventional image case, k-space is sampled in a symmetric manner, that is, with the center of k-space positioned at the center of the data set. When the "no signal aliasing" parameter set, and the FOV kept constant, the scan time is only marginally increased and yet no signal aliasing is seen! The parameter causes k-space to be sampled at a higher density (increased FOV) but in an asymmetric manner such that overall scan time is not increased. While this parameter produces an unaliased image, and scan time is not increased, the disadvantage is that instead of being able to view the extra extent of the view, that image data is discarded by the scanner. In this instance, it would have been better to manually increase the FOV and turn on the partial NEX option.

## K-Space Digital Resolution

All signals that we deal with in MRI are digitally sampled. Unfortunately, this does not represent the data as smoothly as it could. Consider a 1D waveform that is digitally sampled: as the waveform frequency increased, the peaks and troughs get proportionally closer together, and although the digital sampling rate is sufficient to capture this information, the resulting display can appear irregular; that is, even when the correct sampling rate is applied data can be misrepresented. To overcome this limitation of digital sampling, data interpolation can be used. In the case of digitally sampled data, this can make the data appear closer to the true waveform. In Fourier analysis, data interpolation is accomplished by a process known as *zero filling*, and some of the interpolation parameters may reflect this process, such as the "ZIP" option to accomplish Zero filling

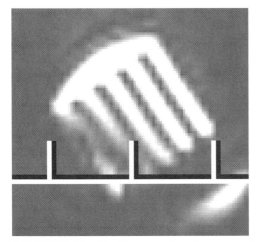
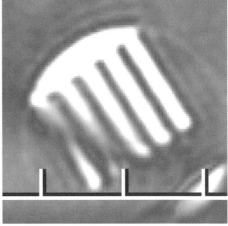

**FIGURE 21-10**   To illustrate the advantage of data interpolation in 3D acquisitions, a "raw", that is, uninterpolated image feature is shown (left), showing the stair-step artifact and compared to the interpolated image (right), which shows a smooth representation all image features.

InterPolation. The data sets that suffer the most from low digital sampling rates are 3D acquisitions. In the 3D acquisition, there are three digitally sampled dimensions. Typically, two of the dimensions are sampled relatively poorly. Therefore, 3D acquisitions are particularly susceptible to "digitization" errors. When data interpolation is applied, image features, especially features at an angle to the major axes, lose their "stair-step" pattern and are represented more smoothly (see Fig. 21-10). The interpolation feature does not affect scan time but helps to make edges appear sharper and less discrete.

## Putting It All Together

In a scan session, all these parameters and more are combined to produce the final product. Depending on the ability of the patient to breath-hold or the resolution sought for feature identification, the parameters are chosen to optimize resolution while balancing scan time and the SNR. In addition to considering spatial resolution, cardiac cine imaging also has to balance temporal resolution, and this is largely dominated by the choice of VPS. As the VPS increases, the scan time decreases but temporal blur progressively increases. Therefore, temporal demands also enter into the equation to obtain diagnostic quality images.

## SUMMARY

K-space has many attributes, and the scanner interface allows these to be controlled in a precise manner. Although rarely seen, k-space is the hidden feature of cardiovascular magnetic resonance (CMR), mastery of which allows excellence in imaging to be achieved, even under adverse conditions.

# CHAPTER 22

# Spin Echo

Mark Doyle

## OVERVIEW

Spin echo (SE) imaging is a class of imaging sequences that utilize an SE to form an image. This will be introduced in the context of k-space imaging requirements (which are briefly summarized). The major application areas of SE imaging include the following:

- Morphology
- Fat or water imaging
- T1 contrast

The property that makes SE most suitable for morphologic imaging is the lack of a blood signal, that is, it is a "black blood" sequence.

## SPIN ECHO IMAGING—BASIC PRINCIPLES

As is common to all imaging sequences, spatial information is encoded by application of magnetic gradients to the spin system. To form an image, it is necessary to acquire an array of data, and it is convenient to arrange the data in the format required by k-space. When arranged in this manner, generation of an image is straightforward, because application of a Fourier transform will produce an image directly. As was described for gradient echo imaging, to encode each k-space line requires application of two separate gradients:

- Frequency encoding gradient, for example, X
- Phase encoding gradient, for example, Y

This terminology is common to other imaging sequences such as gradient echo, and again, there is a requirement for a time delay between slice selection and signal read out, which is required for performing phase encoding. In this case, that delay is achieved by recalling the signal as an SE.

## SPIN ECHO

In an SE, the sequence of events is illustrated in Fig. 22-1:

- Application of an initial radiofrequency (RF) pulse brings the spins into the transverse plane.

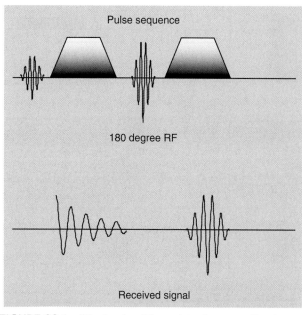

**FIGURE 22-1** The basis of the spin echo operation is shown here. In the top panel, the radiofrequency (RF) and gradients are shown and in the lower panel, the received RF signal is shown. Initially, a 90-degree RF pulse is applied and is followed by a positive gradient that causes the signal to decay as spins dephase. This is followed by a 180-degree pulse, which instantaneously reverses the phase conditions of the spin system. Consequently, when a second positive gradient is applied, it serves to unwind the phase of the spin system. At the midpoint of the second gradient, spins come in to phase alignment and form a spin echo signal.

- Immediately following this, a positive gradient is applied.
- A second RF pulse is applied.
- This is also followed by a positive gradient.
- Spins refocus as an echo during the second positive gradient.

Application of the initial gradient results in signal decay, because spins that are distributed throughout the imaging slice dephase relative to each other. Application of the second RF pulse causes the spins to instantaneously reverse their trajectory (this is elaborated upon in the following section) and therefore application of a gradient with the same polarity as the initial gradient results in signal regrowth as the spins gradually come back into phase. When all the spins are back in phase, the signal is maximal, and an echo peak is formed. As the gradient continues to be applied, spins lose phase coherence, and the signal decays. The echo time, or TE (i.e., time to the echo), is defined as the time from signal origination to the echo peak.

Following application of the first 90-degree RF pulse (in combination with a gradient), the spins dephase. Because the gradient simply adds to or subtracts

from the main magnetic field, spins which experience a net increase in the field strength evolve in phase in a positive manner to their final position, whereas spins that experience a net decrease in the magnetic field evolve in phase in a negative manner. Therefore, following application of the first gradient, spins at different locations experience a net phase difference relative to each other. The essential feature to be aware of in the SE is the action of the second RF pulse. The second RF pulse has the strength to completely flip the spin system through 180 degrees (a so-called pancake flip). Consider the spin that was most advanced in phase, following the 180-degree pulse, it is flipped to the phase conditions that would have been produced under a negative gradient. Similarly, the spin that experienced the most negative gradient, when flipped by the 180-degree pulse acts as if its phase evolved in a corresponding positive gradient. Immediately following the 180-degree pulse, the phase of the entire spin system has been effectively reversed. Therefore, application of a second gradient with the same polarity as the original gradient now serves to "unwind" the spins system. This causes the spins to gradually refocus and form the SE.

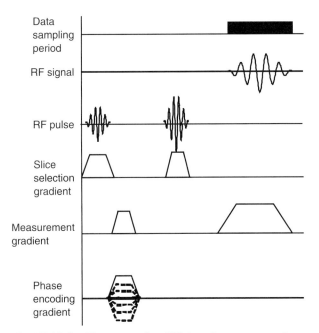

**FIGURE 22-2** The spin echo (SE) imaging sequence is shown. The transmitted radiofrequency (RF) pulses are applied in conjunction with slice selection gradients. The first RF pulse is 90 degrees and brings the spins into the transverse plane, whereas the second pulse is 180 degrees and refocuses spins as an echo signal. The frequency encoding (measurement) gradient is applied in a positive manner, and split to either side of the 180-degree refocusing pulse. The phase encoding gradient is applied in a stepwise manner, and the signal digitized during the formation of the spin echo.

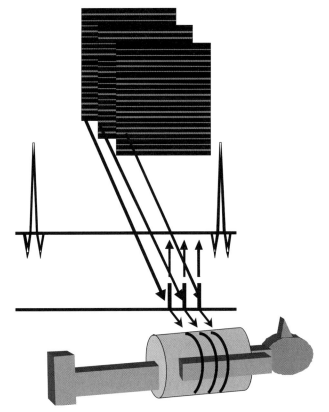

**FIGURE 22-3** When applying the spin echo (SE) sequence in a cardiac triggered manner, it is common to image several slices. Each slice is effectively imaged at a distinct and different portion of the cardiac cycle.

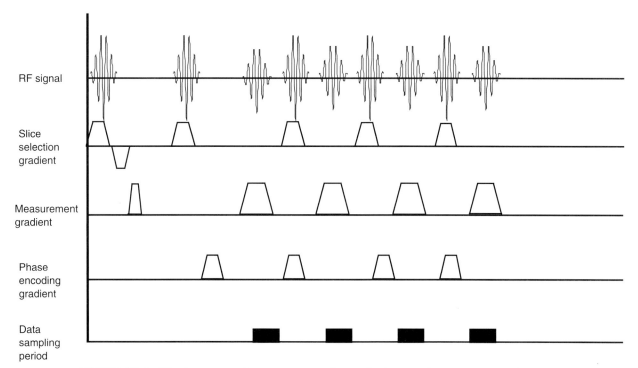

**FIGURE 22-4** The fast spin echo sequence is shown. In this rapid scan, several echoes are recalled, with each one contributing to a different line of k-space. For each echo recalled, a separate 180-degree refocusing pulse is applied in conjuction with the slice selection gradients. Each echo of the series contributes to a separate line of k-space corresponding with data sampling. In this way, upwards of 16 lines of k-space can be acquired from a single excitation of the spin system. RF, radiofrequency.

## SPIN ECHO PROPERTIES

Because the second RF pulse refocuses gradients in the same polarity gradient, any gradients that are present due to inhomogeneities in $\mathbf{B_0}$ will also be refocused. Therefore, the SE signal is diminished by the T2 process, but not by T2*. To contribute to the SE, spins must receive both RF pulses. Therefore, mobile spins will not fully contribute to an SE if each pulse is applied in a slice selective manner. For this reason, SE images are sometimes termed *black blood images*, due to the general lack of blood signal.

## SPIN ECHO PULSE SEQUENCE

The SE sequence comprises the following:

- Slice selection
- First gradient, which forms the first half of the frequency encoding or measurement gradient
- Phase encoding gradient
- Second refocusing RF pulse
- Second lobe of the frequency encoding gradient, during which the signal is digitally sampled for k-space

Note that the phase gradient is applied once to encode each k-space line, and therefore the basic imaging sequence must be applied multiple times to compile a complete k-space matrix (see Fig. 22-2).

## CARDIAC SPIN ECHO IMAGING

To form a series of images triggered to the cardiac cycle, a separate k-space matrix is acquired at each point in the cardiac cycle (see Fig. 22-3). Therefore, the acquisition of each matrix in a cardiac-triggered study requires several cardiac cycles to complete. Typically, SE images are acquired in diastole and are used to identify morphologic features as opposed to examining cardiac function. Consequently, in a grouped acquisition, individual k-space matrices are more typically acquired corresponding to different slices of the body as opposed to one slice imaged at different times in the cardiac cycle.

## FAST SPIN ECHO

For breath-hold approaches, SE images are typically acquired in a "segmented", or "turbo" or "fast" manner. In this mode, for each k-space matrix, during each cardiac

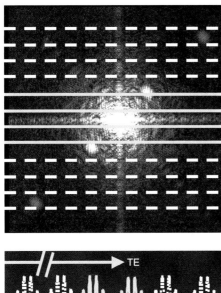

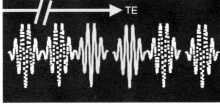

**FIGURE 22-5** The T2 contrast of the image is determined by the echo time (TE) of the system. In a fast spin echo sequence, a train of spin echoes are formed, as illustrated in the lower panel. The TE that is designated for the sequence is determined by the timing of the k-space lines contributing to the central region of k-space. As illustrated here, the solid line echoes encode the central lines of k-space (upper panel), and the echo time of these determines the TE of the sequence. Lines acquired earlier or later (dashed line echos) are assigned to the outer regions of k-space as illustrated.

cycle several lines are acquired. This group of lines, describing a segment of k-space, is characterized by the number of views per segment (VPS), or equivalently by the echo train length (ETL). Typically, the VPS is set relatively high, with values in the range 18 to 24 being common. In a fast SE, each line of k-space corresponds to a separate echo. Therefore, in this variant, multiple echoes are required, each being formed by applying separate refocusing pulses (see Fig. 22-4). For each VPS grouping, a single slice selection is sufficient to service several 180- degree pulses, with a separate phase encoding gradient applied for each echo. Consequently, multiple echo times contribute to each k-space matrix. However, only one image is formed. This raises the questions of which TE best characterizes the sequence, and what factors determine signal contrast.

## IMAGE CONTRAST AND K-SPACE

Image contrast is largely determined by conditions that pertain to lines acquired near the center of k-space.

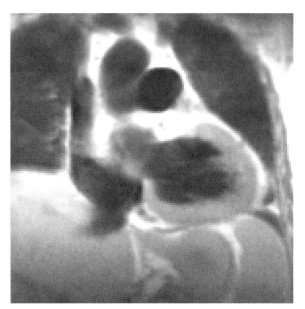

**FIGURE 22-6** A spin echo image of the heart is shown. Blood is seen as a lack of signal, that is black blood imaging, and myocardial signal is of intermediate intensity, whereas the fat signal is bright.

Therefore, the TE for the lines of k-space taken at or near the center of k-space determines the echo time for the image, and this dominates image contrast (see Fig. 22-5). Simply stated, the outer lines of k-space have little influence on image contrast, and thereby acquiring them either earlier or later than the effective TE has little

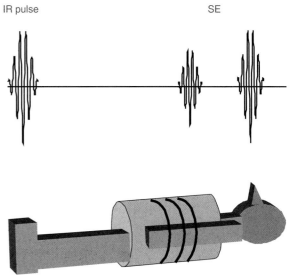

**FIGURE 22-7** The inversion recovery (IR) prepulse is shown in conjunction with the spin echo sequence (only the radiofrequency [RF] pulses are shown). The essential feature is that the IR pulse is applied some time before the spin echo (SE) imaging sequence. The recovery period between the IR pulse and SE imaging, that is, the time for inversion, TI, determines the T1 contrast of the image.

influence on contrast. Conversely, the central k-space lines dominate image contrast. In fast SE, where an extended echo train is acquired, the central k-space lines will be acquired close to the desired TE, with earlier and later echoes assigned to the outer k-space regions.

## SPIN ECHO TERMINOLOGY

The terminology of SE is similar to that of other imaging sequences:

| | |
|---|---|
| TE | Echo time |
| TR | Repetition time of the basic "pulse sequence" |
| Pulse sequence | The imaging procedure, that is, spin echo |
| Relaxation time | Spin-lattice relaxation, T1 and spin–spin, T2 |

Typical values for the imaging sequence parameters are as follows:

| | |
|---|---|
| TR | Long, 600–2,000 milliseconds |
| TE | Long, 20–300 milliseconds |
| Blood | Black, due to spins not refocusing |
| Fat | Bright |
| Myocardium | Intermediate |

SE imaging is typically used to image morphology (see Fig. 22-6), and to aid this, additional contrast mechanisms are used, including inversion recovery (IR) imaging, which provides T1 contrast.

## INVERSION RECOVERY CONTRAST

IR is a prepulse that is applied in conjunction with conventional SE imaging (as well as with other imaging sequences). In IR-SE, an initial 180-degree RF pulse is applied to invert the spin system (see Fig. 22-7). This is followed by a recovery period, when the conventional SE pulse sequence is applied. The SE sequence images the spin system under conditions brought about by the IR sequence. Consider a spin with a short T1, such as fat, and a spin with a long T1, such as, myocardium (see Fig. 22-8). At the initial inversion pulse, both spins are inverted. However, during the recovery period, the short T1 spin relaxes back faster than the long T1 spin. Because the recovery rates are different between the spin systems, the net transverse signal that is seen when the SE sequence is applied will reflect these conditions. In this way, it is possible to preferentially null either the fat signal or the myocardial signal. Because SE requires multiple RF pulses, blood that moves between applications of each pulse will not experience all the pulses that are necessary to contribute to the image.

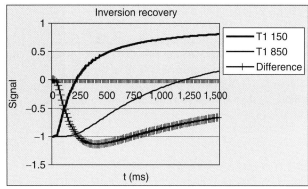

**FIGURE 22-8**    The basic inversion recovery (IR) contrast mechanism is illustrated here. The signal is plotted for two spins, one with a T1 of 150 milliseconds and one with a T1 of 850 milliseconds. On initial application of the IR pulse, both spin systems are inverted (negative 1 signal). As time progresses, the short T1 spins relax rapidly, whereas the long T1 component relaxes back to positive 1 level at a slower rate. Consider applying the SE imaging sequence at approximately 200 milliseconds. At this time, the net signal from the low T1 component is zero, whereas the long T1 component still has a high (negative) value, thereby yielding high contrast between them. The net difference between the two spin systems is plotted, and shows a peak difference at approximately 300 milliseconds, after which time it gradually decays to zero.

Consequently, rapidly moving blood will not contribute to the SE images. It is possible to extend this principle to further suppress blood by applying multiple IR sequences before performing SE imaging, such that even slow moving blood with be suppressed, that is, by employing a double or triple IR sequence (see Fig. 22-9). The IR pulse suppresses either myocardial or fat signal

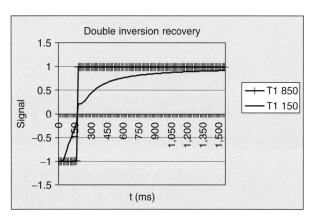

**FIGURE 22-9**    The basis of the double inversion recovery (IR) sequence is shown. Here, the initial IR pulse is followed by a second IR pulse applied at the null time of the short T1 component. The second IR pulse has no net effect on the nulled spins, but reinverts the long T1 spins, back up to positive 1 level.

**FIGURE 22-10** A fat and water phantom is imaged under different inversion recovery (IR) conditions. In the first panel, both fat and water contribute strong signals, whereas in the second panel, the IR delay is selected such that fat is preferentially nulled, while water contributes a strong signal.

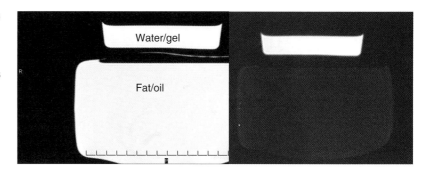

by employing a long or a short IR delay, respectively (see Fig. 22-10).

## SUMMARY

In SE imaging, because blood shows as a lack of signal and fat and myocardial signal are both bright, it is primarily used to image morphologic features. Further, contrast between fat and myocardium can be enhanced and controlled by use of the IR prepulse, which further suppresses blood signal from slow moving blood. SE is not commonly used for cine imaging, and is instead primarily applied to image multiple slices.

# CHAPTER 23

# Fat and Water Properties in Cardiovascular Magnetic Resonance Imaging

Mark Doyle

## OVERVIEW

Fat and water signals are very important in producing contrast in cardiovascular images, allowing differential diagnosis, and identifying cardiovascular features. There are several properties that differentiate fat and water signals including the following:

- T1
- T2
- Resonance frequency

These can be exploited in a number of ways in cardiovascular magnetic resonance (CMR).

- T2 contrast
- Bright versus dark fat and water signal
- Double and triple inversion recovery (IR)
- Phase sensitive IR imaging
- Chemical shift imaging

## T2 Contrast

In general, the echo time (TE) parameter determines the sensitivity to T2. The T2 of myocardium, 80 milliseconds, is relatively low compared to its T1, 850 milliseconds. In contrast, the T2 of fat, 110 milliseconds, is relatively long compared to its T1, 260 milliseconds. In broad terms, for cardiac imaging there are two TE regions of interest:

- Short TE approximately 4 milliseconds
- Long TE approximately 200 milliseconds

The decay curves describing T2 signal for myocardium and fat are such that in the short TE range very little differentiation is realized (the signal decays in each material by approximately 10% for the TE range 0 to 30 milliseconds) (see Fig. 23-1). Further, in the long TE range, although modest differentiation is achieved (fat being approximately 50% brighter), further differentiation based solely on T2 weighting is not easily achieved.

## T2 and Gradient Echo

In general, gradient echo sequences are designed to be sensitive to flow. For this reason the lowest TE is generally the best choice, because it maximizes the sensitivity to flow. In this case, fat and water signals are not strongly differentiated on the basis of T2, but are more influenced by T1 relaxation. Disruption of the blood flow signal is not strongly influenced by T2, but T2* is increased in the presence of turbulence. Effectively, T2* decreases with increasing turbulence and in regions of increasing velocity gradients. Therefore, turbulent and accelerating flow may appear as low signal regions.

## T2 and Spin Echo

The spin echo sequence is predominantly used in the fast spin echo mode: A series of echoes are acquired to produce a segmented scans. In the fast spin echo sequence, TE times can be relatively long, and fat appears brighter than water. However, there is not much further differentiation due to TE in the range 150 to 300 milliseconds.

## FAT, WATER, AND FREQUENCY

Fat and water each contribute a strong signal in the proton resonance. The fat resonance frequency is 1.5 parts per million (ppm) separated from water. At 1.5 T, this evaluates to 224 Hz (i.e., 64 MHz × 1.5 ppm). When the scanner frequency is set to resonate at the water frequency, water is always the "in-phase signal," (see Fig. 23-2). This is accomplished

**FIGURE 23-1** T2 decay of fat relative to water: over the short echo time (TE) range (0 to 30 milliseconds) fat and water signals decay by <10%; as time proceeds, the water signal (e.g., myocardium) decays faster than the fat signal and some appreciable fat–water contrast is generated. However, beyond 150 milliseconds, the contrast between the two tissues changes relatively slowly.

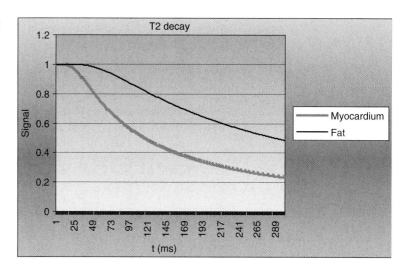

by setting the resonance frequency of the system to 64 MHz (for 1.5 T systems). The scanner detects this frequency as a uniform signal because it compares each signal against this reference frequency. This type of detection is said to take place in the "rotating reference frame," that is, by comparing the detected signal frequency against an internal reference frequency, the detector is effectively rotating in synchronization with the reference frequency. Another term for this is phase-sensitive detection (PSD). At 1.5 T, the reference frequency of water is 64 MHz. As the water and fat resonances are separated slightly in frequency they produce a beat pattern as they drift in and out of phase. This leads to distinct "out-of-phase" and "in-phase" times of 1.8 milliseconds, and 4.2 milliseconds,

respectively. Tissue that is composed of a combination of fat and water can be imaged to appear as:

- Dark (i.e., signals are out of phase)
- Bright (i.e., signals are in phase)

This is most appropriate for gradient echo imaging.

## T1 Differentiation for Fat and Water

The T1 values for fat and water are quite distinct:

- Water 850 milliseconds
- Fat 150 to 300 milliseconds

Because the T1s are distinctly different, IR can be used to generate dramatic contrast. In a single IR sequence, all spins (fat and water) are inverted by

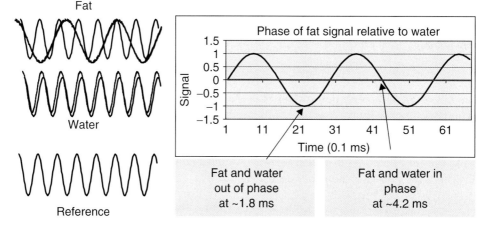

**FIGURE 23-2** Fat and water relative frequencies: the resonance frequencies of fat and water are separated by approximately 250 Hz at a field strength of 1.5 T. When the reference frequency of the scanner is set to water, its signal is essentially detected as a constant (DC) level. Fat, with its slightly different frequency, generates a beat pattern with the water reference frequency and therefore alternates between in-phase and out of phase. The out of phase and in-phase times occur at distinct time points (1.8 and 4.2 milliseconds). For pixels containing a mixture of fat and water, images generated at the out-of-phase and in-phase echo times have dark and bright signals, respectively.

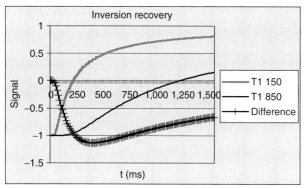

**FIGURE 23-3** Inversion recovery is used to generate fat–water contrast based on the T1 differences. Following an inversion pulse (180 degrees) the short T1 fat signal relaxes back rapidly, whereas the longer T1 water signal relaxes back slowly. When imaging the signal at some time following the inversion (i.e., after a "recovery" time interval, TI), the contrast of fat and water in the image reflects the relative contributions of each signal at that recovery time.

application of a 180-degree radiofrequency (RF) pulse (see Fig. 23-3). The short T1 fat signal immediately begins recovery, and almost completely recovers by approximately 1,000 milliseconds. The slower relaxing water signal on the other hand, relaxes at a much slower rate, and does not return to equilibrium until approximately 4,000 milliseconds. Therefore, at 1,000 milliseconds following the inversion, the water signal has only recovered by approximately 50%. At this special time, half of the water spins point along the positive axis, and half point along the negative axis. By applying an imaging sequence at the 1,000 millisecond time point, the water and fat spins are tipped into the transverse plane, and become magnetic resonance (MR) visible. However, the positive and negative water spins cancel to yield no (or a very low) signal, whereas the fat spins contributes a strong (almost completely relaxed) signal. As can be seen from the IR signal growth pattern, optimum contrast is achieved when negative and positive signals can be differentiated. In general however, images do not differentiate between positive and negative signals, that is, only the absolute signal is seen in the image. This makes the simple contrast curve of the IR sequence follow a more complex pattern, where it increases up to approximately 250 milliseconds, then decreases, and recovers at some later time (see Fig. 23-4).

## PARTIAL INVERSION AND SATURATION

If timings do not allow good contrast to be achieved with an IR sequence, a partial inversion can be used, for example, 120-degree inversion.

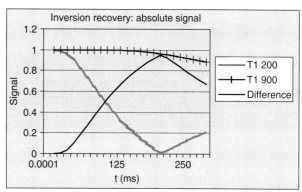

**FIGURE 23-4** Contrast in inversion recovery images may decrease and increase over a short time period. Typically, images do not distinguish between positive and negative signals and only the magnitude signal is represented. This has important consequences for the fat–water contrast in inversion recovery (IR) images. Over the first 300 milliseconds, the magnitude of the contrast between the fat and water signals (*solid dark line*) increases and then decreases, only to later increase again. This is the result of only being sensitive to the magnitude of the signal.

Alternatively, a saturation recovery sequence could be considered, that is, 90-degree pulse.

In these cases, the time of optimum contrast can be altered to some extent.

## MULTIPLE INVERSIONS

If time permits, it is possible to apply multiple IR pulses to achieve the desired contrast at a desired time point, giving more control over the timing of the optimal contrast. Further, this approach is compatible with cardiac triggering. Two major approaches are commonly used, as follows:

- Double IR
- Triple IR

### Double Inversion Recovery

By applying the second inversion pulse at or close to the null point for fat (i.e., the short T1 component), it is possible to make the image have bright fat and bright water (see Fig. 23-5). One advantage of this is that the additional inversion pulse serves to further suppress the blood signal, which, to contribute to the image, must receive all three RF pulses.

### Triple Inversion Recovery

By applying a third inversion pulse at a time designed to null the fat (i.e., the short T1 component), it is possible to have a low fat signal and a bright water

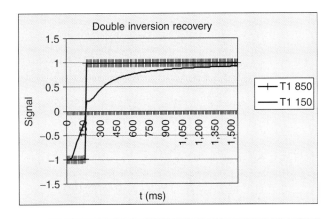

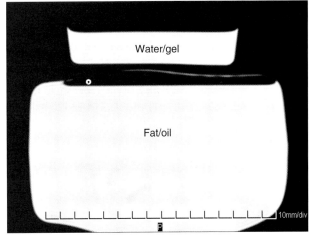

**FIGURE 23-5** In a double inversion recovery (IR) sequence, a second inversion pulse is applied at the time point when the fat (T1 150 milliseconds) signal passes through the "null point." At this point, it has no significant effect on the relaxation curve of the fat signal, because there are an equal number of positive and negative spins. However, the water signal (T1 850 milliseconds) will have relaxed very little by the time of the second inversion pulse, and the effect of the pulse is to convert the negative water spins into positive spins. At this point the water signal is almost fully relaxed. At a relatively short time later, the fat spins have also relaxed, and an image sequence performed at this point results in a bright fat and a bright water signal.

signal (see Fig. 23-6). One advantage of this is that the additional inversion pulses serve to further suppress the blood signal. In the triple IR sequence, a wide range of TEs is possible. However, the TE does not have a major effect on image contrast and TEs ranging from 40 to 140 milliseconds do not significantly affect fat/water contrast (see Fig. 23-7). Note that in the triple IR sequence, you can choose the inversion time (TI) to control image contrast:

- Triple IR, TI 120 (bright water, dark fat)
- Triple IR, TI 300 (dark water, bright fat)
- Triple IR, TI 500 (bright water, bright fat)

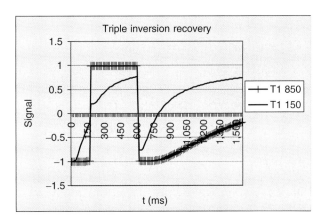

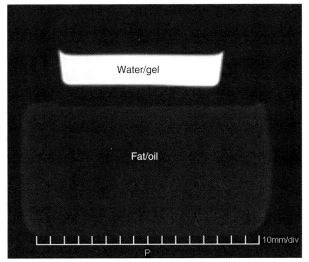

**FIGURE 23-6** In a triple inversion recovery (IR) sequence, the second inversion pulse is applied at the time point when the fat (T1 150 milliseconds) signal passes through the "null point" as for the double IR sequence. Following this, when both the fat and water signals are fully relaxed, a third inversion pulse is applied, and the fat and water spins are allowed to relax from the fully inverted position. By applying an imaging sequence at the point when the fat signal passes through the null point, low fat and bright water signals are seen.

## Multiple Inversion Recovery and Bandwidth

There is plenty of time in the multispin echo multiple inversion recovery (XIR) sequences to increase the sample time, and thereby decrease the sampling bandwidth (BW). By decreasing the BW from 60 to approximately 10 Hz, a signal-to-noise ratio (SNR) advantage can be gained.

## Unshackle the Phase

Just as motion in k-space is represented in the phase of the signal, similarly, signal orientation (i.e., positive or negative) is represented in the phase of the k-space data. To access the signal orientation we must "unshackle the

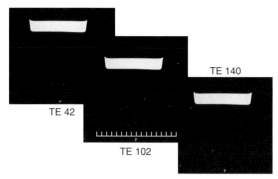

**FIGURE 23-7** Effect of echo time (TE) on triple inversion recovery is minimal over the range 42 to 140 milliseconds. The water remains bright and fat signal is relatively low.

phase." Normally, images reconstructed on the scanner are "magnitude" or "modulus" images. To differentiate positive from negative signal it is necessary to construct an image that is sensitive to the phase of the signal. However, imperfections in the acquisition of k-space disrupt the perfect phase symmetry that is expected. Therefore, disruptions of the k-space phase must be corrected for. Typically, the phase correction is of a low order nature, and it can be corrected by using a minimal k-space data set as a reference (see Fig. 23-8). Applying the phase correction of the minimal reference image to the full image allows positive and negative signals to be differentiated (see Fig. 23-9). In magnitude images, contrast between different tissues drops to zero when the positive signal of one tissue (e.g., water) equals the negative signal of another tissue (e.g., fat). In phase-sensitive images, contrast is high under these conditions.

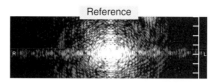

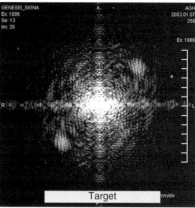

**FIGURE 23-8** Phase-sensitive inversion recovery (IR) is used to identify positive and negative signals in IR sequences. In the magnitude images, the fat–water contrast does not follow a smooth curve over the early time period due to the changes from negative to positive spins. By acquiring the central portion of k-space as a reference (reference), it can be used to correct the phase of k-space for the IR sequence (target). In this way positive and negative signals can be differentiated, thereby allowing easier interpretation of IR contrast.

## CHEMICAL SHIFT

The frequency difference between the fat and water signals can be exploited to preferentially suppress one of them (see Fig. 23-10). Preferential suppression of

Magnitude

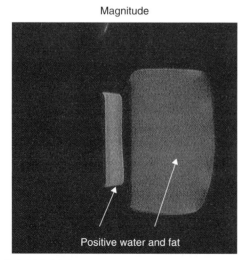

Phase corrected

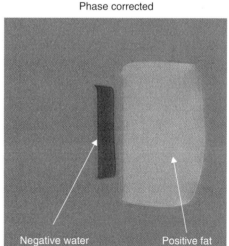

**FIGURE 23-9** At short inversion recovery (IR) times, magnitude images may not successfully differentiate fat and water signals. However, if a phase sensitive IR sequence is used, negative and positive signals can be differentiated, and contrast improved.

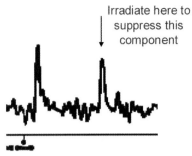

Irradiate here to
suppress this
component

**FIGURE 23-10**   By selectively focusing the radiofrequency (RF) signal on only one of the spectral peaks (fat or water), it is possible to selectively suppress that component. In this case, the image formed following this procedure would only be sensitive to the unsuppressed component.

one spectral frequency is possible if the peaks are well separated. Alternatively, a chemically selective RF pulse can be applied before imaging, to selectively excite only one signal component, such as the fat signal, and can also be used to either saturate or invert the selected signal. These approaches require high main magnetic field ($B_0$) homogeneity and generally, shimming is recommended.

## Chemical Shift Displacement "Artifact"

In the image generation process, the signal echo is read out in the presence of the measurement gradient. The fat/water spectral separation results in a "chemical shift displacement" along the measurement gradient. The BW of the signal readout relates to the spectral width of the signal information, whereas the fat and water signals are separated by a fixed 224 Hz (at 1.5 T). Therefore, as signal readout BW decreases, the fat–water difference becomes an increasingly significant percentage of the

signal space. In general, the fat–water shift increases as BW decreases, and can be very large for sequences that have long signal readouts, such echo planar imaging (EPI) and spirals.

## Dixon Method

A spin echo–based method of producing separate fat and water images was developed by Tom Dixon. Just as for the gradient echo approach, the technique exploits the relative phase difference between fat and water signals at two carefully chosen TEs:

- Fat and water in phase
- Fat and water out of phase

This is achieved by displacing the acquisition of one echo relative to the other in two separate spin echo sequences such that the water and fat signal have evolved to 180 degrees out of phase. Addition or subtraction of the two data sets allows extraction of separate fat and water signals. This two-point approach is a special case of the more general Fourier approaches that allow for increased number of time points to improve spectral definition and SNR.

## SUMMARY

Fat and water are important quantities in magnetic resonance imaging (MRI). They have multiple dimensions to separate them from each other:

- T1
- T2
- Frequency

Specialized imaging sequences and prepulses are available to distinguish fat from water signals.

# CHAPTER 24

# K-Space

Mark Doyle

K-space is the "raw data" for magnetic resonance imaging (MRI). The data acquired by the scanner are assembled and arranged internally into individual k-space arrays. Each individual image is derived from a k-space matrix, for example, for one slice imaged at 20 cardiac phases, there are 20 corresponding k-space arrays. In most imaging modalities, the correlation between the physical property sampled and the manner in which data are arranged to form an image is generally intuitively obvious. In MRI, k-space is acquired and an image generated in a manner that is not naturally intuitive. However, k-space is a feature that may have advantages over other modalities:

- K-space breaks the one-to-one correspondence between the position of the receiver and the orientation of the image.
- It allows arbitrary slice angulation.
- It allows reduction in scan time by post-processing of k-space.
- It allows parallel imaging to reduce scan time.
- It allows image contrast to be altered.

This contrasts with ultrasound:

- Image orientation is directly proportional to the position of the probe
- Operator dependence
- Limited imaging window

And with nuclear medicine:

- Orientation of detector array determines image orientation.
- Projection reconstruction (PR) produces uneven resolution.

## K-SPACE

An appreciation of k-space is central to the understanding of MRI and is explanatory of the origin of its advantages over other modalities. Mathematically, k-space can be succinctly and compactly described by a single equation, which to a mathematician fully explains k-space. However, to a nonmathematician, in general, it is just a series of meaningless symbols. Here we will discuss and explore k-space by means of a series of illustrations, and at the conclusion of this exploration, the equations will be presented. Increased understanding will likely be gained as exposure to the concepts involved occurs.

## K-SPACE DIMENSIONS

Physically, k-space is a matrix of data, with dimensions that are typically square, and typically, these are in powers of 2:

- $128 \times 128$
- $256 \times 256$
- $512 \times 512$

The highest concentration of signal is located towards the k-space center. To generate an image, the k-space data are Fourier transformed (see Fig. 24-1). Sometimes, this operation is referred to as a *fast Fourier transform* (FFT). This is due to a mathematical shortcut that was discovered for matrices with dimensions of powers of 2. The image generated by this mathematical operation has a physical size identical to that of the original k-space matrix:

- $128 \times 128$
- $256 \times 256$
- $512 \times 512$ respectively.

In this respect, there is a one-to-one correspondence between the number of k-space points and the number of image points. Also note that the image features fit within the square (or rectangular) field, termed the *field of view* (FOV).

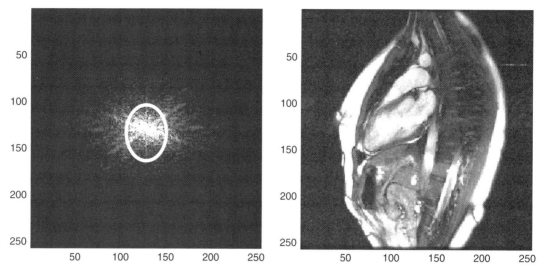

**FIGURE 24-1**    The k-space matrix represented here is a 2D image of signal intensity. The highest concentration of signal is toward the center of k-space (*circled*). In this example, k-space has the physical size of 256 × 256 pixels. The corresponding image is generated by performing a Fourier transform on the k-space data. Note that the dimensions of the image are also 256 × 256 pixels.

## PROJECTIONS

Consider an image of a rectangle within a square FOV. The rectangle has a uniform intensity and no internal detail (see Fig. 24-2). Also, there is no noise in this perfect (if somewhat bland) image. In this case the corresponding k-space matrix exhibits a clear pattern of horizontal and vertical symmetry. An alternative way of viewing the k-space data is to represent the signal intensity as a three-dimensional (3D) surface. When viewed in this manner, it is easier to appreciate that along each major axis the signals represent decaying

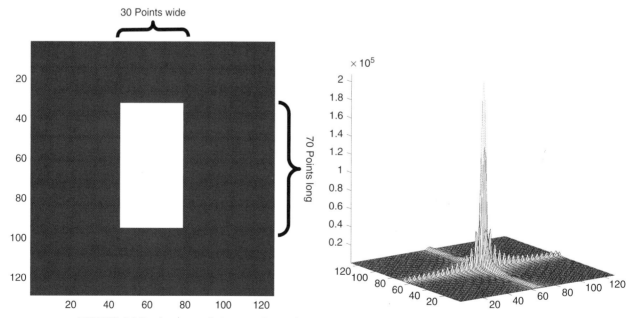

**FIGURE 24-2**    An example image of a uniform rectangular object with no internal detail. In this case, the rectangle is 30 pixels wide and 70 pixels long, within a field of view of 128 × 128 pixels. The corresponding k-space representation is shown here as a 3D surface plot, as opposed to the more common intensity plot of Fig. 24-1. Note that in this case, k-space data lies predominantly along the major axes, with data along one axis demonstrating definite oscillations, whereas data along the other axis appears smoother.

sinusoidal patterns. One property of k-Space is that any line passing through the center can be Fourier transformed to represent a projection of the object corresponding to the orientation of that line (see Fig. 24-3). In the case of the rectangular image, the FFT of the horizontal central line represents a projection through the rectangular object along the horizontal axis, and the FFT of the vertical line represents a projection through the rectangular object along the vertical axis. Therefore, k-space has the property that symmetry in the object is reflected in symmetry in k-space. Consider the k-space representation of a square object; in this case, k-space demonstrates symmetry along both major

axes. Similarly, a circular object results in a k-space pattern that is circularly symmetric, with all lines passing through the center being essentially identical.

## PROJECTION RECONSTRUCTION

In the preceding text, we considered the example of two special lines of k-space

- Horizontal
- Vertical

However, there are an infinite number of lines that pass through the center of k-space, that is, lines not

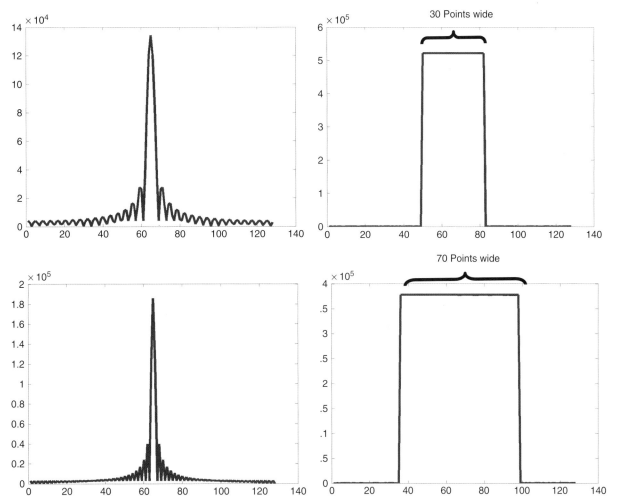

**FIGURE 24-3**    For the k-space data of Fig. 24-2, the central line of k-space along the axis with dominant oscillations is extracted (top left), and the corresponding 1D Fourier transform data presented as a 1D profile (top right). Here, the profile data has a square appearance, with the plateau of the shape being of width 30 points. This corresponds to the width of the rectangle of the original image in Fig. 24-2. The central line along the perpendicular axis of k-space is represented in the lower panel, and the corresponding 1D Fourier transform profile is shown as a square function of width 70 points (lower right), corresponding to the height of the rectangle of Fig. 24-2. It is apparent that the central lines of k-space correspond to projections through the image, which become apparent when viewing the Fourier transformed data.

confined to the two primary axes. By acquiring these lines, enough data can be acquired to generate an image by back PR. To appreciate the relationship between k-space and the gradients applied to the body, consider applying a horizontal gradient to the selected slice: it results in columns of spins with the same frequency. The signal acquired in the presence of this gradient has that frequency information directly encoded in it. When the signal is Fourier transformed into the frequency domain, the data relates directly to projections of the object. The PR method was used in CT and radionuclide imaging and can also be used in MRI. By acquiring multiple lines through the center of k-space and Fourier transforming the magnetic resonance signal, a sufficient number of projections can be generated to form a PR image. The unique features of lines that pass through the center of k-space are that they can be produced by application of one imaging gradient. As a practical aside, we note that a gradient in any direction can be generated by a combination of three orthogonal gradients, which, if applied simultaneously in different strengths, effectively combine to form a single gradient applied at some intermediate orientation. When viewed in terms of k-space, the PR data can be represented as a series of lines, each passing through the center of k-space. In this representation, it is apparent that the highest density of points in the PR data set is toward the center whereas the lines are sparser toward the periphery. PR images have several artifacts, as follows

- Uneven resolution
  - Higher at center
  - Lower at periphery
- Star artifact from bright objects

## SIGNAL INFORMATION

The time domain signal obtained in MRI is digitally sampled (see Fig. 24-4). The digital sampling process is characterized by two variables:

- Sampling rate
- Sampling duration

When sampling data that relates to frequency information, a natural means of assessing the appropriateness of the measuring parameters is to consider the bandwidth (BW) of the measured signal (see Fig. 24-5). The BW of the measured signal is determined by the formula:

$$1/T_{sample}$$

Where $T_{sample}$ is the sampling interval time between individual points. Under conditions that the BW matches or cxcccds the highest frequency component in the signal, the signal is correctly represented. Another parameter to consider is the frequency per point of

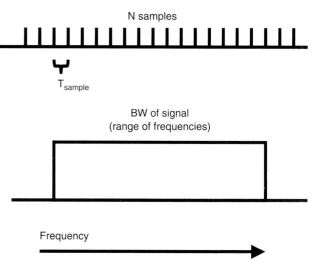

**FIGURE 24-5** The bandwidth properties of the signal sampled in Fig. 24-4 are represented. In this case, N sample points are digitally sampled to represent the time varying waveform, each separated by the time interval, $T_{sample}$. This sampling interval (or rate) determines the bandwidth (BW) of the frequency information that can be adequately represented: BW = $1/T_{sample}$. The important concept is that the rate of sampling data in the time domain determines the response in the frequency domain. Therefore, to adequately represent the frequency information that is present, the BW must match or exceed the highest frequency component.

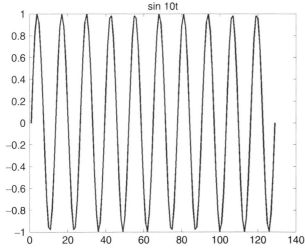

**FIGURE 24-4** Because each point of k-space is digitally sampled, the properties of digital sampling are considered. Here a 1D sinusoidal oscillating time varying waveform is sampled at regular intervals for a total time $T_{total}$. The digital sampling process is fully described by the sampling rate and the sampling duration.

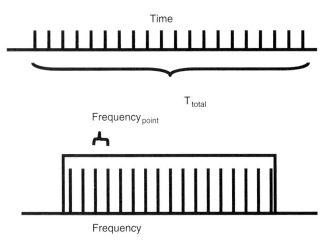

FIGURE 24-6 Because the time domain signal is directly sampled, the digital and discrete nature in this domain is an obvious feature. However, it is less widely appreciated that the digital and discrete nature of the data also extends to the frequency domain signal, that is, signal generated by Fourier transforming the time domain signal produces the frequency domain signal. Here we illustrate the nature of this relationship between the two domains: time and frequency. For a time domain signal sampled for a duration $T_{total}$, the separation of each point in the frequency domain is related to the inverse of this time. As indicated in Fig. 24-5, the bandwidth of the frequency domain signal encompasses all the frequency points and is represented as the enveloping rectangle in the frequency domain.

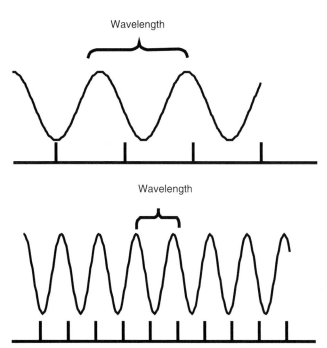

FIGURE 24-7 To correctly sample the time domain signal (represented as a simple sinusoid) there should be at least two sample points per wavelength. This is an expression of the Nyquist sampling theorem. As illustrated in the lower panel, time domain signals with a higher frequency of oscillation requires a higher sampling rate to adequately represent the data.

the frequency domain signal (see Fig. 24-6). This is determined by the total sample interval ($T_{total}$):

$$\text{Frequency per point} = 1/T_{total}$$

To correctly represent a signal at a certain frequency, there should be at least two samples per wavelength (see Fig. 24-7). This is an expression of Nyquist's sampling theorem. These relationships and sampling theory laws have implications for how a signal is digitized. Consider a signal with a predetermined upper frequency component. This frequency component determines the sampling rate (Nyquist). However, the signal can be sampled for a long or a short total time duration. The long sample time necessitates that many sample points are generated, leading to a narrow BW for each frequency point (i.e., frequency resolution is high) (see Fig. 24-8). Conversely, applying the same sampling rate, but sampling the signal for a short duration, only generates a few sample points. In this case, the BW for each frequency point is wide (i.e., frequency resolution is low) (see Fig. 24-9). Note, that in the previous examples, the BW of the frequency domain signal was identical, because it was fully determined by the individual sample interval of the time data. Additionally, in each case, the high-frequency information was correctly sampled and therefore correctly represented in the data.

The short sample time resulted in the frequency per point being very wide and the long sample time resulted in a narrow frequency per point. These features of digital sampling will have profound consequences for k-space.

## SPATIAL FREQUENCIES

The very central point of k-space is by far the highest intensity point. Generally, intensity falls off dramatically from the center of k-space to the periphery. The form of k-space can be better appreciated when viewed as a 3D surface. There is a correlation between k-space and image space, as follows:

- The center of k-space relates to low spatial frequencies.
- The periphery of k-space relates to high spatial frequencies.

Therefore, different regions of k-space relate to the spatial frequency content of the image, with fine image detail (high spatial frequencies) tending to the periphery of k-space and broad contrast features (low spatial frequencies) tending toward the center of k-space (see Fig. 24-10).

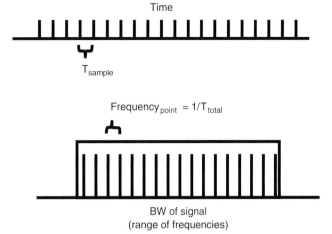

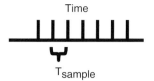

FIGURE 24-8 The relationship between sample time, signal bandwidth, and the resolution of frequency domain points is illustrated. For a fixed sample interval for the time domain signal, the Nyquist sample rate is fully determined, which fully determines the bandwidth of the frequency domain representation (visualized by performing a Fourier transform on the time domain signal). However, the duration of the time domain sampling is not determined by these considerations. In the case illustrated here, the time domain sampling is represented as sampling the signal for a long overall time ($T_{total}$). Because the number of frequency points must match the time domain points, it follows that the frequency domain points are tightly packed in the bandwidth available to them. Therefore, a long total sample time generates frequency points with fine resolution.

## TIME AND FREQUENCY DOMAIN

Although not explicitly stated until now, k-space is a time domain signal and the image is a frequency domain signal. The units of time are seconds and the units of frequency are events per second, that is, there is an inverse relationship between k-space and image space. To explore this relationship further, consider a 1D time signal and its corresponding 1D Fourier transform (FT) (frequency signal). When the sampling characteristics of the time data match the frequency information, the frequency data is well represented. However, when there is a mismatch it is possible to alias the frequency signal, that is, signal "fold over" will occur. From sampling theory, signal aliasing occurs when the sampling rate is not sufficient to adequately represent the highest frequency information. For a fixed sample period this is equivalent to considering the sampling density, which is the number of sample points per unit time (see Fig. 24-11). In a completely analogous manner, 2D k-space also exhibits aliasing if the data sampling rates are too low. In the 2D case, sampling density is typically limited only in the number of lines per unit k-space but is not limited by the number of sample

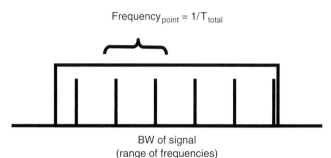

FIGURE 24-9 The relationship between sample time, signal bandwidth (BW), and the resolution of frequency domain points is illustrated for a relatively short sample time. With reference to Fig. 24-8, the sample interval for each time domain data point is identical, and therefore the bandwidth of the frequency domain data is identical. However, in this case, the time domain sampling is only carried out for a short total duration. Therefore, the frequency per point of the frequency domain signal is very wide compared to the Fig. 24-8 example. This corresponds to coarse resolution in the frequency domain.

points per line (note, each axis of k-space has the units of time). To illustrate this, consider a "normal" k-space data set and the corresponding "normal" image (see Fig. 24-12). In the normal image no signal aliasing is seen, and we can be assured that the sampling density along both k-space axes was adequate. We can effectively halve the k-space sampling density along one dimension by removing every other line. In this case, we see that the corresponding image exhibits severe signal aliasing in that half of the image is folded over to the other half. The aliased signal region is sometimes referred to as a fold-over artifact, because the data from one edge "folds in" at the opposite edge. From this example, we can appreciate that k-space obeys the laws of data sampling and that any mismatch in sampling conditions results in generation of fold-over artifacts.

## K-SPACE REPRESENTATION

In the treatment of k-space thus far it is apparent that it is a 2D representation of a time domain signal, and this time domain signal is composed of sine and cosine waves of varying frequency and amplitude. To extract this frequency information, an FT is performed, allowing the amplitudes of the frequency information to be extracted

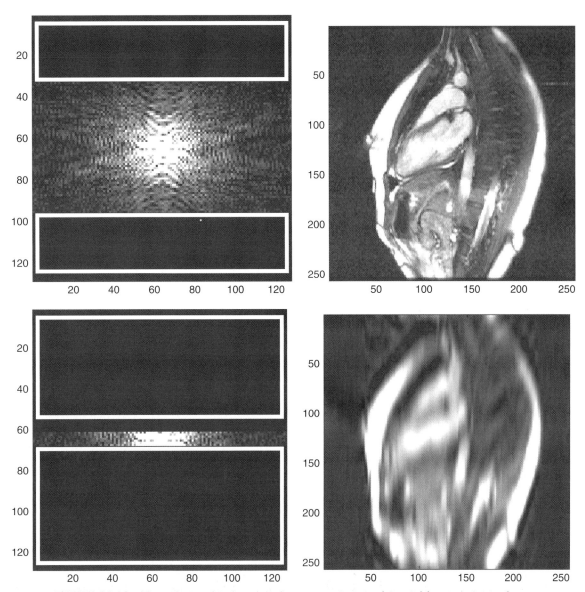

**FIGURE 24-10**  The relationship between k-space regions and spatial frequencies in the image domain is illustrated. The top panel shows k-space being truncated by removing lines symmetrically from the top and lower sections. Compared to the previously shown cardiac image, the corresponding image appears to be slightly blurred. In the lower panel, this process is taken to an extreme, and severe blurring is noticeable. The image feature being affected is termed *spatial frequency*, that is, a high spatial frequency expresses that pixel intensities change rapidly over the image, whereas a low spatial frequency expresses that pixels change intensity gradually over the image. In the lower case, only low spatial frequencies are present. Therefore, it is apparent that the outer regions of k-space represent finer detail information in the image.

and interpreted as an image when suitably arranged. However, this interpretation may not be immediately apparent from the appearance of the k-space data. The usual presentation of 1D time domain data is that it is simply presented as a waveform plot, with excursions up and down the page representing signal amplitude. However, that same 1D signal can be more compactly represented as an intensity plot, where the intensity of

the signal amplitude is represented as a brightness feature (see Fig. 24-13). In this case, the 1D signal is compactly represented as a single line of intensity variations (similar to a bar-code representation). When the signal is a simple sine or cosine wave, the connection between the two representations is easy to appreciate. However, for more complex waveforms, consisting of multiple frequencies, the pattern may be more difficult

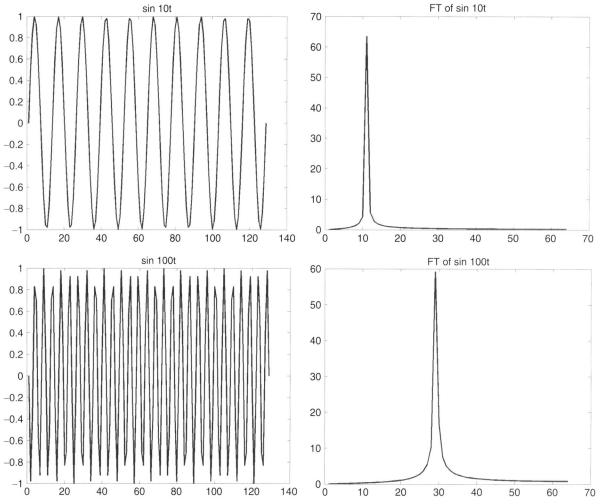

**FIGURE 24-11** The relationship between the time domain and frequency domain signal is illustrated, with a demonstration of signal aliasing. In the top panel, a 10-Hz sinusoidal time domain signal is digitally sampled (confirmed by counting waveform peaks of the sample interval). In the top right panel, the corresponding Fourier transform (FT) signal is seen. In this case, the peak of the frequency domain signal is centered at the 10-Hz signal point. Note that the upper limit of the signal bandwidth is 64 Hz. Here the Fourier transform correctly identified that frequency component of the time domain signal. In the lower panel, the time domain signal is a 100-Hz oscillation, but in this case, the Fourier domain signal incorrectly represented the peak of the data at 30 Hz. This is a case of signal aliasing. The 100-Hz signal was sampled at too low a sampling interval, and therefore the bandwidth of the signal (64 Hz) was too narrow to correctly represent the data. The aliased signal effectively wrapped around the frequency domain data, disappearing off the higher end and reappearing from the lower frequency end to position at approximately 30 Hz (i.e., 64 Hz + 30 Hz ~100 Hz).

to interpret, but is nonetheless still valid. Further, we have seen that the central lines of k-space correspond to projections through the object. Although while we can now appreciate that the other lines of k-space (i.e., those not passing through the center) also contain frequency information, and that this time domain signal is commonly represented as an intensity plot, we have not addressed the issues of what information these other lines (regions) contain and how this information

is encoded. To accomplish this, we must now consider the influence of magnetic gradients.

## K-SPACE AND GRADIENTS

In MRI, frequency information is encoded by the application of imaging gradients. Along one axis of k-space, this information is rapidly encoded over a

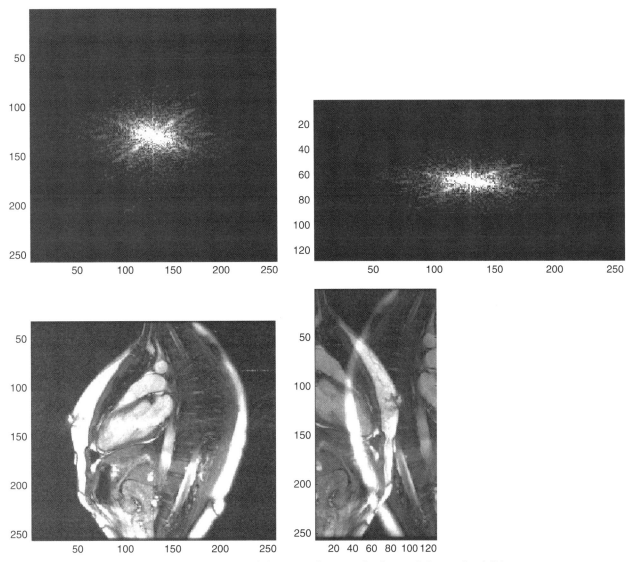

**FIGURE 24-12** Demonstration of aliasing in k-space. In the top left panel, a full k-space matrix is represented, and the corresponding image is shown in the lower left panel, with all image features correctly visualized. In the k-space matrix on the right, every other line has been removed. This is equivalent to reducing the data sampling rate along the vertical direction by a factor of 2. The corresponding image below it demonstrates signal aliasing, that is, signal regions are represented in an overlapping manner. This illustrates that the sampling density in k-space effectively corresponds to the field of view in the image space.

few milliseconds. This direction is referred to as the *measurement* or *frequency encoding direction*. In this dimension, signal data comprising multiple frequencies is efficiently encoded and digitally sampled. However, the second axis of k-space cannot be as rapidly encoded, and requires successive iterations of the basic MRI sequence. This direction is referred to as the *phase encoding direction*. Therefore, it can be appreciated that there are two distinct data sampling directions (e.g., X and Y), and that each requires a separate approach to correctly encode data. To illustrate the need for this separate treatment of each encoding axis, consider

the result of applying two gradients at the same time; they would simply combine to form a single gradient at an intermediate angle. Therefore, the two k-space encoding gradients must be applied at different points in time and never applied simultaneously. To appreciate the information that is encoded by each gradient (either applied continuously or in a stepped manner), consider the k-space signal of a square object (see Fig. 24-14). Its k-space representation has both vertical and horizontal symmetry, and in this case the vertical and horizontal k-space central lines are identical. Therefore, because the k-space pattern along each major axis looks the same

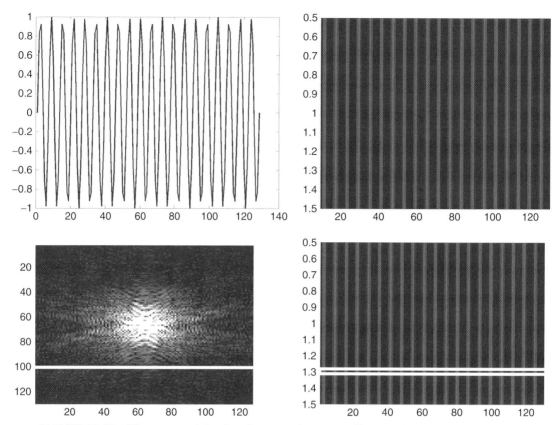

**FIGURE 24-13** The nature of the data format in k-space is illustrated. In the top left panel, a sinusoidal signal variation is represented. In the top right panel, the same sinusoidal pattern is represented as an intensity variation. In this case, the intensity variation (*brightness and darkness*) represents the signal amplitude, and the same pattern is repeated for all lines of the figure. In the lower left panel, a k-space matrix is shown. Note that the similarity of one line of k-space (*white*) is similar to one line of the 1D sinusoidal pattern. This shows that k-space data is a compact representation of a series of lines representing sinusoidal patterns of differing complexity, dependant on the number of sinusoidal signals present in each line.

for a spatially symmetric object, we might suspect that fundamentally the phase encoding and measurement gradients are performing identical data encoding tasks. To explore this possibility, consider the phase evolution that occurs in the presence of a measurement gradient applied for 80 units of time at level 100 (see Fig. 24-15). In this instance, the phase accumulation experienced by a spin at one physical location linearly increases until the gradient is terminated. In this case, the spin experienced a phase accumulation of 8,000 units (e.g., degrees, radians). In this context, phase accumulation is experienced by the magnetization vector rotating in the transverse (x-y) plane, and the net angle rotated through by this spin is regarded as the "phase accumulation." Now consider the phase accumulation experienced by the same spin in the presence of a pulsed phase encoding gradient (see Fig. 24-16). For one application of the phase encoding gradient, whereby a low gradient amplitude is employed, only a moderate

amount of phase accumulation is achieved. Further, when the phase encoding gradient is terminated, no further phase accumulation is experienced. Consider a second application of the phase encoding gradient, but in this instance, it is applied at a higher gradient strength and for the same short time duration. In this case, the phase accumulation is much higher, and again, is fixed after the gradient is switched off. The difference that is observed between the phase encoding gradient and the continuously applied gradient is that the stepped gradient only generates one specific phase accumulation amount per application, whereas the continuously applied gradient generates a range of phase accumulations overtime. However, the similarity between the two gradients is that for each phase accumulation point, the net result is the same from the spin's perspective (see Fig. 24-17). In other words, the stepped phase encoding gradient achieves the same phase encoding as does the continuously applied

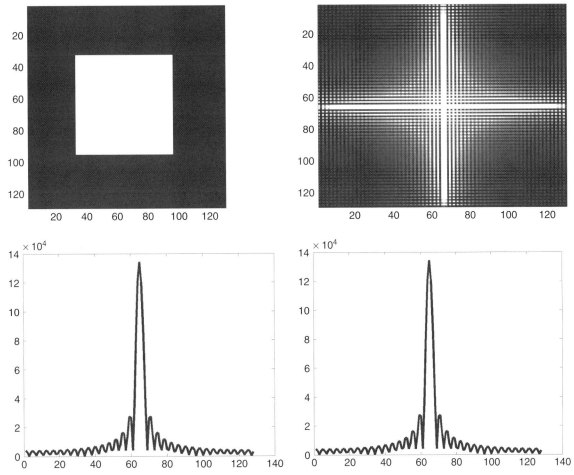

**FIGURE 24-14**   An image of a square and the corresponding k-space pattern is shown. Note the symmetry of the image and the k-space pattern. In the lower panel, the signal patterns corresponding to the vertical and horizontal lines of k-space are shown. Note that they are identical to each other. Given that each horizontal line of k-space is produced by an imaging gradient and each vertical line of k-space is encoded by successive application of a phase encoding gradient, it is reasonable to conclude that there is a commonality of the information encoded by each gradient type, that is, there is a simple relationship that exists between the measurement gradient and the phase encoding gradient.

measurement gradient, with the difference being that only one phase point is achieved for each separate application of the phase encoding gradient. It can be appreciated that the same linear range of phase accumulation can be realized by successive application of the phase encoding gradient as is achieved by a single application of the measurement gradient. The important feature for the encoded signal includes not only the final phase that is achieved (i.e., after all gradients have been applied), but that at each sampled time point, the appropriate phase accumulation level is sampled. Therefore, in summary, k-space is really a measure of phase accumulation at each sampled point, and that phase accumulation in each direction can be achieved equivalently by applying a gradient either continuously or in a stepped manner.

## K-SPACE MATHEMATICAL FORMULISM

A 1D FT is suitable for processing a simple waveform consisting of several sine and cosine waves. In this case, it is apparent that the FT process extracts the amplitudes of each component frequency. By direct extension, k-space is the 2D version of such a signal data set, and therefore requires a 2D FT to produce the amplitudes of the frequency components, which in this case directly correspond to an image of the object.

To relate the k-space signal to the physical reality of the scanner, consider the following variables and their relationships:

- $B_0$ = main magnetic field
- G(t) = time dependant gradient in the z-direction
- Z = distance along z-axis of a particular spin

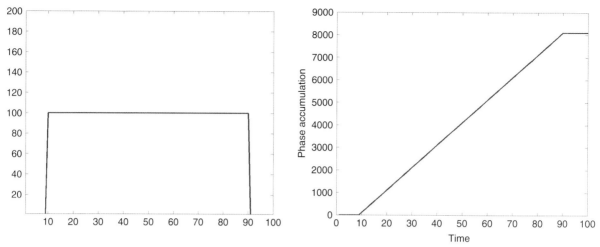

**FIGURE 24-15**   The relationship between imaging gradients and phase accumulation is illustrated. On the left, an imaging "measurement gradient" is shown. It is applied at a level 100 and applied for 80 time units, starting at time 20 and ending at time 90. The corresponding phase map of an individual spin is shown on the right. In this case, the spin undergoes multiple complete revolutions (each revolution being 360 degrees) and during application of the gradient it accumulates 8,000 degrees in a linear manner. In a k-space acquisition, data are acquired during the total time that the gradient is applied.

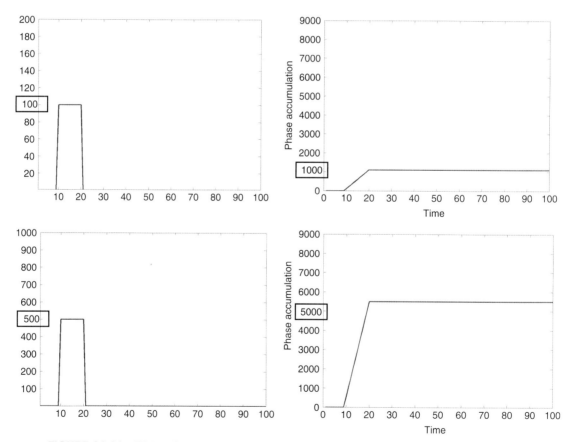

**FIGURE 24-16**   With reference to Fig. 24-15, the phase accumulation due to the application of the phase encoding gradient is shown. In the top panel, the phase encoding gradient is applied for duration 10 time units, at a level of 100. The corresponding phase accumulation is 1,000 degrees, and then this level is unchanged when the gradient terminates, because there is no further gradient applied. In the lower panel, the phase encoding gradient is applied for duration 10 time units, at a level of 500. The corresponding phase accumulation is 5,000 degrees, and then this level is unchanged following termination of the gradient.

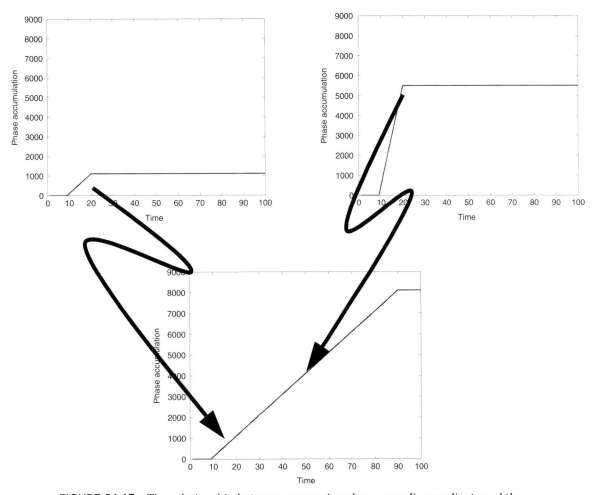

**FIGURE 24-17** The relationship between successive phase encoding gradients and the measurement gradient is shown. With reference to Figs. 24-15 and 24-16, the phase encoding achieved by the two separate applications of the phase encoding gradient are shown to be two points on the phase accumulation achieved by application of the continuously applied measurement gradient. Because the data are digitally sampled, the discrete nature of applying the phase encoding gradients has no noticeable effect. Therefore the successively applied phase encoding gradient achieves exactly the same phase evolution as the continuously applied measurement gradient, and the nature of the information encoded by each gradient is identical.

It follows that the magnetic field experienced at each point along the z-axis is given by:

$$B(z, t) = \mathbf{B_0} + Z \times G(t)$$

The Larmor equation links the precession frequency of a spin to the magnetic field strength experienced by that spin. Therefore, in the case of the applied gradient, the angular frequency of a spin ($\omega$) is given by:

$$\omega(z, t) = \omega_0 + \omega_G(z, t)$$

It is convenient to consider the case where linear gradients are applied, therefore

$$\omega_G(z, t) = \gamma \times Z \times G(t)$$

For a gradient applied for a time t, the accumulated phase is given by

$$\varphi_G(z, t) = -\int_0^t dt \times \omega$$

$$\varphi_G(z, t) = -\gamma.Z \int_0^t dt \times G(t)$$

For a sample region with spin density $\rho$, the signal is given by

$$s(t) = \int_0^t dz \times \rho(z)e^{i.\varphi_G(z, t)}$$

Using standard notation:

$$e^{i\varphi} = \cos(\varphi) + i\sin(\varphi)$$

Substituting for $\varphi$

$$s(k) = \int_0^t dz \times \rho(z)e^{-i2\pi k(t)z}$$

Where

$$k(t) = \gamma \times \int_0^t G(t) \times dt$$

By inspection, the signal s(k) is written in the form such that it is the FT of the spin density distribution, $\rho(z)$. For linear gradients the function for k simplifies to

$$k = \gamma \times G(t) \times t$$

The formula developed so far has dealt with a 1D distribution of spins and gradients that are applied in one dimension. To extend the process to 2D (or higher dimensions), simply express the integrals over 2D (or higher dimensions)

$$s(k) = \int_x dx \int_y dy \times \rho(x, y)e^{-i2\pi(k_x x + k_y y)}$$

## SUMMARY

K-space is produced by application of gradients in a highly controlled manner. The measurement gradient imposes phase accumulation that is read out in a single rapid sequence. The phase gradient produces the same affect by successive step-wise application. When expressed mathematically, k-space has the exact form of an FT. This is exploited in imaging to efficiently encode image information directly.

# CHAPTER 25

# Magnet Design

Mark Doyle

## OVERVIEW

Magnets and magnet design are central to the field of magnetic resonance imaging (MRI), and although the main magnet is the dominant feature of the MRI system, there are several other magnets, each with their own design and performance characteristics, that determine the performance level of the system. Topics covered in this chapter are as follows:

1. Field strength, 1.5 T versus 3 T
2. Determinants of signal-to-noise ratio (SNR)
3. Specific absorption rate (SAR)
4. Design of magnets
   ○ Static field
   ○ Gradients
   ○ Radiofrequency (RF)

## 1.5 T VERSUS 3 T FIELD STRENGTH

Historically, the 1.5 T magnetic systems have dominated the market for commercial systems, and this situation has prevailed for approximately 15 years. Currently, 3 T systems are vying for the position as the new standard, and there is rapid adoption of this field strength for neurologic and body imaging applications. However, at the time of writing, the advantages for cardiovascular magnetic resonance (CMR) applications are not as straightforwardly appreciated. There are several aspects that can be considered in comparing 1.5 T and 3 T systems:

- SNR and field strength
- T1 and field strength
- Gradient-recalled echo (GRE), spin echo (SE), SNR, and field strength
- Steady state free precession (SSFP), SNR, and field strength

*SNR and field strength.* As the field strength increases, the number of spins that are "unmatched" increases and thereby the signal increases. For a fully relaxed imaging sequence (i.e., a proton density–weighted imaging sequence) the effective SNR increases linearly over the range 0.1 to 5 T (see Fig. 25-1). Therefore, the gain in SNR from 1.5 to 3 T for this sequence is effectively 100%.

*T1 and field strength.* The T1 relaxation process involves energy exchanges between the spin system and the lattice. The energy required to achieve the T1 exchange is dependant on field strength; however the lattice only possesses a finite amount of energy, in the form of bodily heat, and therefore the T1 time increases with field strength (see Fig. 25-1). From 1.5 to 3 T the T1 increases by approximately 50%.

*GRE, SE, SNR, and field strength.* The SNR in gradient and SE imaging sequences (but not SSFP) depends on the ratio TR/T1.

Taking the signal gain and the T1 dependence of GRE and SE sequence into account, the observed SNR improvement becomes muted compared to the gains expected purely from signal strength considerations. Comparing 3 to 1.5 T the effective SNR should increase by approximately 40% (see Fig. 25-1).

*SSFP, SNR, and field strength.* The SNR in SSFP is dependent on $\sqrt{(T2/T1)}$.

Because the T2 relaxation process is energy independent, the T2 characteristic is field strength independent. Taking the signal gain and the T1 dependence of SSFP sequence into account, the observed SNR should increase by approximately 70% when comparing 3 to 1.5 T (see Fig. 25-1).

## SPECIFIC ABSORPTION RATE AND FIELD STRENGTH

SAR is the measure of how much RF power is deposited in the body. Power is the rate of doing or absorbing work. In the United States, the U.S. Food and Drug

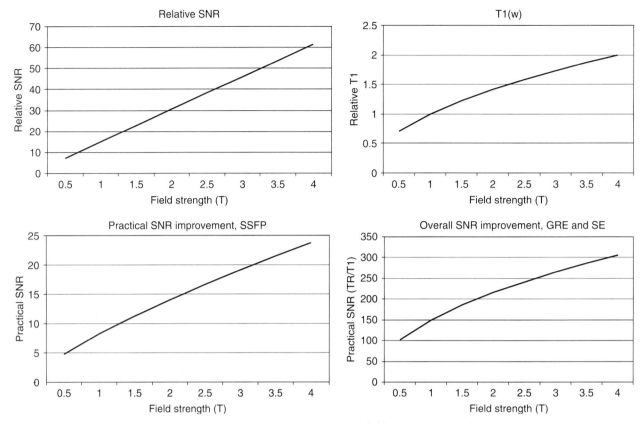

**FIGURE 25-1** Spin properties change with magnetic field strength: signal-to-noise ratio (SNR), T1, SNR of steady state free precession (SSFP), SNR of gradient-recalled echo (GRE) and spin echo (SE).

Administration (FDA) guidelines limit the SAR, as follows:

- 3 W per kilogram over the whole body
- 8 W per kilogram over a local region

Because the RF power level increases as the square of the field strength, a 90- degree pulse at 3 T requires four times the amount of power compared to 1.5 T. Therefore, at 3 T, duty cycles may have to be reduced to avoid overheating.

## MAGNETS

In an MRI system there are several distinct magnetic fields in use:

- Main static magnetic field
- X, Y, Z magnetic gradients
- Transmitter RF coil
- Receiver RF coils

All of these magnets (with the possible exception of the main magnetic field, which in rare systems is a permanent magnet) are typically of the electromagnetic

design. The basic physical principle that allows the design of electromagnetic coils is that current flowing in a conductor will generate a magnetic field in the surrounding volume. The Biot-Savat law is the law describing the strength and direction of the magnetic field, **B(X)** at all points, X, due to the current, I, a distance, r, away in a medium with permeability, u, and is given by:

$$dB = u \times I \times dl \times r/(1 \times \pi \times r^3)$$

One of the most basic coil designs is that of the simple circular loop, consisting of a loop of wire which can be regarded as a continuum of wire elements which all combine to produce a magnetic field. For a circular wire loop that is oriented in the X-Y plane, the field produced is predominantly oriented along the Z direction (see Fig. 25-2). The next level of complexity is to consider two simple circular loops (see Fig. 25-3). Wire loops can be positioned on axis with each other to produce fields in the Z direction that combine to increase the strength of the magnetic field at the midpoint between the two coils. A special case of such a design is termed a *Helmholtz pair*, and can be arranged to produce an extended region with an approximately uniform field between the two coils. In this case, the spacing of the

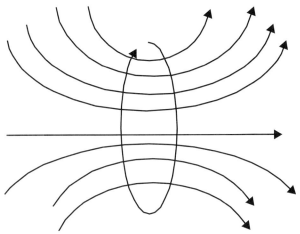

**FIGURE 25-2** The magnetic flux lines generated by a circular loop of current carrying wire. Toward the central axis of the circular loop, the magnetic flux lines approximate to a uniform magnetic field.

coils is twice the radius of each coil. The spherical region with the approximately uniform magnetic field has a diameter close to the diameter of one coil. To strengthen the field from the basic Helmholtz coil configuration, additional coils can be added. Ideally, these coils should be positioned to lay on a surface with spherical geometry (see Fig. 25-4). However, spherical coil designs are not very practical, and present considerable challenges for

allowing the human body to enter such a magnet. A more practical design for including multiple circular coils is to add coils based on a cylindrical geometry, which allows for human entry into the magnet (see Fig. 25-4). The cylindrical design can be achieved by adjusting the current through each circular loop as opposed to changing the radius of each circular loop with a constant current. Note, that in this scenario, the strength of the central spherical field is increased, not its size.

## Practical Main Magnet

The coil windings using the cylindrical geometry can be made to emulate a spherical current distribution by increasing the number of windings toward the edges of the cylinder. Note that from the Biot-Savat law, magnetic fields are not confined to the central region, but extend in all directions from the magnet. These, often unwanted, fields are termed *fringe fields*. The magnetic field falls off under an inverse cubed relationship, which represents a steep decrease with distance. A field of 5 G is generally considered a safe field for people with pacemakers and for sensitive equipment such as cathode ray tube (CRT) computer screens, and so on. For a main magnetic field of 1.5 T (15,000 G), the 5-G field corresponds to 0.00005 T. Therefore, given the inverse cube law, the 5-G line occurs at approximately 15 m from the magnet center. Consequently the environmental impact of the large fringe field

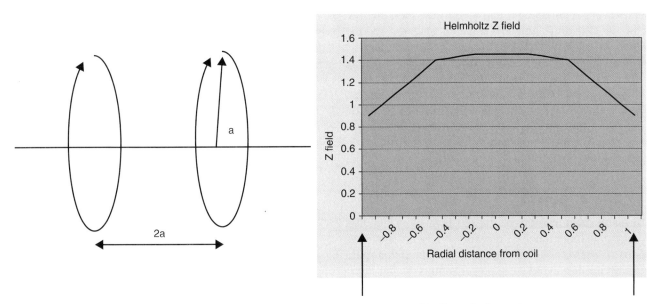

**FIGURE 25-3** An approximately uniform magnetic field is generated in the region between two circular current carrying wires, each of radius "a", and separated by a distance "2a." This is termed a *Helmholtz configuration*. The magnetic field along the Z-axis is shown in the graph, where each coil element is positioned at −1 and +1. The magnetic field on axis increases as distance from the coils increases because the effects of each coil reinforce toward the center of the configuration where the field is approximately uniform.

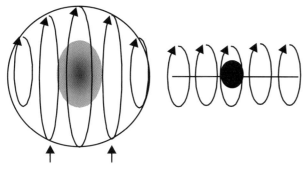

Original coils

**FIGURE 25-4** A strong uniform magnetic field is produced by extending the concept developed for the Helmholtz pair. In the first instance, additional coils are wound on a spherical surface (it can be appreciated that the original Helmholtz configuration includes only two of these coils indicated by arrows). Note that the volume of the uniform region is not increased relative to the original configuration. The concept can also be extended to a cylindrical geometry; in this case instead of decreasing the radius as in the spherical case, the strength of the current in the outer coils is increased to compensate for the relative increase in radius while currents decrease towards the center.

produced by a standard cylindrical magnet is generally considered too great for most settings. Considering that this extends in all three directions, many floors of a building may be affected. To overcome the large fringe field, magnetic shielding is employed. One such method is active shielding. Actively shielded magnets are designed with a counter wound magnet surrounding the original magnet (see Fig. 25-5). Given that the magnetic field falls off with an inverse cube relationship, the outer counter wound magnet only minimally affects the inner, primary magnet, whereas it has a large effect on decreasing the external fringe field. Active shielding of magnets typically produces a 5-G region that does not extend much further than the foot of the scanner table.

## Coil Characteristics

The major parameter describing electromagnetic coils is inductance. Inductance, L, measured in Henries is analogous to resistance. Consequently, inductance should be minimized to avoid large power requirements. Physically, inductance is related to the amount of magnetic flux lines that pass through the coil; therefore larger coils have larger inductances. Voltage is generated across the terminals of the coil when current through the coil changes:

$$V = L \, dI/dt$$

From this formula it can be seen that high voltages are required whenever a magnetic coil is switched on or off,

but no voltage (in practice a low voltage, due to a small resistance) is required to drive a steady current through a coil. Therefore, switching current in coils becomes a major design criteria for the coils and power supplies required to drive them.

## Gradient Coils

Just as uniform magnetic fields are generated by electromagnetic coils, gradient coils can be produced by rearranging the design. The features to optimize for gradient coils are as follows:

- Maximize extent of linear gradient
- Minimize inductance

There are the following three primary gradients in the MRI system:

- Z gradient
- X gradient
- Y gradient

## Z Gradient

To form a Z-direction gradient, the basic pair of circular coils is combined with reversed polarity current to form a gradient from two opposing fields (see Fig. 25-6). For the two circular loop design, the most linear gradient is formed when they are separated by:

$$\sqrt{3} \times \text{radius}$$

This optimized version is termed the *Maxwell configuration*, and is usually the most efficient of the three gradient coils. Note that the Maxwell gradient is linear

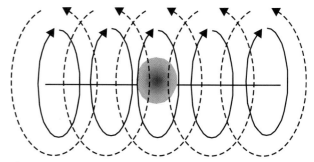

**FIGURE 25-5** The idea behind the self-shielded magnet is illustrated for the cylindrical geometry. The primary magnet is represented by the inner (*solid*) set of winding, and a counter wound, but weaker, magnet is constructed at a wider radius (*dashed*). The uniform region of field is indicated as a sphere in the center of the coils. The counter wound magnet has a proportionately larger effect on the external fringe field compared to the central field and therefore only minimally affects the main magnetic field, although dramatically decreasing the external fringe field.

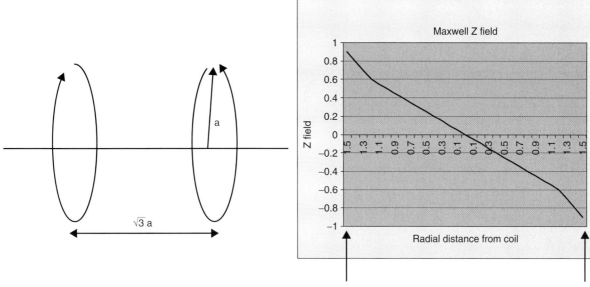

**FIGURE 25-6**   The elements of the Z gradient coils are shown. Two circular current loops, each of radius "a" and separated by a distance $\sqrt{3}$ a, but with current flowing in opposing directions generates an approximately uniform gradient between the coils as indicated in the field plot on the right (coil positions are at $+1$ and $-1$). This configuration is termed a *Maxwell coil set.*

over a greater region than the uniform field produced by the Helmholtz coil.

## X and Y Gradients

The basis of the design of X or Y gradients is based on the Helmholtz circular coil pair with the difference that the coils have a missing section, which creates the required gradient in either the X direction or the Y direction. The fundamental problem to be solved with this design is how to create a break in the coils. This is achieved by constructing the spilt Helmholtz coil in four sections, with the "return path" of each section set away from the central region (see Fig. 25-7). The basic design of the X or equivalently Y gradients is termed the *Golay coil.* In the Golay coil, the field from a straight wire element that is inherent in the return path generates a circular field. Because this field is perpendicular to current direction, there is no field component in the Z direction, which is the important direction for each of the gradient coils (see Fig. 25-8). Note that the gradient from each coil is in the Z, X, or Y directions, but the field from each is in the Z direction, such that they add to or subtract from the main magnetic field along the Z direction. The essential features of the Golay coils are as follows:

• Split circular loop design
• Straight wires are parallel to $\mathbf{B_0}$ and do not contribute to Z field

• Remote curved sections are far away from central field and do not contribute to the gradient

The basic Golay coil configuration can produce an X gradient. A second configuration rotated by 90 degrees is required for the Y gradient, but otherwise the design is exactly the same. The gradient from the Golay coil is linear over approximately 60% of the radius. In general the inductance of the Golay design is higher than the Z gradient design, and consequently, the X and Y gradients require more power.

## High Performance Gradients

Cardiac imaging demands the highest performance from the gradients. In this optimization strategy, some degree of linearity can be sacrificed because it is possible to correct nonlinearity through post-processing of the image. However, a fundamental difficulty with all switched gradients is the generation of "eddy currents." Eddy currents are generated because the switching gradients cause changes in the magnetic flux, which in turn generate a voltage, termed an *electromotive force* (*EMF*), in the metallic infrastructure of the scanner. The EMF causes current to flow in the metallic structure, which in turn generates a magnetic field. The EMF is only present when gradients are switched:

$$\text{EMF (V)} = d\text{flux}/dt$$

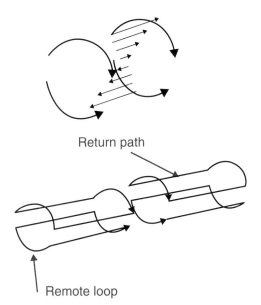

**FIGURE 25-7** The basic design of a Y gradient coil is indicated. The primary coil sections are indicated in the top panel, which are essentially two split Maxwell coil sets. The split design allows each section of the coils to be powered with opposing currents to generate a Y gradient as indicated. In the lower panel, the practical construction of the coil set is shown complete with the current return paths necessary to generate a complete circuit. The straight wire sections do not contribute to the Z field, and the return circular sections are too remote to affect the field.

Therefore, when a magnetic field gradient changes, a secondary field is set up, and proceeds to die down within a matter of milliseconds. This transitory spurious magnetic field is the eddy field. Because eddy fields are transitory, they are difficult to accommodate. Eddy currents are set up in the cylindrical metal shells that are integral to the magnet system that are, generally, outside of the gradient coil structure. One way to prevent eddy currents is to physically keep the gradients away from the rest of the magnet. This can be accomplished by utilizing specialized insert gradient coils, which are generally only large enough to scan a patient's head. A second approach, more applicable for body imaging systems, is to shield the scanner infrastructure from the changing magnetic fields. This is accomplished by using self-shielded gradients.

## Shielded Gradient Coils

Self-shielded gradient coils have two main structures, as follows:

- An inner main gradient shell
- An outer gradient shell

The outer gradient has a coil winding that produces a magnetic field that opposes the main gradient field at that position. By powering the shielding gradient with the reverse polarity current of the main gradients system, the metallic infrastructure of the scanner does not experience any change in magnetic field, and therefore no (or greatly reduced) eddy currents are generated, typically $<1\%$.

## Distributed Coil Designs

Up to this point we have considered eddy currents in an entirely negative light, that is, as something to be eliminated. However, it is possible to harness them to improve gradient coil design. The coils considered so far are based on classical, analytical, solutions of the Biot-Savat formula. A more distributed design is generated when coils are designed with the aim of mimicking the current path set up eddy currents for a given field configuration. Distributed coils are designed by setting up (in the computer) the desired field, that is the "target field," and considering the eddy currents that would be set up in a metallic shell or surface surrounding the target field region. By assuming (in the computer simulation) that the metallic shell is superconducting, any currents established in the surface will continue without decay. In many cases, the complicated current paths thus designed are etched in a copper material rather than being wound in the traditional sense.

## Shimming

As we have seen, there are many compromises made in the design and manufacture of a practical magnet system. For instance, it is impractical to design a $\mathbf{B_0}$ magnet with sufficiently high homogeneity for MRI. For this reason, shim coils were introduced. A typical magnet has approximately 20 shim coils included to correct the field. Shim fields are applied in a static manner, and are typically fixed during installation of the system. Each shim coil produces a certain order of correction:

- First-order X, Y, Z linear gradients
- Second-order, $X^2Y$, $Y^2X$ gradients
- Third-order $Z^3$, and so on

Most systems allow adjustment of the first-order shim gradients to correct inhomogeneities that are introduced by the patient. Typically, real-time correction using higher order shim gradients is impractical, and generally unnecessary.

## Radiofrequency Coils are Magnets Too!

The main magnetic field, $\mathbf{B_0}$, is static (in reality it experiences a very gradual "drift"). The gradient coils

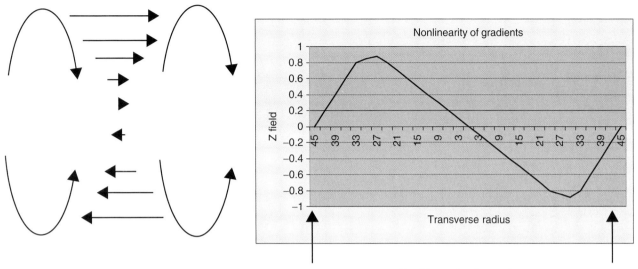

Position of primary loops

**FIGURE 25-8**   The essential elements of the Y gradient are drawn in isolation from the return current paths. Note, that although the gradient is in the Y-axis, the field direction is along the Z-axis. This configuration is termed a *Golay coil set*. The X gradient is achieved with a similar design, which is rotated through 90 degrees. The form of the gradient is indicated in the graph on the right.

require that the fields be switched on the order of 0.25 milliseconds, which puts them in the kHz range (i.e., audio frequency). The transmitter and receiver RF coils are sensitive to magnetic fields that change in the MHz range (i.e., radiofrequency). A basic RF coil produces (or equivalently is sensitive to) magnetic fields in the transverse plane, for example, the X or Y directions, as opposed to the Z direction. For initial design considerations, consider a Helmholtz coil pair that produces a uniform field over a spherical region between the coils, and in the case of RF coils, this pair would be oriented perpendicular to the **B₀** direction (see Fig. 25-9). In the case of a cylindrical magnet structure, this RF coil pair would be further bent over a cylindrical former to better fit in the scanner.

## Body Coil

The body RF coil is one that can excite spins uniformly over an extended region of the body. The modified Helmholtz design can be used to accomplish this because of its suitability for large volumes. Body coils are designed for uniformity of excitation, often at the expense of efficiency.

## Quadrature Detection

Note that the ideal elemental coil of an RF detection system is only sensitive to one component of the magnetic field. However, a rotating magnetic field (i.e., emanating from precessing spins) can be broken down into two orthogonal components. Quadrature detection

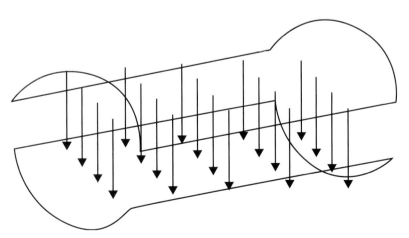

**FIGURE 25-9**   The design of a radiofrequency (RF) transmitter coil is illustrated. Conforming to a cylindrical geometry, the basic design is that of a Helmholtz coil pair, in this case oriented to produce a field in the vertical direction (field of arrows).

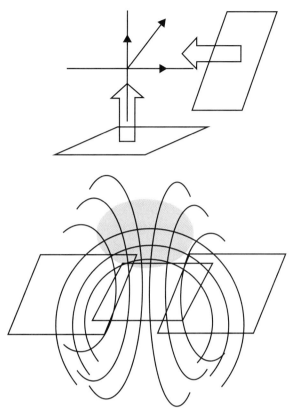

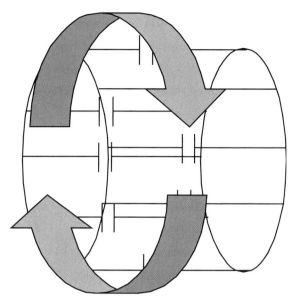

**FIGURE 25-11** The current path of the highly efficient birdcage radiofrequency (RF) coil is shown. Each leg of the birdcage coil has a capacitor to tune the leg to the correct phase, such that a net circular current path is achieved as indicated.

**FIGURE 25-10** Quadrature signal detection. In the top panel, the signal source is indicated as a spin precessing in the transverse plane. One coil positioned below is sensitive to the spin component along the vertical axis, and the coil to the side is sensitive to the spin component along the horizontal axis. In this case, sensitivity to each primary component of the spin (i.e., quadrature detection) is achieved with two orthogonal coils. In the lower panel, a practical realization of quadrature detection is shown using a coil configuration wound on a flat plane. The flux lines from the outer linked coils are shown intersecting the flux lines from the single central coil. At the region indicated by shading, the flux lines are approximately orthogonal, and therefore achieve quadrature detection for this region of the body. The advantage of quadrature detection is that the signal-to-noise ratio (SNR) is improved compared to a coil system sensitive to only one component.

possible to balance positive and negative flux such that the net flux cancels to zero.

## Phased Array Design

Phased array coils are arranged such that the net flux from one coil to the others is zero. Further, the penetration (or sensitive region) of each coil element is approximately equal to the radius of one coil and therefore it is apparent that an array of smaller coils allows greater coverage of the body, with good sensitivity achieved for each body region. In this mode, each element requires its own receiver electronics for optimal performance.

## Birdcage Design

The birdcage design of RF coil is a highly efficient design. Each "leg" of the coil is tuned relative to the others such that the current travels around the coil (i.e., between each leg) in a sinusoidal manner, effectively simulating a wide circular loop, which is achieved with minimum current requirements (see Fig. 25-11). Quadrature detection is possible with this design. Head coils are typically of this design at 1.5 T.

## Radiofrequency Coil Quality

The quality, or Q, factor of an RF coil describes the "lossyness" of the system:

- Q is frequency dependant
- $Q = \omega \times$ energy stored/power lost

describes the ability to be sensitive to each component simultaneously (see Fig. 25-10). Quadrature detection results in the SNR improving by $\sqrt{2}$. Quadrature detection requires that two coil elements be positioned such that their fields are orthogonal in the region of interest. One feature of quadrature designs is that the elements should ideally not interact with each other; this condition is said to be described as *zero mutual inductance*. Remember, that inductance is a function of the net flux that passes through the coil. Therefore, by arranging for coils to overlap to some extent, it is

When the body is positioned near the RF coil, it absorbs energy from the RF in the form of heat:

- Power to body $= P(1 - Q_{loaded}/Q_{unloaded})$

SAR is the measure of how much power is deposited in the body. SAR is the specific absorption rate.

Power is the rate of doing (absorbing) work. FDA guidelines limit the SAR:

- 3 W per kilogram over the whole body
- 8 W per kilogram over a local region

Regulations are constantly changing, reflecting the evolving understanding of magnetic resonance (MR) and application of technology.

## SUMMARY

There are many magnet systems used in an MRI system

- Static $\mathbf{B_0}$
- RF $\mathbf{B_1}$

- Receiver coils
- X, Y, and Z gradients

Gradient performance dominates scanner performance:

- Slow gradients—low performance

Optimization of RF coils for signal reception requires that each RF coil element has its own receiver channel. Systems are being built with increasing numbers of channels and the processing power to integrate the high stream of data generated by CMR.

# CHAPTER 26

# Parallel Imaging

Mark Doyle

## OVERVIEW

Parallel imaging, sometimes referred to as *reduced field of view* (FOV) *imaging*, is a means to rapidly acquire k-space data by exploiting the spatial relationships that exist between several imaging receiver coils. Alternatively, parallel imaging can be used to acquire high-resolution k-space matrices in a conventional scan time. Parallel imaging is a feature unique to magnetic resonance imaging (MRI) because it exploits special properties of k-space.

## REDUCED FIELD OF VIEW BASIC PRINCIPLES

An understanding of the basic properties of k-space is central to appreciating the mechanism of parallel imaging. Each magnetic resonance (MR) data set is acquired in the k-space domain, which is achieved by application of a frequency encoding gradient, in combination with successive applications of a phase encoding gradient to encode each line of k-space separately. Once assembled, the k-space data are Fourier transformed to generate an image. Normally, the number of lines acquired in k-space is determined by a combination of the FOV of the body region being imaged and the resolution required. When the FOV is made smaller and resolution maintained, the net scan time is reduced, but signal aliasing may result as the FOV becomes smaller than the body region. Usually, some degree of signal aliasing is permissible, especially if the region of interest is toward the center of the image, and this region is unaffected by the folded over signal. Further, resolution is uniform throughout the image, such that image regions contaminated by fold-over data, and regions not obscured by signal aliasing are represented at the same resolution as in a higher FOV scan.

## PARALLEL IMAGING APPROACH

Parallel imaging is an FOV reducing strategy that avoids the fold-over artifact that is associated with conventional reduced FOV approaches. There are two features that make parallel imaging possible when k-space data are acquired corresponding to a small FOV:

- Signals corresponding to spatially distinct receiver coils are separately acquired.
- Special image processing is applied.

A key feature of parallel imaging is the use of several receiver coils. Coils are typically configured with 4, 8, 16, or even more elements. Each coil element primarily receives a signal from a localized region of the body. In this scenario, coil elements close to a slice region receive the strongest signal from that region, whereas coil elements that are more distant receive relatively little signal. Further, some coil elements, which have sensitivity to regions outside of the selected FOV, will contribute strongly to alias artifact (see Fig. 26-1). As is common to alias artifact, the aliased signal appears at a region remote from the source of the signal (see Fig. 26-2). Each coil element generates a complete image, and these are typically combined to form an image with increased signal-to-noise ratio (SNR). However, by the simple addition of multiple images form the multiple coils, the image contribution from some coil elements may introduce substantial fold-over artifact to a region that, when imaged by a separate coil element, did not previously have a significant artifact. In this way, addition of the separate images may serve to distort some regions while improving the SNR in others.

Fold-over artifacts originate from tissue outside of the FOV, but within the sensitivity range of the receiver element(s). Depending on the sensitivity characteristics of the receiver coil, the fold-over artifact may be very faint if the region is physically remote from the coil

Coil element on chest

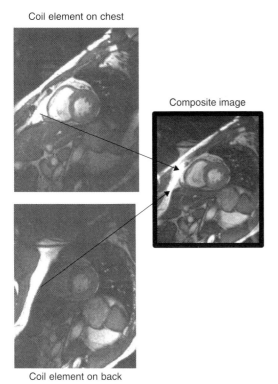

Composite image

Coil element on back

**FIGURE 26-1** The coil element on the chest wall images the heart region well, with minimal contribution from artifact (top left), whereas the coil element closest to the back contributes a large signal alias over the heart (lower left), which dominates the heart region in the composite image (right). The alias signal originates from the field of view being set too small relative to the sensitivity of each element.

element or bright if close. Stated mathematically, each separate receiver coil contributes the following two features of interest:

- A range of sensitivities over the body
- A range of contributions to fold over artifacts

In the final image, which is a composite of each separate image, all these features are apparent, and only prior knowledge of the coil sensitivities allows the details of the fold-over artifact to be appreciated.

## REDUCED FOLD-OVER APPROACH

To avoid aliasing artifact, we could consider a first-order approximation approach, whereby a composite image is compiled only from regions of the separate images in which each region is best observed, with good SNR and without appreciable signal alias. In this (generally unworkable) approach, the signal sensitivity is reduced, because no signal averaging occurs, and the final image looks like a patchwork with sharp intensity transitions. This is an unsatisfying approach because not all the coil information is used.

Coil element on chest

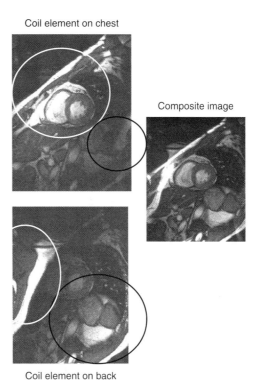

Composite image

Coil element on back

**FIGURE 26-2** The separate contributions from two coil elements are shown, one positioned on the chest wall (top left) and one positioned on the back (cover left). There is only one field of view (FOV) for the entire composite image (right). However, the chest coil has high sensitivity to the heart (*light circle* on chest coil image) and low sensitivity to the back (*dark circle* on chest coil image). Conversely, the back coil has high sensitivity to the back (*dark circle* on back coil image) and low sensitivity to the chest. However, the back coil contributes a large artifact signal (*light circle* on back coil image) originating from the back region but appearing over the chest wall.

## K-SPACE AND THE FIELD OF VIEW

Another, more general, approach can be used, which exploits some of the properties of k-space. There is a relationship between k-space and the FOV. When k-space is "fully sampled," it means that the sampling density in k-space matches the FOV, that is, the number of lines sampled and the line spacing is such that the FOV is correctly encompassed. To increase the FOV, the sampling density of k-space must be increased. Conversely, to reduce the FOV, the k-space sampling density must be reduced (see Fig. 26-3). Consider reducing the FOV by a factor of 2. This is achieved by removing every other line of k-space. In this special case, compared with the full image, the half FOV image is simply the superposition of the two halves of the original image, one placed on top of the other. This is a result of the body region and the coil sensitivities extending beyond the FOV. Note that in

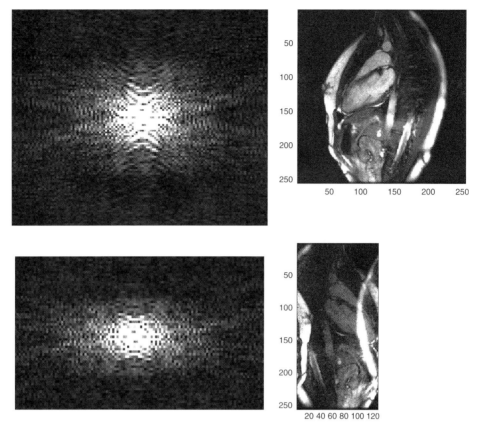

**FIGURE 26-3**   The influence of k-space coverage on field of view (FOV) is illustrated. The top panel represents a fully resolved k-space matrix and the corresponding image. The lower panel represents k-space with every other line removed, showing the resulting image with a reduced FOV, in this case reduced by a factor of 2, with severe signal aliasing readily apparent.

this procedure the resolution of the reduced FOV image is identical to that of the full FOV image.

## ADDITIONAL INFORMATION

If the half FOV image was all that we possessed, then the two halves of the image could not be unambiguously disentangled, and the severely aliased image would be the final result that we could extract. However, by using two or more separate coils, each with a separate spatial sensitivity, then we can consider disentangling the information, and producing a fully resolved and unaliased image. Consider a two-coil system:

- Coil 1—top section
- Coil 2—lower section

In Fig. 26-4, coil 1 is most sensitive to the top region of the object (each pixel is represented by the letters A, B, C, and D) but it also has some sensitivity to the lower section (with pixels represented by the letters Q, R, S, and T). Similarly, coil 2 is positioned over the lower

section of the same object, and has high sensitivity to pixels Q, R, S, and T, and diminished sensitivity to pixels A, B, C, and D. In the case where the FOV is reduced by a factor of 2 (i.e., removing every other line of k-space), signal aliasing occurs such that pixel A exactly overlays pixel Q, pixel B overlays pixel R, and so on (see Fig. 26-5). Further, note that this overlapping set of pixels is imaged twice, once by coil 1, and simultaneously by coil 2. Thus, at this point what we have achieved is the acquisition of two aliased images.

## DECONVOLUTION

Consider the situation expressed mathematically for a single pixel, in which pixel "A" overlaps pixel "Q." The signal of this pixel from coil 1 is:

Coil-1sensitivity@ A × A + Coil-1sensitivity@ Q × Q

And from coil 2 is :

Coil-2sensitivity@ Q × Q + Coil-2sensitivity@ A × A

where Coil-1sensitivity@ A stands for the sensitivity of coil 1 at pixel A, and "A" represents the signal

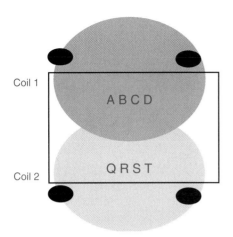

FIGURE 26-4   The sensitivities of two coils are shown: coil 1 has high sensitivity to regions marked A, B, C, D and coil 2 has high sensitivity to regions marked Q, R, S, T. In this example, we will treat A, B, C, and so on, as if they were individual pixels in the fully resolved image. Note that although coil 1 has the highest sensitivity to A, B, C, D it has some sensitivity to Q, R, S, T and vice versa for coil 2.

originating from pixel "A," and so on. Note that these two (simultaneous) equations have six unknowns, as follows:

- "A"
- "Q"
- Coil-1sensitivity@ A
- Coil-1sensitivity@ Q
- Coil-2sensitivity@ Q
- Coil-2sensitivity@ A

Therefore, they cannot be solved unless we know the sensitivity of each coil at each pixel position.

## SENSITIVITY MAPPING

The sensitivity of each coil at each pixel position can be determined using a specially designed prescan.

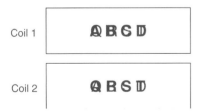

FIGURE 26-5   When alternate lines of k-space are not sampled, it effectively reduces the field of view (FOV) by a factor of 2. In this case, the pixels A and Q exactly overlap in the aliased image, and so on. Additionally, there are two distinct images formed, one from coil 1 and one from coil 2. Note that in the coil 1 image, A, B, C, D is represented at higher intensity than Q, R, S, T and vice versa for coil 2.

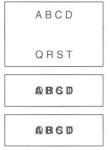

FIGURE 26-6   The two aliased images (lower panels) can be deconvoluted (resolved into a full image, upper panel), if the sensitivities of each coil to each pixel are known. With this knowledge, the intensity at A and Q could be disentangled due to possession of two folded over images with complementary data regarding sensitivity.

This is generally a rapid, low-resolution scan, which may encompass a slice or (more generally) a volume. The sensitivity information from this prescan is stored for use during the post-processing stage, to allow deconvolution of the half FOV image (see Fig. 26-6). The parallel imaging process can be made more general than presented here, and higher reduction factors can be used, but a factor of 2 is one that is commonly used. In the limit, the criterion governing the maximal reduction factor is that there is at least one coil element per reduction factor, e.g. 32 coils could allow a reduction factor of 32.

## PARALLEL IMAGING

With a sensitivity map and separate receiver coils (the electronics for the receiver coils are often called *channels*), parallel imaging can be performed. Parallel imaging gets its name from acquiring two halves (or less) of k-space in a parallel manner, that is, by acquiring only 50% of k-space lines; the remaining 50% are effectively filled in by the mathematic process indicated in the preceding text. The processing can occur in the k-space domain or in the image domain. Parallel imaging is also referred to a *reduced FOV imaging*.

## PARALLEL IMAGING EXAMPLE

An original scan of a water phantom, imaged using the cardiac phased array coil, will experience some intensity variations, which are not artifacts, but simply reflect the sensitivity variations of the coil configuration (see Fig. 26-7). In the parallel image of this phantom (see Fig. 26-7), some artifacts are apparent that mostly relate to edge features that would have resulted in signal aliasing, but are not fully eliminated by the parallel imaging processing. It is interesting to compare the performance

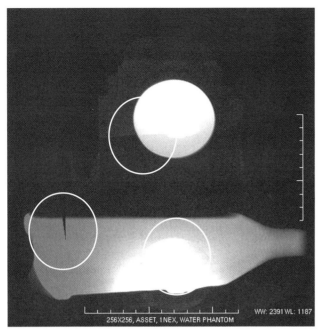

**FIGURE 26-7** A water phantom imaged with a parallel imaging factor of 2. In this case, some residual artifacts are apparent. These are related to incomplete suppression of aliased features (*circled*). The wedge-shaped region that is missing has no obvious source of alias, and is probably related to a masking procedure of signal regions contaminated by noise.

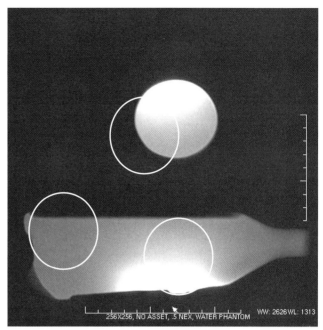

**FIGURE 26-8** A comparable image to Fig. 26-7 is shown. In this case, the scan times were the same although the image here was acquired using a number of excitations (NEX) factor of 0.5. Note the lack of artifacts in comparable regions to the image in Fig. 26-7 (*circled* regions).

of parallel imaging using a reduction factor of 2 with a partial number of excitations (NEX) scan using a factor of 0.5. The scan time of the two approaches is identical, although the partial NEX scan has fewer artifacts (see Fig. 26-8). In the 0.5 NEX scan, no residual fold-over artifacts are present, and further, the scan resolution is identical, and no prescanning sequence is required to obtain a sensitivity map.

## PARALLEL IMAGING WATER AND FAT EXAMPLE

Consider another phantom, consisting of separate water and fat based objects, again imaged using the phased array cardiac coil (images available on CD). Some intensity variations are present, reflecting the interface between solid and liquid fat, and the intensity variations of the separate coils. In the parallel imaging example, additional edge artifacts are present relative to the pure water phantom. The origin of the fat- or water-specific artifacts is from the different resonance frequencies of water and fat (3.5 parts per million frequency shift, or approximately 250 Hz at 1.5 T). This frequency difference leads to a fat shift that may be different between the sensitivity scan and the final scan, due to differences in the gradient strengths used for each

scan. Again, a 0.5 NEX scan has a similar scan time to the parallel image, and produces no additional artifact due to the presence of water and fat signals. As with most acceleration features, multiple strategies can be combined to reduce the scan time further, such as combining parallel imaging with partial NEX. However, the law of diminishing returns, and the scanning overhead associated with each approach, limits the practical scan time reduction that can be routinely achieved.

## MAJOR APPLICATION AREAS

The major application area for parallel imaging is that of rapid imaging, although increasing the scan resolution is less widely used. The parallel imaging methods in common use now are as follows:

- SMASH
- SENSE
- ASSET

When applied *in vivo*, parallel imaging may generate noticeable artifacts, especially when a small FOV is employed. Naturally, other sources of signal artifact (e.g., respiratory motion and pulsatile blood) may still be present in parallel images. One feature of parallel images is that the SNR is diminished as a consequence of

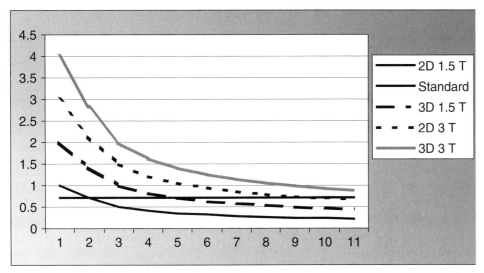

**FIGURE 26-9**   The benefits of parallel imaging will likely increase with 3D imaging and higher field strengths. Plotted here are signal-to-noise ratio (SNR) estimates for various scans against increasing parallel imaging factors. For the case of 2D imaging at 1.5 T, the SNR drops to 70% when a factor of 2 is used. This is represented by the straight horizontal line, and is generally considered to be the lower level of acceptable SNR. At 1.5 T, 3D has a higher inherent SNR, and two phase encoding directions are applied. Parallel imaging can be applied along each phase direction and higher factors can be used while still maintaining the SNR above the lower limit of acceptability (e.g. a factor of 4 in this example). When 3 T fields are considered, higher parallel imaging factors are feasible, as indicated for the 2D and 3D scans.

acquiring fewer data points. When only half the number of lines are acquired compared with a full scan the SNR is reduced by a factor of $1/\sqrt{2}$ ($\sim$70% of the full scan). In general, the reduction factor is dependent on the number of coils that are combined. Imaging systems are available with >32 channels, and therefore the potential for decreased scan time is high, limited only by the SNR that is acceptable.

## PARALLEL DIMENSIONS

Because the SNR increases with the number phase encoding steps performed and the field strength used, the reduction in SNR inherent in parallel approaches may be offset by increasing the number of scan dimensions imaged, such as is possible with three- dimensional (3D) imaging, and increasing the inherent SNR by increasing the main magnetic field strength, as is achieved using a 3 T compared with a 1.5 T system. Consider that an im-

age produced at 1.5 T using a parallel imaging factor of 2 produces an acceptable SNR, and that this represents the lower limit of acceptability, then 3D imaging, and higher field strengths have potential to allow reduction factors of up to 32 without SNR falling below this limit. Therefore, at the time of writing, it appears that the major benefits of parallel imaging are yet to be realized, and involve 3D imaging approaches, possibly at higher field strengths (see Fig. 26-9).

## SUMMARY

Parallel imaging can be used to reduce the scan time if separate channel coils are used. Higher scan dimensions, such as 3D, may have more opportunities for scan time reduction compared with 2D, and higher field strengths may allow parallel imaging to be applied to greater benefit. Application areas such as angiography, volume imaging, and cine imaging can all potentially benefit from incorporating parallel imaging.

# CHAPTER 27

# Steady State Free Precession

Mark Doyle

## OVERVIEW

Steady state free precession (SSFP) imaging is the means of combining all three echo types: gradient, spin, and stimulated; to form a very efficient, signal rich image. Here we will quickly review the basic properties of k-space and the role of gradients, and develop the mechanism utilized in SSFP imaging. The major application area discussed here for SSFP is cardiac functional imaging.

## K-SPACE

The magnetic resonance imaging (MRI) data space is termed *k-space*. Briefly, each image requires a two-dimensional (2D) arrangement of signal data, termed *k-space*. To form an image, the k-space data undergoes Fourier transformation. Here we represent k-space as a series of parallel lines, each line corresponding to an individual acquisition of an MRI echo signal. Most conventional MR imaging sequences fill k-space one line at a time. To encode each k-space line requires application of two separate gradients:

- Frequency encoding, for example, X
- Phase encoding, for example, Y

Magnetic gradients are applied to accomplish frequency encoding and phase encoding.

## SIGNAL PREPARATION AND ENCODING

A basic property of nuclear spins is that an individual nuclear species precess at a field-dependent frequency, $\omega$, given by the Larmor equation:

$$\omega = \gamma \times \mathbf{B_0}$$

A magnetic gradient applied to the body causes nuclear spins in different locations to process at field-dependent frequencies:

- Low field strength, low precession rate
- High field strength, high precession rate

The phase encoding gradient is applied before signal detection, and therefore the signal is required to be delayed from the slice selection time point to the time when it is measured. Although this time is only a matter of milliseconds, it is nevertheless required, and requires special treatment. The signal echo is the means of delaying the signal to allow spin preparation to take place before sampling of k-space. Here we discuss the stimulated echo, which is one component contributing to SSFP.

## STIMULATED ECHO

In a stimulated echo, the initial radiofrequency (RF) pulse is followed by a positive gradient; after some time a second RF pulse is applied with no gradient; after a second delay, a third RF pulse is applied, which is followed by a positive gradient. Under these conditions, spins

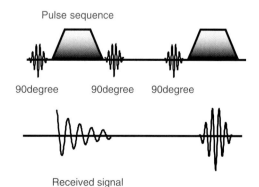

**FIGURE 27-1** The basic elements of the stimulated echo are first radiofrequency (RF) pulse, gradient, second RF pulse, delay, third RF pulse, gradient. Following the third RF pulse, a stimulated echo is generated.

Pulse sequence

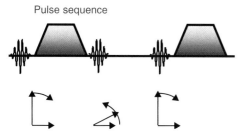

**FIGURE 27-2** The first radiofrequency (RF) pulse (*horizontal arrow*) brings the magnetization vector, **M₀** (*vertical arrow*), into the transverse plane, and a free induction decay (FID) signal is seen. The spins are dephased by the imaging gradient. The second RF pulse (*horizontal arrow*) puts the spins back up along the Z-axis, and therefore no signal is generated. The third RF pulse (*horizontal arrow*) brings the spins (*vertical arrow*) back to the transverse plane, where the second gradient refocuses the spins, and an echo signal is seen.

refocus as an echo following the third RF pulse (see Fig. 27-1). Therefore, in a stimulated echo the essential features are as follows:

- Apply an initial 90-degree RF pulse
- Time delay
- Apply the second 90-degree RF pulse
- Time delay
- Apply the third 90-degree RF pulse
- Imaging gradients are balanced after the first and third RF pulses

One way of thinking about the stimulated echo is to consider the combination of the second and third 90-degree RF pulses to be equivalent to a single 180-degree refocusing RF pulse, as used in spin echo imaging (see Fig. 27-2). The significance of splitting the pulse into two components with a time delay between them will become apparent in the following discourse.

## STIMULATED ECHO EFFICIENCY

Following the initial 90-degree RF pulse, all spins are brought down into the transverse plane. During the delay following this pulse, spins dephase because of the application of a magnetic gradient. However, at the time of application of the second RF pulse, only 50% of spins are effectively put back along this axis. To appreciate this, consider the spin system resolved into X and Y components in the transverse plane (see Fig. 27-3):

- The first RF pulse brings down the coherent **M₀** magnetization into the transverse plane.
- The applied gradient dephases spins until no net signal is seen. At this point, resolving spins along the

Pulse sequence

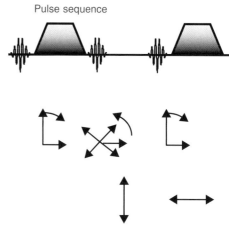

**FIGURE 27-3** The efficiency of the stimulated echo is limited by the percentage of spins returned to the Z-axis by the second radiofrequency (RF) pulse. The first RF pulse acts on 100% of the signal along the Z-axis (*vertical arrow*). Owing to the dephasing action of the first gradient, at the time of the second RF pulse, the spins are completely dephased. At this stage, they can be resolved into X and Y components (*crossed arrows*). The second RF pulse (*horizontal arrow*) only affects the component that is orthogonal to it. Thus, immediately following the second RF pulse, only 50% of the spins are aligned along the Z-axis (*vertical arrows* in lower panel). The third RF pulse acts on 100% of the signal along the Z axis, and brings it down to the transverse plane (*horizontal arrows* in lower panel).

X- and Y-axes, we see that there are equal spin components along the positive and negative X- and Y-axes.
- The second RF pulse only acts on the spin component that is perpendicular to the RF magnetization, and therefore if the RF is applied along the Y-axis, only the component of **M₀** along the X-axis will be affected by the RF pulse. In this case, this corresponds to 50% of the signal.
- The third RF pulse brings down the component of **M₀** positioned along the Z-axis, completing the conditions for the spins to refocus in an echo in the third time period.

An important aspect of the stimulated echo is that spins are realigned along the Z-axis faster than the T1 relaxation process achieves the same Z-level magnetization. This is advantageous under certain imaging conditions, especially if rapid pulsing is required. However, the loss of 50% of signal diminishes enthusiasm for the stimulated echo sequence in this form.

## STIMULATED ECHO REFOCUSING

It is possible to improve the efficiency of the stimulated echo by refocusing the spins before application of the second RF pulse, such that all the spins are sent back

Pulse sequence

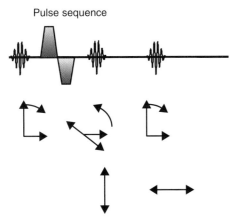

**FIGURE 27-4** The efficiency of the stimulated echo sequence is improved by refocusing the spins at the time of the second radiofrequency (RF) pulse. In this case, the gradient following the first RF pulse has equal positive and negative lobes, and therefore spins are refocused at the time of application of the second RF pulse. The second RF pulse (*horizontal arrow*) puts all the spins along the Z-axis (*vertical arrows* in lower panel of figure). The third RF pulse acts on the Z-axis spins (100%) to bring them into the transverse plane to contribute to the stimulated echo (*horizontal arrows* in lower panel).

along the Z-axis (see Fig. 27-4). This is achieved by balancing gradients between the first and second RF pulses. In this case, the refocused spins only generate one component in the transverse plane. Because there is only one component, the action of the second RF pulse acts on the complete spin system, yielding 100% efficiency in spins contributing to the final echo signal. The optimum condition for stimulated echo imaging is to use 90 degrees for each of the three RF pulses.

## COMBINING ECHOES

Going beyond this efficiency gain in the stimulated echo sequence, it is possible to realize even further gains in signal to noise by combining echoes (see Fig. 27-5):

- Gradient
- Spin
- Stimulated

Combining all three echo types in each image requires that each echo is generated following each RF pulse, and that the echoes are coincident with each other. To accomplish this, the RF pulse strength must be compromised compared to the optimum for each echo type, with a 45-degree to 60-degree pulse angle being typical. Additionally, the train of RF pulses must be applied at a constant rate, so as not to disrupt the continuity of the signal conditions. Under these conditions, the first RF pulse and gradient generates a pure gradient echo, the second RF pulse and gradient,

Pulse sequence

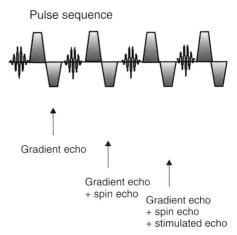

**FIGURE 27-5** The first radiofrequency (RF) pulse and balanced gradient generates a pure gradient echo, the second RF pulse generates its own gradient echo and forms a spin echo in combination with the first RF pulse. The third RF pulse generates its own gradient echo, a spin echo with the second RF pulse, and a stimulated echo due to interaction with the spins excited by the first and second RF pulses. All subsequent RF pulses will generate all three echoes.

form not only a gradient echo, but combine with the "spin memory" of the first RF pulse to form a spin echo. Similarly, the third RF pulse forms a gradient echo, a spin echo, and a stimulated echo. There are no other types of echoes, and therefore the fourth RF pulse and successive pulses, generate these three types of echoes. By keeping the train of RF pulses regular, each of the three echo types are superimposed on each other, realizing the combination of echoes required for maximizing the signal. The signal does not settle to a constant level immediately, and a period of preparation is required to achieve the steady state signal level. This can be as long as two heartbeats in duration. However, if the RF flip angle is varied up to the steady state level, then the preparation time can be dramatically reduced.

## STEADY STATE FREE PRECESSION PULSE SEQUENCE

The SSFP echo sequence has the following components (see Fig. 27-6):

- Slice selection
- Gradient echo
- Frequency encoding (or measurement)
- Phase encoding

Note that the gradients have to be balanced within each interval between RF pulses. Following each RF pulse interval, the next RF pulse interval immediately commences, with the gradients even being continuous

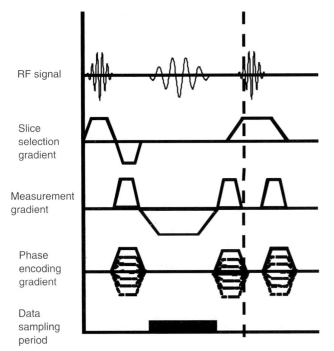

RF signal

Slice
selection
gradient

Measurement
gradient

Phase
encoding
gradient

Data
sampling
period

**FIGURE 27-6** The pulse diagram of the steady state free precession (SSFP) sequence is shown: radiofrequency (RF) pulse; slice selection gradient; measurement or frequency gradient; phase encoding gradient; data sampling. Note that the gradients are balanced between positive and negative components within each cycle (i.e., the interval between each RF pulse). The *vertical dashed line* indicates where the gradients for the next application of the sequence start, with some gradients being continuous from one application to the next.

from one interval to the next. In SSP imaging the echo time (TE) is quoted for the gradient echo portion of the sequence only. This can be a misleadingly low time, when it is considered that the spin and stimulated echo components have TEs, which are factors of 2 and 3 longer, respectively. To avoid spin dephasing, the whole sequence is repeated rapidly:

- Repetition time (TR) ~4 milliseconds
- TE ~2 milliseconds

In SSFP imaging a steady state must be established and maintained. This requires a train of >20 RF pulses and gradients before a steady state is achieved, and nothing should disrupt the train of pulses, not even the requirement of electrocardiogram (ECG) triggering.

## STEADY STATE FREE PRECESSION AND CARDIAC TRIGGERING

Because the SSFP sequence cannot be disrupted by ECG gating requirements, such as waiting for the R wave

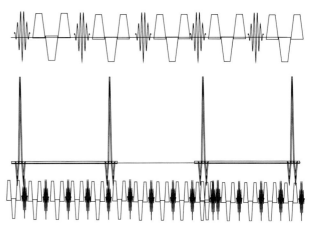

**FIGURE 27-7** The relationship of the steady state free precession (SSFP) sequence to the electrocardiogram (ECG) cycle is indicated. On the top line is indicated the uniform timing of the radiofrequency (RF) pulses and the balanced nature of the gradients. On the lower line, the sequence is represented as uniformly applied over successive cardiac cycles.

before advancing the k-space lines for the next cardiac cycle (see Fig. 27-7). Therefore, advanced ECG triggering is employed to keep the train of pulses constant. For this reason, cardiac triggered SSFP images usually span the cardiac cycle fully, that is, starting at the R wave, and with the last acquisition completed immediately before the next R wave.

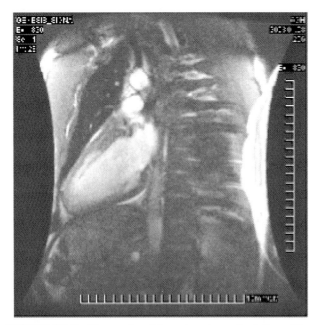

**FIGURE 27-8** The contrast to noise characteristics of the steady state free precession (SSFP) sequence applied to cardiac imaging are seen here. Note that fat and blood are bright, whereas myocardial and muscle signals are of intermediate intensity.

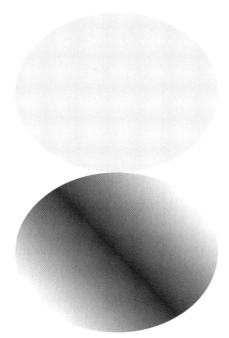

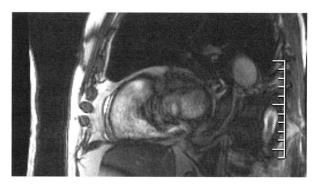

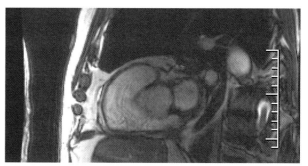

**FIGURE 27-9** Ideally, the phase of the image should be uniform across the entire image field (top figure). Illustrated in the lower figure is the variation in phase that might be expected because of a linear variation in the magnetic field homogeneity. These features affect the appearance of the SSFP image.

## STEADY STATE FREE PRECESSION PROPERTIES

In SSFP imaging, because all three echoes contribute to each signal, the signal-to-noise ratio (SNR) is inherently high. Additionally, because there are many RF pulses applied in a short time interval, the specific absorption rate (SAR), a measure of energy deposited in the body, is also quite high. This may present a problem at high fields. The contrast to noise ratio (CNR) in SSFP is dependent on the ratio of T2 to T1:

$$CNR \propto \sqrt{(T2/T1)}$$

To contribute to the SSFP signal, spins must receive all three RF pulses, and therefore very fast moving spins may generate motion artifacts, or may not contribute to the signal.

## MYOCARDIAL BLOOD CONTRAST

The SSFP signal intensity is dependent on the ratio of T2/T1, and the values and contrast for myocardium, fat, and blood are as follows:

Myocardium
- ○ T1 850 milliseconds
- ○ T2 70 milliseconds
- ○ T2/T1 = 0.08

**FIGURE 27-10** In the top figure, there is obvious disruption of the flow signal in the middle of the image. This is due to the selected resonance frequency of the acquisition not accurately representing the actual resonance frequency in this part of the image. In the lower figure, the acquisition was repeated with the reference frequency adjusted to better represent the resonance frequency in the region of flow. Here, the flow artifact has disappeared.

Fat
- ○ T1 260 milliseconds
- ○ T2 110 milliseconds
- ○ T2/T1 = 0.43

Blood
- ○ T1 1,000 milliseconds
- ○ T2 400 milliseconds
- ○ T2/T1 = 0.40

Therefore, it can be appreciated that myocardial signal is relatively dark compared to either fat or blood (see Fig. 27-8).

## STEADY STATE FREE PRECESSION ARTIFACTS

Because the SSFP is sensitive to spin phase interactions, a common artifact is the appearance of a "phase roll" in the image (see Fig. 27-9). Usually this phase roll occurs in the periphery of the image where the artifact makes what should be a bright region alternate between bright and dark. The origin of this artifact is the interplay between the reference frequency of the system and inhomogeneities within the body. Sometimes, these phase roll artifacts manifest as severe disruptions of blood flow (see Fig. 27-10). To remedy this, it is possible to alter the reference frequency of the scanner (performed at the resonance frequency operation in the prescan) and the repeated scan may be free of this artifact.

## SUMMARY

SSFP imaging combines all three echo types to produce an inherently high SNR image. The sequence requires short TR, TE, and no interruption of the signal train. This requires specialized ECG gating, usually resulting in good coverage of the complete cardiac cycle in cine imaging. The SSFP imaging sequence is primarily used for functional imaging. It is a bright blood sequence, and has good myocardial-blood contrast by virtue of the relatively low level of the myocardial signal against a background of bright fat and blood signals.

# CHAPTER 28

# Cardiac Tagging

Mark Doyle

Because there are very few fixed reference points in the heart, detection of relative motion is inherently difficult to assess. Cardiac tagging provides a gridded reference frame from which to assess relative motion throughout the cardiac cycle for all regions of the myocardium. Initially, the grid is imposed on the heart at the start of the cardiac cycle and deforms with the myocardium throughout the cycle.

## PRINCIPLE OF TAGGING

Tags can be applied by the spatial amplitude modulation method (SPAMM) technique.

The essence of the SPAMM approach is to sinusoidally vary the signal across the image plane (see Fig. 28-1). When viewed as an image, this directly translates to an alternating dark–light stripe pattern across the entire image. To achieve this sinusoidal pattern, it is not necessary to vary the amplitude of the signal, only its phase (see Fig. 28-2). Tags are implemented by the following two operations:

- Inverting the spin system
- Varying the phase of the inversion signal cyclically

Application of a gradient across the body imposes a progressive accumulation of phase angle for all excited spins. In SPAMM tagging, a gradient is applied which imposes the required sinusoidal variation in phase across the image plane. In the SPAMM sequence, spins are initially tipped over using a 90-degree radiofrequency (RF) pulse (see Fig. 28-3). Next, a gradient is applied to vary the phase of the spins in a sinusoidal manner. Following this, a second RF pulse is applied which rotates in phase spins back along the positive axis and further tips the out-of-phase spins toward full inversion.

## SPATIAL AMPLITUDE MODULATION METHOD

The combination of a 90-degree RF-gradient-90-degree RF combination was the arrangement used in the original implementation of SPAMM. This combination of RF-gradient-RF is referred to as a *1-1 pulse*, because the amplitude of each RF pulse is the same (i.e., 1), which corresponds to 90 degrees in this case. The basic SPAMM sequence produces a series of stripes across the image plane. A grid can be simply produced by applying a second SPAMM sequence, with the gradient oriented in the orthogonal direction. The two sets of overlapping stripe patterns produce the tag grid (see Fig. 28-4).

## GRID PROPERTIES

The gradient area determines the stripe spacing and width. Stripes persist longest when the spins are inverted. As the cardiac cycle advances, tag contrast diminishes because of recovery of the spin system toward equilibrium. The stripe or grid tags are typically applied at the start of the electrocardiogram (ECG) R wave. However, the placement of tags inserts a time delay between the R wave and the first image that can be acquired.

## IMPROVED TAG DEFINITION

The basic 1-1 pulse only allows formation of sinusoidal tags, which means that the tag lines are not sharply defined. It transpires that the 1-1 pulse is the first order case of a binomial expansion. Higher order expansions such as a 1-3-1 or 1-3-9-3-1 series of RF pulses allow sharper definition of tag lines. The numbers refer to

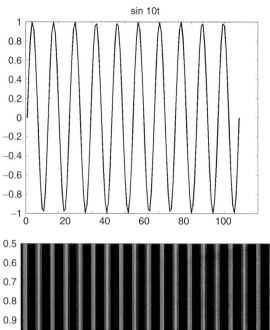

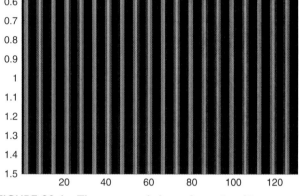

**FIGURE 28-1**   The top panel shows how signal is modulated in a sinusoidal manner across the image plane. In the lower panel, this sinusoidal variation in signal phase manifests as a series of alternating bright and dark lines across the image.

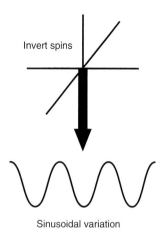

Invert spins

Sinusoidal variation

**FIGURE 28-2**   The basic principles of spatial amplitude modulation method (SPAMM) tagging are shown conceptually. The top panel shows the process of signal inversion, and in the lower panel the alternation of this inverted signal is illustrated, resulting in an alternating inverted and noninverted pattern of spins.

## CARDIAC TAGGING PROBLEMS

Common problems with tagging include the following:

- Tags do not persist sufficiently long into the cardiac cycle to assess diastole.
- At key cardiac phases, such as end-systole, the tag lines merge or become indistinct.

the relative strength of the RF pulses. The sum total of the pulses should add up to 180 degrees to result in spin inversion. The higher order SPAMM pulses allow separate control of tag width and spacing. Although higher order SPAMM pulses produce sharper tags, there are some potential disadvantages:

- Preparation time is increased compared to a 1-1 pulse.
- Imaging time in the cardiac cycle is reduced.
- Higher resolution is almost always associated with higher noise.

Good intrinsic scan quality is required to realize a practical advantage for these higher order pulses. Tags that are more densely packed potentially allow better delineation of cardiac motion. However, by setting the SPAMM tags very close to each other, a point may be reached whereby the tags become indistinct from each other throughout the cardiac cycle. Therefore, a compromise has to be reached between tag spacing and resolution.

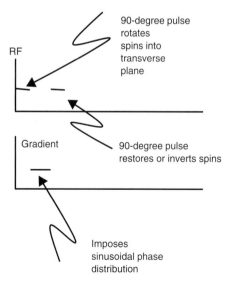

RF

90-degree pulse rotates spins into transverse plane

Gradient

90-degree pulse restores or inverts spins

Imposes sinusoidal phase distribution

**FIGURE 28-3**   The physical process of producing spatial amplitude modulation method (SPAMM) line tags is shown. A combination of radiofrequency (RF) pulses and gradients are used. Initially, a 90-degree RF pulse tips spins into the transverse plane. Following this, the gradient imposes a sinusoidal phase variation across the image plane. The second 90-degree RF pulse inverts some spins while tipping others back to the fully relaxed position.

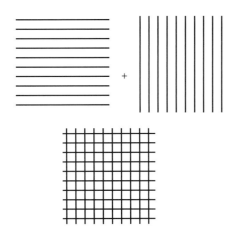

**FIGURE 28-4** Grid tags are produced by a simple combination of a series of horizontal tags with a series of vertical tags.

- The tag application time is long and the tags are applied at a time considerably past the ECG R wave.

Early in the cardiac cycle, tag contrast is maximal, being the difference between fully inverted spins and fully relaxed spins. Later in the cardiac cycle, the inverted spins relax whereas the fully relaxed spins remain constant, which leads to diminished contrast. To minimize

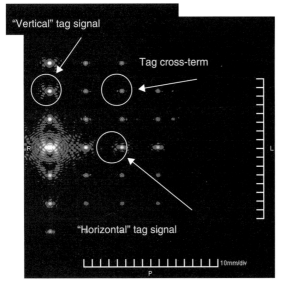

**FIGURE 28-5** The k-space pattern of a conventional grid tag image. In this k-space map, the very bright center is displaced to the left-hand side of the image. The vertical series of spots along the primary vertical axis (passing through the bright center of k-space) define the vertical tag lines. The horizontal spots along the primary axis passing through the center of k-space define the horizontal tag lines. The off axis "cross-terms" are responsible for defining the corners (*intersection points of lines*) of the tags.

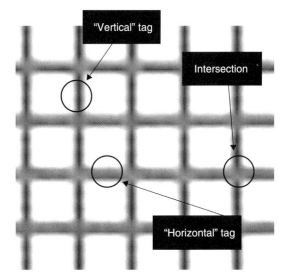

**FIGURE 28-6** The image domain tags formed by the conventional approach of first applying the horizontal lines and secondly by applying the vertical lines. The intersection points at the corners of each grid tag therefore receive a double inversion, and may appear brighter than the line tag sections (either vertical or horizontal).

tag fade, a low excitation flip angle of approximately 10 degrees should be used for the gradient echo imaging sequence used to read out the tags.

Complementary spatial amplitude modulation method (CSPAMM) is an approach that maintains tag contrast throughout the cardiac cycle. In CSPAMM, two tagged data sets are acquired, each differing in phase of the RF pulse, which is changed by 180 degrees between each separate application. By subtracting the two data sets from each other, the effects of signal regrowth due to T1 relaxation tend to cancel. However, in CSPAMM, although contrast is maintained throughout the cardiac cycle, noise increases toward the end of the cycle, effectively reducing the contrast to noise as the cycle progresses. The disadvantages of the CSPAMM approach to tag fade are that it doubles the scan time, owing to combining two separate acquisitions, and therefore a high degree of motion compensation is required because the scan is typically extended beyond a breath-hold. Additionally, formation of the grid pattern requires application of two tag preparation pulses, thereby delaying the tag application relative to ECG R wave and diminishing the ability to track tags during early systole.

Another solution to the tag fade problem is presented in the common k-space tagging approach. To appreciate the common k-space approach, it is necessary to consider tagging from the perspective of k-space. In conventional tagging, two orthogonal tag series are applied, resulting in distinct concentrations of signal in k-space (see Fig. 28-5). The patterns formed are a series

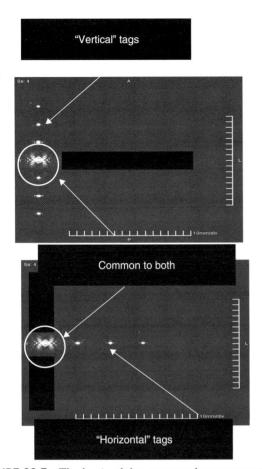

**FIGURE 28-7**  The basis of the common k-space approach is shown. In the top panel, only vertical tags are applied. In the lower panel, only horizontal tags are applied. Note the absence of cross-terms. The center of k-space is common to both data sets, and only need to be sampled once.

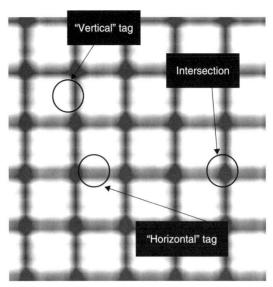

**FIGURE 28-8**  The appearance of grid tags in the common k-space image. The vertical and horizontal tags are well defined, and the corners are equally or even better defined.

of concentrations of signal along the major vertical and horizontal axes. However, because the two tag series are applied consecutively, they also generate cross-terms in k-space, that is, the formation of signal concentrations off the main axes along the diagonals. These cross-terms are responsible for defining contrast at the tag intersection points, that is, the corners of the tags. Conventionally, these intersection points are brighter than the nonintersecting tag regions, because effectively the corners (or intersections of the horizontal and vertical lines) are doubly inverted and may therefore even become fully reinverted or effectively equivalent to fully relaxed spins (see Fig. 28-6).

The common k-space acquisition approach allows tags to persist longer into the cardiac cycle and is based on the observation that the "central" region of k-space is the same when either "vertical" or "horizontal" tags are applied, that is, it is common to both series (see Fig. 28-7). Because the central region is common, it is possible to acquire it either during application of vertical

tags or horizontal tags. During each cardiac cycle in the common k-space acquisition, only the "horizontal" tags or "vertical" tags are applied, never both. Because the "vertical" and "horizontal" tags are applied separately, no cross-terms are generated, and this effectively conserves signal energy in k-space, confining it to the vertical and horizontal tag positions. Physically, tag intersection points only receive a single inversion pulse in each cardiac cycle and so should be correctly inverted. In common k-space images, tag intersection points are typically darker than nonintersecting tag regions (see Fig. 28-8).

## COMMON K-SPACE VERSUS CONVENTIONAL TAGGING

In conventional tagging, the interference between horizontal and vertical SPAMM pulses causes some general disruption of the signal, leading to increased noise (see Fig. 28-9). In common k-space tagging, noise tends to be lower, and this is especially noticeable in the blood pool signal (see Fig. 28-10). It is possible for conventional and common k-space tagging images to be acquired with identical parameters. Typically, the signal-to-noise ratio (SNR) advantage of common k-space tagging is seen in higher definition of the compressed tag pattern at the end-systolic time frame. At the end of the cardiac cycle, tag lines tend to fade in the conventional series, whereas in the common k-space images the tag intersection points are particularly distinct. In conventional tagging,

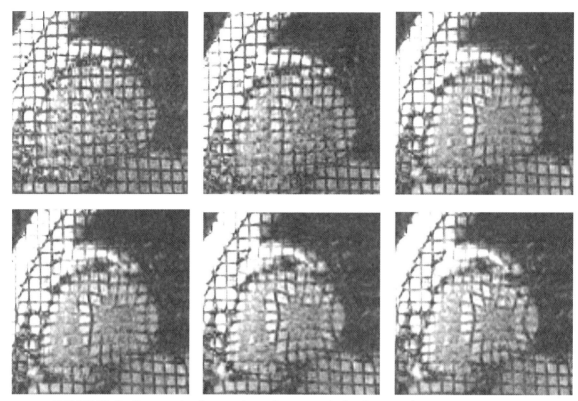

**FIGURE 28-9** Consecutive frames throughout systole for the conventional tag sequence are shown. Note the relatively dark blood pool, the high degree of tag fade at end-systole, and the general high level of noise.

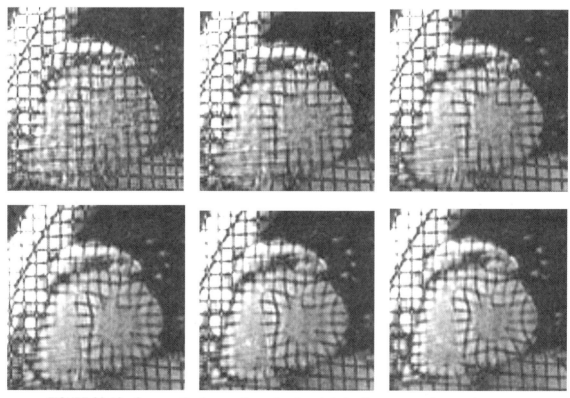

**FIGURE 28-10** Consecutive frames throughout systole for the common k-space tag sequence are shown, corresponding to the views shown in Fig. 28-9. Note the relatively bright blood pool, the low degree of tag fade at end-systole, especially at the tag intersection points, and the general low level of noise.

the blood pool is dark due to the application of two tagging pulse sequences. In the common k-space images, the blood pool is brighter, and provides increased contrast between the myocardium and blood pool.

## SUMMARY

Cardiac tagging produces a deformable reference grid that allows visualization and quantification of myocardial motion. The main problems of tagging are the lack of tag persistence toward the end of the cycle and the increase in noise when cross tags are used. A number of approaches have been developed to address these issues, and tag imaging is now widely available on commercial scanners.

# CHAPTER 29

# Perfusion and Viability

Mark Doyle

## OVERVIEW

Myocardial perfusion and viability imaging both involve imaging contrast conditions following administration of a bolus of contrast agent. There is little or no inherent signal characteristic of myocardium that differentiates normally perfused tissue from tissue at risk of ischemia. For this reason, an exogenous contrast agent is required. At rest, it is used to detect the presence or absence of resting ischemia, and under vasodilatation conditions it is used to detect high-grade coronary artery stenoses by provoking a transitory ischemia.

## PARAMAGNETISM

Most contrast agents reduce the tissue T1 when they come in close contact with the tissue. Commonly, agents exhibit the property of paramagnetism, which results in a slight increase in the local magnetic field. Although water has a natural T1 relaxation time in the range of 700 to 1,000 milliseconds, the addition of paramagnetic impurities can dramatically reduce the T1 relaxation time (i.e., increase the relaxation rate). Gadolinium (Gad) is a paramagnetic agent that possesses unpaired electrons. These paramagnetic particles tumble and rotate at frequencies close to the Larmor frequency of protons, resulting in reducing the T1 of protons (see Fig. 29-1).

## CONCENTRATION AND RELAXIVITY

The reduction in T1 relaxation is proportional to the concentration of Gad

$$1/T1 = 1/T1_{w/o} + R(Gad)$$

where $T1_{w/o}$ is the T1 without Gad and R(Gad) is the concentration of Gad (see Fig. 29-2). The relaxivity of Gad is in the range 4 to 10 mm/sec/kg. Gad is a heavy metal, which is naturally toxic, but is rendered inactive by the process of chelating, effectively surrounding the Gad particle with a molecular cage. Gad is commonly chelated with diethylenetriaminepentaacetic acid (Gd-DTPA), which has a molecular weight of approximately 600, and a blood half-life of approximately 40 minutes.

## REGION OF OPERATION

Gd-DTPA is an extracellular agent and is not confined to the blood pool. It is not taken up by cells and is excreted by the kidneys and liver. In most cases, the administration of Gad occurs without adverse incident; however, there are some side effects to be aware of:

- Headache <10%
- Coldness at injection site <5%
- Severe reaction <1%

To confine Gad to the blood pool, it has to be bound to a larger agent such as albumin, with a molecular weight of 70,000 to 100,000. The clearance time for this formulation is several weeks, and due to the long residency time, there are concerns with toxicity.

## NANOPARTICLES

Nanoparticles are increasingly being used to deliver Gad contrast agents. A common nanoparticles delivery agent is 19-Fluorine, which forms the core of the particle (see Fig. 29-3). The core is surrounded by a lipid membrane to which are attached upward of 100,000 Gad particles. The diameter of the particle is on the order of 250 nm and has a relaxivity value in excess of 20,000. Nanoparticles can be designed to target specific sites, and be activated by a number of mechanisms, including the following:

- Functional activated agents
- Enzyme activated agents
- Reporter agents

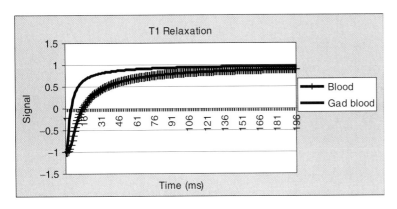

**FIGURE 29-1** Following an inversion pulse (−1), spins relax back to the equilibrium signal level (+1) following an exponential curve, with the half-life characterizing the T1 of the tissue. In the presence of gadolinium contrast (Gad), the T1 of blood is reduced compared to unexposed blood.

The advantage of nanoparticles is that a low-dose overall is delivered but it can have a large, but localized effect on contrast. One nonoparticle that has a very high paramagnetic effect is the superparamagnetic iron oxide (SPIO). It has to be used with more caution because it never clears the body. Its diameter is approximately 50 nm.

## CONTRAST VISUALIZATION

When contrast media is present, it reduces the T1, and in the case of SPIO particles, can also reduce T2 values. Generally, the gradient echo sequence is used to image the presence of the agent, and although this sequence has some inherent sensitivity to T1, contrast differences are generally enhanced by incorporation of the inversion recovery (IR) prepulse.

## INVERSION RECOVERY

In equilibrium, spins are aligned with the main magnetic field. Following inversion by application of a 180-degree radiofrequency (RF) pulse, spins relax back to realignment with $\mathbf{B_0}$. However, during the basic IR process, no signal is detected. To image the spin system, it is necessary to apply an imaging sequence before complete recovery has been accomplished. Signal is then detected from the net magnetization vector component that is knocked into the transverse plane: Consider a two-spin system, one spin with a short T1, and one with a long T1 (see Fig. 29-4). After the initial inversion and recovery period, application of a 90-degree RF pulse (in conjunction with an imaging sequence) images the spin system, and because the recovery rates are different between the two spins, the net transverse signals are also different. This is the origin of the IR signal contrast. Typically, a single IR sequence is used. The T1 of

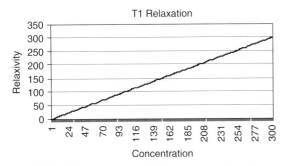

**FIGURE 29-2** The inverse of T1 is expressed as the "relaxivity." The relaxivity of blood increases linearly with concentration of the gadolinium agent. An upper limit to this linear relationship exists (not shown), where the addition of more contrast agent does not produce an increase in relaxivity. Ideally, perfusion scanning should be performed with concentrations well within in the linear range.

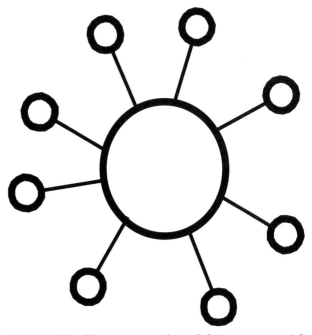

**FIGURE 29-3** The structure of a gadolinium nanoparticle is illustrated. The core material is a fluorine compound that is surrounded by a lipid membrane, and embedded in the membrane are upward of 100,000 gadolinium molecules.

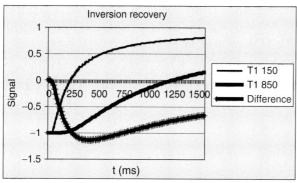

**FIGURE 29-4** The dynamic nature of contrast between pure blood (T1 850) and blood in the presence of contrast agent (T1 = 150) is shown. At the time of the initial inversion, there is no net contrast between the two blood pools, and as time proceeds, the contrast increases and goes through a maximum. Notice that to achieve this contrast it is necessary to distinguish between negative and positive signals. If this type of acquisition is not available, the time course of contrast is more complicated.

myocardium is approximately 850 milliseconds and in the presence of a contrast agent this may fall by a factor of 2 to 4, to approximately 150 milliseconds. Under these conditions, the inversion time suitable to generate contrast is in the range of 150 to 200 milliseconds. At this recovery time, the short T1 tissue appears bright relative to the long T1 tissue. In perfusion imaging, the natural T1 of the tissue is never altered, but what is seen is the temporary reduction in T1 due to the proximity of the contrast agent.

## INVERSION RECOVERY AND PERFUSION IMAGING

By introducing a Gad contrast agent, the T1 of myocardium is shortened only during passage of the agent. The agent is administered as a bolus, and rapidly imaged using the inversion recovery–gradient-recalled echo (IR-GRE) sequence. Imaging is performed during first pass of the agent. Recirculation of the Gad makes further evaluation of the perfusion data invalid (see Fig. 29-5). In myocardial perfusion imaging, multiple slices are imaged as the contrast agent passes through the cardiovascular system:

- Right ventricle
- Left ventricle
- Myocardium

## MYOCARDIAL PERFUSION ANALYSIS

Software is required to extract time intensity curves from the myocardial perfusion images (see Fig. 29-6).

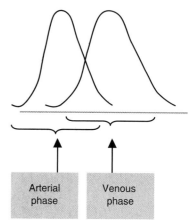

**FIGURE 29-5** The gadolinium contrast agent is administered as a tight bolus. This allows differentiation of well perfused tissue and tissue perfused in a tardy manner. Further complicating this administration issue is that as contrast enters the venous system, recirculation occurs. Therefore, a bolus of short duration allows a clear distinction between well perfused and poorly perfused myocardium.

After registering myocardial frames for respiratory motion, time intensity curves are extracted from the myocardium and left ventricular (LV) blood pool regions. These data can be quantitatively evaluated. To normalize the signal to accommodate different bolus injection conditions, the myocardial uptake slope is divided by the LV uptake slope (see Fig. 29-7). Using this normalized data, several properties may be used to evaluate myocardial perfusion:

- Normalized myocardial perfusion slope
- Time-to-peak perfusion signal
- Net signal increase from the baseline value

## REST-STRESS PERFUSION TESTING

As in other modalities, perfusion imaging can be performed at rest and at stress (by infusion of a vasodilatation agent such as adenosine). Comparison of the normalized rest and stress uptake slopes of myocardium allows calculation of the perfusion reserve or coronary flow reserve (CFR) (see Fig. 29-8). A low CFR, <1.5, is associated with low sensitivity for detecting high-grade stenosis, whereas in a patient with an adequate CFR, high-grade stenoses are seen more distinctly. In the example in Fig. 29-9, each patient had similar high-grade stenoses, but the inducible perfusion deficit was more clearly seen in the patient with a high CFR.

## VIABILITY

Approximately 10 minutes following administration of the Gad contrast agent, the Gad becomes trapped

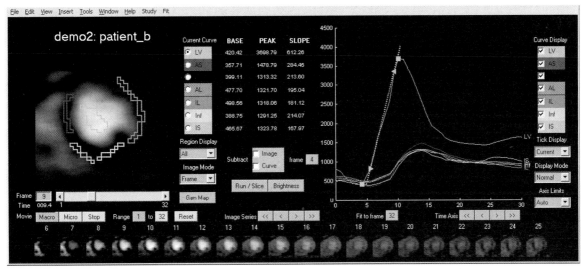

**FIGURE 29-6** Software is required to extract quantitative myocardial perfusion information. The main steps of most approaches are shown here. Along the lower panel are shown a series of successive myocardial frames, which show the contrast entering first the right side, then the left, and finally perfusing through the myocardium. In the main left panel, regions of interest are drawn in the myocardium and left ventricular (LV) blood pool. The right panel shows the time intensity curves corresponding to the LV blood pool and the myocardial segments. Relative differences in these curves indicate perfusion anomalies.

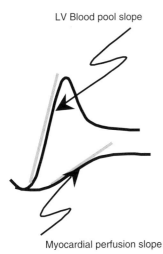

**FIGURE 29-7** Because many factors affect the administration of the contrast bolus, it is necessary to normalize the myocardial time intensity curve by division of the slope of the left ventricular (LV) time intensity curve.

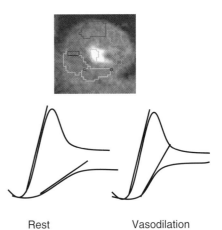

**FIGURE 29-8** Comparison of the normalized time intensity slopes for the resting and vasodilatation (stress) states allows an index of the coronary flow reserve (CFR) to be obtained. Typically, the stress slope is increased compared to the rest.

## Adequate CFR

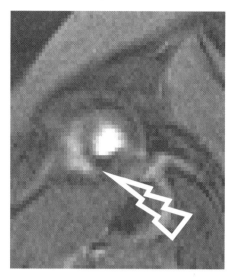

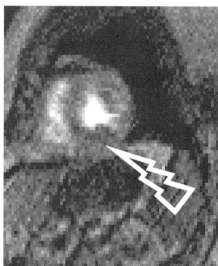

## Inadequate CFR

FIGURE 29-9  In a study of the adequacy of the coronary flow reserve (CFR), it was observed that in patients exhibiting an adequate CFR it was easier to detect the presence of high-grade coronary artery stenoses (arrows).

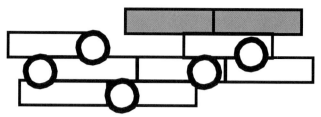

FIGURE 29-10  The principle of viability imaging is illustrated. Approximately 10 minutes following administration of the gadolinium contrast agent, the agent (circles) becomes trapped in the interstitial debris of dead cells (open rectangles). In this way, the presence of contrast agent corresponds to nonviable myocardium.

in the debris of dead cells. Therefore, accumulation of Gad at the delayed time stage is associated with nonviable myocardium (see Fig. 29-10). Viability imaging can occur under steady state conditions, as opposed to dynamically during first pass of the agent, and can therefore be imaged with greater clarity and resolution.

## SUMMARY

Administration of an exogenous contrast agent is required to detect myocardial perfusion conditions. Real-time imaging is required to detect the first pass of the agent when assessing perfusion. Viability imaging can be performed in the steady state, approximately 10 minutes after injection of contrast.

# CHAPTER 30

# Phase Velocity Mapping

Mark Doyle

## PHASE INFORMATION

In phase velocity mapping, the velocity of spins in each voxel is represented in the phase of the spin system. In most instances, the images that we see contain only magnitude information, in that they only represent the magnitude of the spin system. However, each spin is a vector, and can be described in terms of the following two unique quantities:

- Magnitude
- Phase

Typically, there is no requirement to be sensitive to phase information, and images are reconstructed in such a manner that the phase of the signal does not affect image appearance. Consider the net magnetization vector ($\mathbf{M_0}$) that describes the spin system, possessing both magnitude and phase (see Fig. 30-1). When encoding k-space data, the phase of the $\mathbf{M_0}$ vector is affected by the applied gradients in a controlled manner, and we note the following two features:

- The central point of k-space corresponds to the signal acquired without application of any gradients, that is, all spins are in phase with each other at this single point.
- The "phase" of the corresponding image reflects the phase conditions pertaining when the central point is acquired.

## PHASE BASICS

The possible range of phase information is as follows:

- 0 to 360 degrees
- 0 to $2\pi$ radians

Values of phase $>2\pi$, or $<0$, are not uniquely represented and are therefore aliased into the range 0 to $2\pi$ radians. Ideally, the phase image should be flat, and have the value of zero for all pixels. However, k-space data are rarely this perfect due to a number of sources, including the following:

- Nonidealized gradients
- Time dependent eddy currents
- $\mathbf{B_0}$ field inhomogeneities

Therefore, the "phase information" rarely forms the flat, featureless, image that we might expect (see Fig. 30-2). Distortions of the phase information are typically a function of nonideal phase increments between k-space lines, and between points along the frequency encoding direction.

## EDDY CURRENT COMPENSATION

The most disruptive features affecting phase information are time-dependent eddy currents. With each

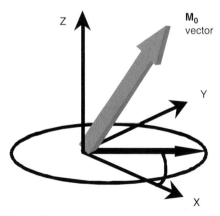

**FIGURE 30-1** The net magnetization vector, $\mathbf{M_0}$, possesses both magnitude and phase information. Although the phase information of the spin is integral to the k-space encoding mechanism, the phase information is rarely represented in the final image, which is dominated by the magnitude data.

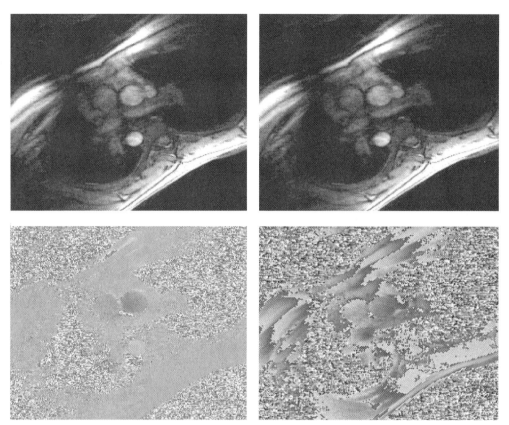

**FIGURE 30-2** The left panel shows an idealized magnitude image (top) and phase image (lower). In the phase image, velocity is represented as bright and dark information. The right panel shows corresponding magnitude (top) and phase (lower) images where the phase information is disrupted. This is more typical of the phase that is normally achieved. Notice that the magnitude image is not appreciably influenced by the phase information.

gradient transition, there is an associated eddy current, which is a current induced in the magnet superstructure (see Fig. 30-3). Eddy currents are transitory electrical currents that oppose the field that generated them. Self-shielded gradients are employed to reduce eddy currents, but these are only partially effective. Eddy current compensation is an additional approach that adds a time-dependant counter current to the gradient waveform, and is applied at each gradient transition point. However, even when employing eddy current compensation and shielded gradients, phase information remains disrupted.

## REFERENCE PHASE IMAGE

It can be appreciated that any process that requires sensitivity to phase information must be able to accommodate the nonideal phase variations present. One way to accomplish this is to obtain a reference image (with nonideal phase variations) and use this to correct the phase encoded image. Therefore, phase

subtraction of the reference and encoded images can be used to undo the effects of phase variations, effectively allowing a flat baseline for the phase information to be obtained.

## MOVING SPINS AND PHASE

Consider a static spin. Application of a positive gradient followed by a negative gradient forms a gradient echo. The echo peak is the point where all spins (less T2 effects) are in phase with each other. In contrast, a spin moving along the direction of the applied gradients (positive and negative components) will not come back into phase at the echo peak due to the change of position that occurs while the gradients are applied (see Fig. 30-4). Therefore, it can be appreciated that static and moving spins can be differentiated from each other by the phase conditions present at the echo peak. It is possible to design gradient waveforms to control this phase difference such that the difference is linearly proportional to velocity.

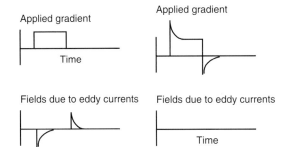

**FIGURE 30-3** The left panel shows an applied gradient (top), and the corresponding induced eddy currents (lower panel). Notice that the induced eddy currents are initiated when the main gradient is switched on or off, and that the direction of each eddy currents is dependent on whether the gradient is switched on (negative) or off (positive). The right panel shows the principle of eddy current compensation. In this instance, the waveform of the applied gradient (top) is deliberately distorted to counteract the eddy currents. Following this procedure no, or dramatically reduced, eddy currents are generated.

## BIPOLAR GRADIENTS

In a bipolar gradient, equal areas of the positive and negative gradients are applied. When a bipolar gradient is applied:

- Static spins undergo a net zero phase evolution.
- Moving spins undergo a nonzero phase evolution.

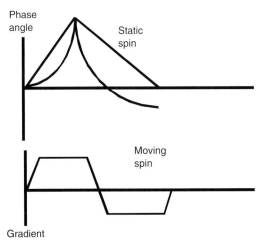

**FIGURE 30-4** The spin phase accumulation for a static and moving spin is shown in response to a bipolar gradient. In the case where the positive and negative gradient areas are balanced, the net phase accumulation for static spins is zero, corresponding to the echo peak position (where all spins are in phase with each other). In contrast, the phase accumulation of a moving spin undergoes a curved time evolution. At the time of the conventional echo peak, the moving spin has acquired a net phase value that is proportional to its velocity.

Consider the relationship between spin phase and velocity in the presence of the bipolar gradient:

$$X(t) = X(0) + V \times \text{time} \tag{1}$$

$$\omega = \gamma \mathbf{B_0} \times G(x) \times \rho(x) \times X(t) \tag{2}$$

$$\omega = \gamma \mathbf{B_0} \times G(x) \times \rho(x) \times (X(0) + V \times \text{time}) \tag{3}$$

Where $X(t)$ is position as a function of time, V is the velocity of the spin, $\omega$ is the angular frequency, $\gamma$ is the gyromagnetic ratio, $\mathbf{B_0}$ is the main magnetic field, $G(x)$ is the gradient that varies as a function of position, $\rho$ is the spin density (as a function of position). Equation 1 simply states that the position of a spin depends on where it started, $X(0)$, at time position 0, and where it moves to due to its velocity. Equation 2 is an expression of the Lamor equation, relating the spin signal to the spin density, position, and gradient strength. Equation 3 is a result of substituting Equation 1 into Equation 2. The phase of each spin is calculated by integration. Integration takes into account the shape, duration, and time origin of each of the gradients applied. In Equation 3, two distinct components are seen, one that is dependent on the starting position of the spins ($X[0]$), and one that is dependent on the velocity of the spins (V). In the case of applying a simple bipolar gradient, $G(X)$ is applied first in a positive manner, then in a negative manner. It can be easily appreciated that if the positive and negative gradients are applied for equal times, then for static spins the net phase accumulation is zero. This feature is termed the *zeroth order moment* of the gradient (i.e., net sum of the product of gradient strength and time of application). The second term involves two terms—velocity and time. In this case, it is somewhat less obvious, but the equal positive and negative gradients do not cancel out to zero, primarily because of the time component. This is termed the *first-order moment*. The first-order moment is responsible for encoding velocity information. Therefore, in the presence of time varying bipolar gradients, moving spins will either gain or lose phase evolution compared to static spins. A set of bipolar gradients can be added to any imaging axis to control the phase accumulation along each of the three primary directions:

- X
- Y
- Z

Therefore, compared to an image without the bipolar gradients, applying a bipolar pair will encode velocity as phase information.

## ADDITIVE GRADIENTS

Adding bipolar gradients to an imaging waveform can be performed in a superposition manner (see

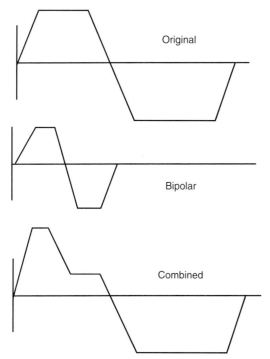

**FIGURE 30-5** Here the original gradient represents the conventional gradient-recalled echo that is used in an imaging sequence. The bipolar gradient used to encode velocity information is shown in the middle plot. Note that the bipolar gradient is confined to the time of the first lobe of the imaging gradient. The lower plot shows the composite gradient that would be applied to accomplish both (a) gradient echo imaging and (b) velocity encoding. Note that the composite gradient is simply the sum of the two original gradients.

Fig. 30-5). This produces the desired effect as long as no radiofrequency (RF) pulses are being applied or measurements performed during the period when the bipolar gradients are added. Further, when using a triphasic gradient, it is possible to refocus (i.e., bring into phase) moving **and** static spins. It can be appreciated that a triphasic gradient allows for the possibility (mathematically) of simultaneously forming a zero value for the zeroth order moment and the first-order moment, achieved by matching positive and negative areas (a function of gradient shape) and the time-gradient integral (a function of gradient strength and time), respectively.

## PHASE VELOCITY IMAGING

With the ability to arrange for moving and static spins to simultaneously come into focus or make moving spins preferentially exhibit additional phase information we are in a position to design an imaging approach to quantify velocity. The system imperfections require

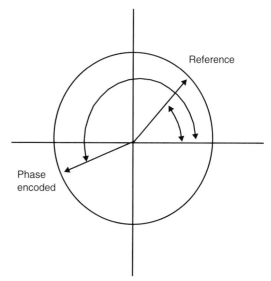

**FIGURE 30-6** The principle of comparing phases is illustrated. The reference vector is subtracted from the velocity encoded vector. Because both vectors have the same residual phase accumulation, the difference between them gives the velocity-related component directly.

that two images be compared to extract velocity information:

- Velocity compensated (tripolar gradients)
- Velocity encoded (bipolar gradients)

Phase subtraction can be used to undo the effects of the phase variations (see Fig. 30-6). When using a reference image, the phase of the reference image (on a pixel basis) is subtracted from the velocity phase encoded image. In this instance, the maximum phase information is limited to the range:

- 0 to 360 degrees
- 0 to $2\pi$ radians

Similarly, when encoding velocity in only one direction (e.g., through plane flow) it is possible to encode phase using two separate bipolar gradients, each applied using opposing polarities. In this instance, the maximum phase range is doubled:

- −360 to 360 degrees
- −2 to $2\pi$ radians

The signal-to-noise ratio (SNR) of a phase encoded velocity image is proportional to two features:

- Magnitude
- Phase

Therefore, even for a phase image, it is important to maximize signal strength as well as minimize dynamic range. Regions where there are no or little magnitude signals (e.g., background air or lungs) are characterized by high noise in phase sensitive images.

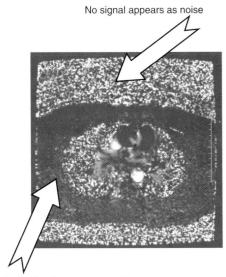

No signal appears as noise

Static signal, appears as midgray

**FIGURE 30-7**   One commonly used convention to represent positive and negative velocities in a gray scale image is illustrated: midlevel gray represents static tissue, with brighter regions representing positive velocity and darker regions representing negative velocity. Regions of noise appear as speckled intensity. This is because the signal-to-noise ratio (SNR) of a velocity image is dependant on both magnitude (low for noise) and phase (random for low signal).

## POSITIVE AND NEGATIVE VELOCITY

On the basis of the phase information, it is possible to distinguish positive from negative velocities. However, an image can only represent positive numbers. Therefore, to represent positive and negative values in an image, a display convention is required. One possibility is the use of color (e.g., blue positive, red negative) or in the case of a gray scale image, intensity offset can be used:

- Negative velocities are represented in the range 0 to 2,048.
- Positive velocities are represented in the range 2,049 to 4,096.

   In this scheme, static tissue has the appearance of a midlevel gray (see Fig. 30-7).

## PROPERTIES OF PHASE VELOCITY IMAGES

Importantly, each velocity direction has to be separately encoded. A minimum of three velocity directions are required to completely describe the velocity of each pixel (assuming that the directions are mutually orthogonal). Therefore, to image all three velocity directions requires a minimum of four image sets (one reference and three velocity encoded images). Further, the velocity sensitivity range and direction have to be determined before scanning (just as is the case for echo Doppler), otherwise aliasing or low dynamic range could result. The most common problem seen is related to signal "aliasing" in the velocity dimension (see Fig. 30-8). Velocity aliasing results when the velocity encoding limits are set too low. Unless sophisticated unaliasing software is available, the only alternative is to repeat the scan with the velocity limit increased, say by 50%.

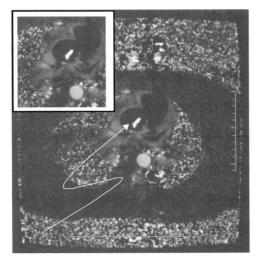
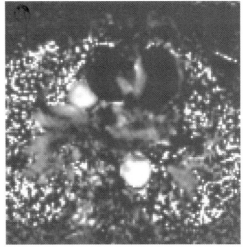

**FIGURE 30-8**   Aliased flow appears as a sharp transition in the flow signal from bright to dark or *vice versa* (*arrows* in left panel and inset). The right panel shows the same vessel after the velocity sensitivity has been increased, showing no evidence of aliasing.

## SEGMENTATION

Commonly applied imaging procedures may have profound influence on phase velocity images. One such procedure is segmentation. Segmentation is the means whereby cardiac cine imaging data are rapidly acquired by grouping a series of k-space lines at each nominal position in the cardiac cycle. Typically, we aim for a segmentation interval of approximately 50 milliseconds or less. In flow imaging, it is common to encode the reference and the flow encoded data within each cardiac cycle. This expediency effectively extends the segmentation length for the basic sequence. The extension factor is directly dependent on the number of flow directions encoded. It can be appreciated that this affects the temporal resolution of the phase velocity image series. Consider using a basic repetition time (TR) of 7 milliseconds. A conventional cine sequence could employ a segmentation value of 8, resulting in a temporal resolution of 56 milliseconds. However, if flow encoding in only one direction were employed, we require a reference and one encoded data set, therefore a segmentation value of 4 is required to obtain a time resolution of 56 milliseconds. Similarly, if flow encoding is to be performed in all three directions, we require a reference and three encoded data sets, therefore a segmentation value of 2 is needed to obtain a time resolution of 56 milliseconds. Therefore, the acceptable segmentation value is lower for phase velocity imaging compared to conventional imaging.

## VELOCITY AND FLOW

In phase velocity imaging, although the velocity is the property that is directly encoded, it is possible to extract flow rate by application of some minimal image processing. The calculation of flow rate involves the integration of velocity over pixels and time:

$$\text{Flow} = \Sigma \text{ Velocity} \times \text{time} \times \text{no. of pixels}$$

To extract flow rate from a velocity image, the vessel/region of interest is outlined, and software integrates the velocity and time per frame. The integral over the cardiac cycle of flow rate is equal to the forward stroke volume. Even when phase subtraction is performed, it is possible that there remain systematic errors in the phase information over the image. Typically, if errors are present, these are most noticeable as a gradient of intensity in the phase/velocity image. To accommodate this, it is conventional to "subtract" the phase from a nearby "static" region (see Fig. 30-9). To calculate flow volume, it is essential that the processing software subtract the data directly (because the calculation involves an integral). However, it is not always possible to find a suitable static region close to the flow region of interest. In such cases, it is important to note the format of any systematic error in the phase information. If (as is typical) the phase information varies in a linear manner, it may be possible to select a static tissue region at the same level but parallel to the gradient direction. However, such attempts at correcting for phase should

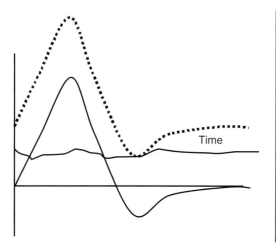
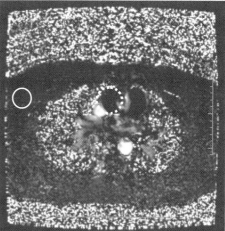

**FIGURE 30-9** The principle of correcting a linear intensity gradient in the velocity image. Notice in the static muscle regions that there is a gradient of intensity present in the vertical direction. The vascular region with flow is outlined (*dashed circle*) and the velocity profile is observed (*dashed line*). This velocity curve can be corrected by subtracting the background velocity measured in the static region parallel to the vessel (*solid circle, solid approximately constant offset line*). As long as the static background region is chosen to be orthogonal to the intensity gradient, the correction should be valid (*pulsatile solid line*), although the static tissue is remote from the vessel.

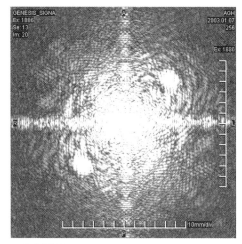 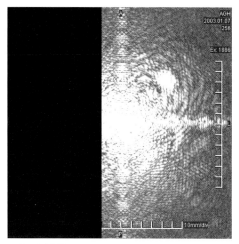

Full TE 4 ms                              Partial TE 3 ms

**FIGURE 30-10**    A full k-space matrix (left panel) and a partial echo k-space matrix (right panel) are shown. Symmetry in k-space is exploited to allow a partial echo to be acquired (right panel), allowing a shorter echo time (TE) to be realized for phase contrast approaches.

be used sparingly. Ensuring that adequate spatial and temporal resolutions are obtained at source are the best approaches to achieve accurate information.

## FLOW SENSITIVITY

Short echo times (TE) are required to obtain the best sensitivity to flow. This minimizes errors due to a number of common flow features, including the following:

* Phase dispersion due to velocity gradients
* Sensitivity to flow acceleration

In general the gradients are maximized, and no further reduction in TE is possible. However, the symmetry of k-space that was previously used to acquire data in an asymmetric manner for partial number of excitations (NEX) imaging, can be exploited to reduce the TE. In velocity imaging, the same symmetry of k-space can be used to reduce the TE, that is, by employing partial echo imaging. In partial echo imaging, only a short portion of the buildup of an echo is sampled,

which reduces the TE and thereby increase sensitivity to moving spins (see Fig. 30-10). However, it follows that if partial echo imaging is used, the symmetry cannot be exploited to reduce scan time reduction by employing partial NEX. Given all these constraints, it is apparent that velocity imaging leads to inherently long acquisition times.

## SUMMARY

Spin phase is used to encode quantitative velocity information. To obtain this information, inherently longer scans and additional scan information are required. In general, shorter scan segmentation values have to be used due to the requirement to obtain reference and velocity encoded scans, partial NEX cannot be used due to the use of partial echo, and because additional gradients are required, the TR is relatively long. Therefore, because scan times are inherently long, rapid imaging approaches will likely enhance the performance of phase velocity imaging approaches in future applications.

# CHAPTER 31

# Slice Selection

Mark Doyle

## OVERVIEW

Slice selection is a fundamental operation applied in almost every imaging sequence. It requires an interacting between the spins in the magnet, the applied gradient and radiofrequency (RF) pulses.

## SPINS IN A MAGNET

In the natural (i.e., unmagnetized state) spins are aligned in random orientation and do not produce a net magnetization. When placed in a magnetic field, spins fall into one of two possible orientations:

- Aligned
- Antialigned

The population of these two energy states is almost equal and is governed by the Boltzman energy distribution. In this way, the magnetization from each aligned (i.e., positive) spin is canceled by the antialigned (i.e., negative) spin. However, at a field strength of 1.5 T there are approximately 3 per 1,000,000 that do not cancel (see Fig. 31-1). Because there are trillions of spins, there is therefore a detectable net magnetization, $M_0$, generated in the body. However, spins never truly align (low energy state) or antialign (high energy state) with respect to the magnetic field; instead, spins can be considered to orient at a slight angle to the main magnetic field, $B_0$ (see Fig. 31-2). This slight angle and the intrinsic spin property become very important for magnetic resonance imaging (MRI), and in particular for slice selection.

## ANGULAR MOMENTUM

Spins have the property of angular momentum. Consider that a bicycle resists falling over when in motion due to the properties of the forces of angular momentum,

gravity, and tipping forces. The wheels resist tipping over, because perpendicular forces are established in response to the tipping action and the pull of gravity (see Fig. 31-3). Similarly, spins misaligned with $B_0$ will experience perpendicular forces, which in this case are magnetic in nature. The interaction of the spins and the magnetic field causes the spins to precess. Nuclear spins precess at a field-dependent frequency, $\omega$, given by the Lamor equation:

$$\omega = \gamma \times B_0$$

However, in the body there is not just one spin, but there are trillions, each spin precessing in random phase with respect to the others. What we observe is the net result of combining all spins, which becomes resolved into the magnetization, $M_0$, which is oriented along the direction of the main magnetic field.

## RADIOFREQUENCY PULSE AND $M_0$

To experience a signal from the net magnetization, $M_0$, we must tip it into the transverse plane. To see how this is accomplished, consider that individual spins precess about $B_0$ at a slight angle. Under this condition, a rotating magnetic field in the transverse plane applied at this precessional frequency will attract spins to the transverse plane (see Fig. 31-4). This applied field is referred to as the *RF pulse*, because it only need be applied for a short duration on the order of 1 millisecond. Once the $M_0$ magnetization is tipped over into the transverse plane, it will freely precess, again due to the interaction with the main magnet.

## SIGNAL DECAY

As individual spins progressively precess, they fall in and out of phase with each other and consequently

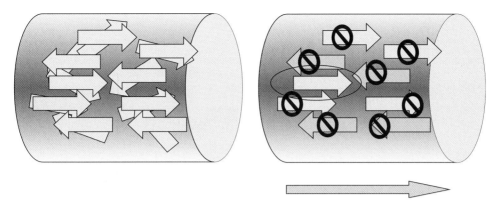

**FIGURE 31-1**   Outside of the magnetic field, spins are aligned randomly within the body (left panel). When placed in a magnetic field (right panel), spins will either become aligned or antialigned (parallel or antiparallel) with the main magnetic field. The population of the two energy states is almost equal, and therefore each positive spin tends to be canceled by a negative spin. However, a few spins per 1,000,000 (*circled*) remain unpaired. These unpaired spins are the only ones that contribute to the net magnetization vector. Because there are trillions of spins involved, the net magnetization vector, although small, is in the detectable range and results in a small net magnetization vector.

lose coherence, leading to signal decay. This loss of coherence can be thought of as being formed by spins initially spanning a small range of orientations relative to each other, with the most advanced spins describing the leading edge, and the lagging spins describing the trailing edge, and all other spins spanning the range between them. As time progresses, the net signal observed is seen to decay in a smooth manner as the range spanned by the spin system gradually widens. The curve describing the signal decay pattern is exponential in nature, with T2 describing the half-life of the spin coherence decay curve.

## SIGNAL DETECTION

A conducting coil placed near a rotating (precessing) magnet will experience a voltage termed an *electromotive force* (EMF). In other words, the precessing magnet induces a voltage in the conductor, without any direct physical contact occurring. Similarly, the process by which the MRI signal is detected is termed *signal induction*. From the instant the spin is tipped in to the transverse plane, it freely precesses and can therefore induce a voltage in a conductor placed in its

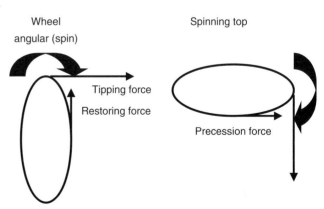

**FIGURE 31-3**   A vertically aligned wheel, such as on a bicycle, when it turns will resist tipping over due to a perpendicular restoring force set up as a result of its spinning property (angular momentum). Similar reasoning applies to a spinning top (right panel). Similarly, spins, oriented at an angle to the main magnetic field, $B_0$, experience a restoring force, which in this case, causes the spins to precess about the magnetic field.

**FIGURE 31-2**   When placed in a magnet, the so-called "aligned" spins are not truly aligned, and orient at a slight angle to the main magnetic field, $B_0$. The interaction between this angle and the spin property results in generation of forces that cause the spins to precess.

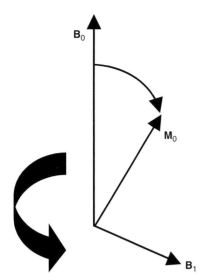

**FIGURE 31-4** Initially, the net magnetization, $\mathbf{M_0}$, is aligned with the main magnetic field, $\mathbf{B_0}$, but is composed of individual spins that precess at a slight angle to $\mathbf{B_0}$. Applying a rotating magnetic field, $\mathbf{B_1}$, attracts the $\mathbf{M_0}$ magnetization toward the $\mathbf{B_1}$ field. When the magnetization vector $\mathbf{M_0}$ reaches the transverse plane, the $\mathbf{B_1}$ radiofrequency (RF) field is switched off, leaving the $\mathbf{M_0}$ vector precessing in the transverse plane.

vicinity. However, as the spins lose coherence with each other, the signal decays. Consequently, the MRI signal is termed a *free induction decay*, (FID):

- Free, because it freely precesses, that is not a forced precession
- Induction, because that is the means of detection
- Decay, because the signal decays due to the T2 process

## MAGNETIC GRADIENTS AND SPINS

A magnetic gradient applied to the spin system results in altering the magnetic field at each location. Because the precessional frequency of each spin is linearly dependent on the magnetic field experienced, a range of precessional frequencies is established in the body by application of the gradient. This linear range of frequencies is dependent on spatial location along the gradient:

- Low field strength, low precession rate
- High field strength, high precession rate

When a gradient is applied along the body, slices of spins are thereby established, each infinitesimally thin, and each slice defined by a unique frequency (see Fig. 31-5). Therefore, to excite a slice of finite width we need to simultaneously apply a gradient and excite a thin band of spins, with the band directly corresponding to the slice location and width. In signal processing terms, a thin band of frequencies is referred to by the technical

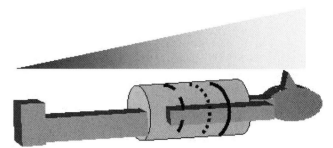

**FIGURE 31-5** When a linear gradient is applied along the body, slices of spins precess at unique frequencies, indicated here by *solid, dotted,* and *dashed stripes*. As the gradient increases in strength across the body, the spins increase in frequency, from a low frequency (*dashed slice*) to through higher frequencies (*dotted and solid*).

term of a *top hat function*. The mathematical manner to deal with such functions involves an understanding of Fourier theory. Here, we take a detour to discuss Fourier theory.

## FOURIER THEORY

Fourier theory states that any mathematic shape (e.g., a top hat function) can be formed from a series of sine and cosine waves, that is, by adding together sine and cosine waves of appropriate frequencies and amplitudes it is possible to generate the original more complex waveform (e.g., the top hat function). In principle, a band of frequencies can be simultaneously excited by adding all the frequencies in the desired range. In the case of the top hat function, all the frequencies in the range have the same amplitude, and summing them generates a shape called a *Sinc function* (see Fig. 31-6). Therefore, a band of spins can be excited by modifying the RF pulse amplitude using a Sinc function. Naturally, Fourier theory would not be very practical unless there were mathematical ways of generating the desired functions, and fortunately the mathematics has been worked out

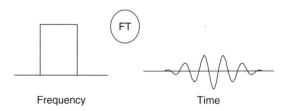

Frequency           Time

**FIGURE 31-6** Shapes in the time domain and the frequency domain are related through the mathematical process of the Fourier transform (FT). In this instance, a "top hat" function in the frequency domain is related to the time domain signal of a "Sinc" function. By shaping the radiofrequency (RF) pulse as a Sinc function, we are able to excite a band (i.e., a top hat function) of spins in the frequency domain.

and implemented on the scanner computer. When a function is decomposed into its component frequencies using Fourier theory, it is said to be Fourier transformed. Another way of thinking about this is that a Sinc function can be generated by Fourier transforming the top hat function, and conversely the top hat function can be generated by Fourier transforming the Sinc function.

## SLICE SELECTION PRINCIPLE

Slice selection is achieved by applying a linear magnetic field gradient to the body to set up a linear range of frequencies. The RF pulse is applied at the central resonance frequency and the shape of the RF pulse is that of a Sinc function, that is, it is designed to excite a narrow range of frequencies (see Fig 31-7). The range of frequencies is described by its bandwidth (BW), that is there is a range or, band, of frequencies that describe the outer edges of the slice, extending from the lowest frequency through the highest frequency in the range.

## BANDWIDTH OF RADIOFREQUENCY PULSE

The RF pulse that is applied to achieve slice selection in the presence of the gradient has a characteristic central frequency, which dictates where the slice is centered along the body, and a BW, which determines the slice width. The BW of the RF pulse is inversely proportional to the duration of the pulse:

- BW = 1/T pulse
- Short pulse—wide BW
- Long pulse—narrow BW

Note that the relationship between the application time of the RF pulse and the effects of this pulse in the frequency signal is expressed in inverse terms (see Fig. 31-8). This is a feature of Fourier theory, for example, if the Sinc function and top hat function are related by the Fourier transform (FT), the units of these functions are also inversely related to each other: The Sinc function is a time signal, whereas the top hat function is the inverse of time, which is frequency. Because the RF pulse is applied in time, a short duration pulse is preferred, to keep the imaging sequence short and achieving short echo times (TEs), which give better sensitivity to flow and more immunity from artifacts. However, because of the inverse relationship between RF pulses and the excitation profile in the frequency domain, short RF pulses necessitate that a wide BW is excited. Consequently, because the BW of frequencies is directly proportional to the applied gradient, a strong gradient is required to produce a thin slice. Consider the requirement to excite a slice of width 8 mm, if a long RF pulse is used, the BW is narrow, and therefore only a small gradient is required to produce this distribution of frequencies over the body; conversely if a short RF pulse is used, the BW is wide, and a strong gradient is required to compress this wide range of frequencies into a physically small space. In each case, the same slice width, for example, 8 mm, can be achieved.

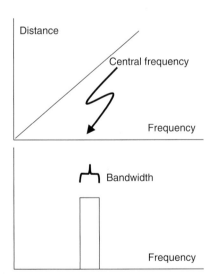

**FIGURE 31-7** By applying a linear magnetic field gradient (*sloped line* in top panel) to the body, a range of frequencies are imposed on the body. The radiofrequency (RF) pulse is applied at the central resonance frequency corresponding to the desired spatial position of the slice. The special Sinc shape of the RF pulse ensures that a small band of frequencies are excited, corresponding to the slice thickness.

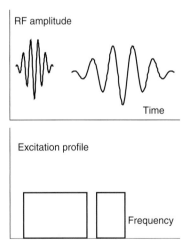

**FIGURE 31-8** The bandwidth (BW) of the radiofrequency (RF) pulse is inversely proportional to pulse duration, with a short pulse exciting a wide BW and a long pulse exciting narrow BW.

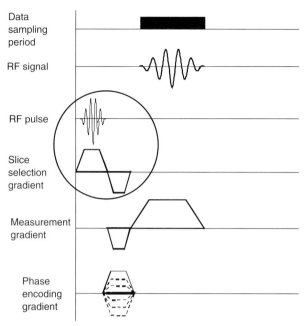

FIGURE 31-9   In the gradient echo imaging pulse sequence, the slice selection section is circled. The two components of slice selection are the gradient, to produce the linear distribution of frequencies, and the Sinc-shaped radiofrequency (RF) pulse.

## SLICE SELECTION

To excite spins in a slice we need two components (see Fig. 31-9):

- A gradient applied to produce the linear distribution of frequencies
- An RF pulse, modulated in shape by the Sinc function

However, following slice selection, we note that the spins have been exposed to a gradient. Naturally, the

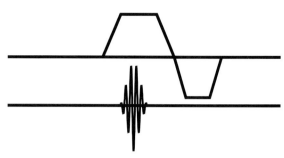

FIGURE 31-10   The slice selection gradient partially dephases spins, yielding a lower signal than optimum. To focus the spins the slice selection process is followed by a rephasing gradient, seen here as a negative gradient applied following the slice selection section.

gradient causes spins to dephase, and therefore they yield a lower signal than is optimal, compared to all spins being in phase. Spin focusing can be accomplished by following the slice selection process by a rephasing gradient (see Fig. 31-10). The rephasing gradient is applied such that it occupies half the area of the initial slice selection gradient.

## SUMMARY

Although only a small percentage of spins contribute to the MRI signal, spin presession occurs naturally in the magnet. Application of an RF pulse is required to excite the spins and bring them into the transverse plane. A gradient applied to the spins imposes a distribution of spin frequencies. A Sinc-shaped RF pulse applied in conjunction with the gradient excites a sharp-edged slice. The shape of the RF pulse is governed by Fourier theory.

# CHAPTER 32

# Rapid Cardiovascular Magnetic Resonance Imaging

Mark Doyle

## MOTIVATION

In the context of cardiovascular (CV) applications, rapid magnetic resonance imaging (MRI) is required primarily for two purposes:

- To image the CV system in times less than physiologic time scales
- To increase scan efficiency and patient throughput

There are several physiologic time scales that present a challenge to MRI, as follows:

1. Respiratory motion
   a. Breath-holding; requires patient co-operation
   b. Respiratory monitoring and synchronization; time consuming
2. Cardiac motion
   a. Cardiac triggering; requires good electrocardiogram (ECG) signal
   b. Real-time imaging; currently suffers from low resolution and/or contrast
3. Blood motion
   a. Myocardial perfusion; contrast has a 20-second transit time
   b. Contrast angiography; contrast has a 20- to 40-second transit time

Currently, conventional imaging applied to maximize speed is capable of providing diagnostic information, often of high quality. For example, in the area of angiography, a bolus of gadolinium–based contrast agent is imaged while in the arterial phase, allowing generation of a three-dimensional (3D) angiogram of a wide region. The acquisition time for this sequence is in the order of 20 to 30 seconds. In the area of myocardial perfusion imaging, the change in myocardial contrast as a contrast agent passes through is dynamically visualized. This requires a time resolution of one to two heartbeats, and is achieved while imaging multiple slices. One of the standard examinations performed by

MRI is functional evaluation of the left ventricle (LV). This is typically accomplished in a breath-hold time to obtain a temporal resolution within the cardiac cycle of approximately 50 milliseconds.

Given this background, it may be queried why there is a requirement for yet more rapid imaging, because clearly, MRI can be used to acquire CV images of diagnostic value. Consider each of the major application areas itemized in the preceding text:

- For angiography, correct synchronization of the angiographic imaging sequence with the arterial phase of the contrast agent is crucial to obtain good image quality. To this end, an angiographic timing sequence is typically run before the full acquisition. In the timing run, a small bolus is injected to calculate the time for contrast to reach the arterial system. This knowledge is used to activate the 3D acquisition. When the 3D acquisition is timed well, arterial blood contrast is excellent. However, when the 3D acquisition is timed badly, arterial blood contrast is poor. When poor contrast is obtained, at best, this may require a delay of several minutes to allow clearing of the agent, or at worst, the vascular information may not be acquired during that scan session (see Fig. 32-1). Sometimes, contrast is low due to aberrant flow patterns, and in these cases there is no single "correct" imaging time. The availability of rapid imaging would allow continuous imaging, thereby reducing setup time and improving reliability with the availability of time-resolved angiographic data.
- For myocardial perfusion imaging, additional time is required in the cycle to generate contrast. Optimal contrast is not always generated due to acquisition time constraints, which often place an upper limit on the inversion time for the contrast pulse. Rapid imaging would allow improved contrast to be realized.
- Although cine imaging of the LV can be accomplished in a breath-hold, the patient's idea of a "comfortable

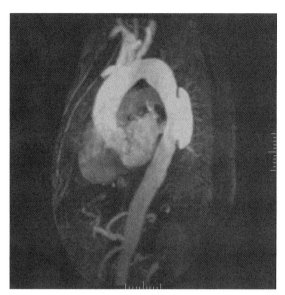 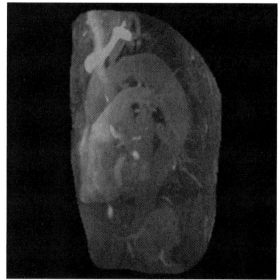

**FIGURE 32-1**  Example of adequate (left) and inadequate (right) vascular contrast for a 3D angiographic study using a bolus injection of contrast agent. The scan time and acquisition parameters for each scan were identical, the major difference being the timing of each scan relative to the passage of the contrast agent. This illustrates the sensitivity of the angiographic approach to timing.

breath-hold" may be dramatically abbreviated from the "ideal" required for imaging. Therefore, rapid imaging can at the least reduce the breath-hold time, or at best eliminate the need for breath-holding if adequate quality could be obtained with a real-time approach.

## RAPID IMAGING APPROACHES

High-resolution images are usually preferable for diagnostic purposes. However, lower resolution images may yield "sufficient" information, the advantage being that lower resolution images can be obtained in less time. Further, it is possible to reduce the scan matrix while maintaining the resolution by the use of partial number of excitations (NEX). However, this approach reduces the signal-to-noise ratio (SNR). Alternatively, a partial phase field of view or rectangular matrix can result in fold-over artifacts. When using the multielement phased array coils it may be possible to deactivate one or more of the elements. This expediency can be used to reduce the effects of fold-over artifact, by removing the signal source. Special placement of active element(s) of the coil may be required for optimal imaging.

## ECHO PLANAR IMAGING

Echo planar imaging (EPI) is a rapid gradient echo technique that employs a train of echoes, each one relating to a line of k-space. EPI can produce an image in approximately 50 milliseconds. EPI requires high performance gradients due to the multiple gradient switches required. However, because of the inherently long read out time for EPI, short T2 components tend to be blurred. A single-shot EPI image is generally of relatively low resolution, with matrices typically ranging from $64^2$ to $128^2$. The major application of single-shot EPI to date has been in functional brain imaging, where the high T2 values, leading to strong T2 weighting, are an advantage. Currently however, application to cardiac use is limited.

## MULTISHOT ECHO PLANAR IMAGING AND MULTIPLE ECHO GRADIENT ECHO

While gradient echo requires multiple applications of the basic imaging sequence to compile multiple lines of k-space, single-shot EPI generally has too long an echo train for cardiac applications. Therefore, a hybrid of the two has evolved, which acquires several lines of k-space for each basic imaging sequence. Echo train length (ETL) imaging utilizes a short train of echo signals, typically with values of 4 to 8. A series of four echoes (i.e., four lines of k-space) can be acquired with a repetition time (TR) of approximately 10 milliseconds. This is approximately a factor of 2 faster than the traditional gradient-recalled echo approach. The ETL approach can be combined with segmented scanning for CV imaging. Segmented ETL imaging is often used to perform the rapid scanning required for myocardial perfusion imaging.

## SPIRAL SCANNING

A spiral trajectory in k-space can be accomplished by use of gradually increasing sinusoidal and cosinusoidal gradients (see Fig. 32-2). In principle a spiral scan could be obtained in a single shot, but more commonly, multiple interleaved shots are used. In the interleaved version, each spiral arm is approximately 20 milliseconds long, which is quite long for T2 blurring considerations. The spiral data requires regridding to accommodate the regular k-space matrix, which makes reconstruction times longer.

## PARALLEL IMAGING APPROACH

The parallel imaging approach to reduce scan time relies on the use of a number of receivers positioned around the region of interest. Time reduction factors of 2 are common. Although a reduced field of view is used, the advantage to this approach is that no signal aliasing occurs (when properly applied).

## K-SPACE SYMMETRY

K-space has the property of complex conjugate symmetry through the center (see Fig. 32-3). Using this property of symmetry, reduced scan times can be accomplished by acquiring reduced portions of k-space and filling in the portion not acquired by knowledge of the symmetry. Such an approach is exploited when a partial NEX value is used.

## CARDIAC-SPECIFIC RAPID IMAGING

For breath-hold approaches, cine images are typically acquired in a "segmented", or "turbo" manner (see Fig. 32-4). Each cardiac view is composed of a grouping of acquisitions or views per segment (VPS). In cardiac imaging, one of the determinants of scan time is the number of VPS. For instance, for a matrix with 256 phase encoding lines, scan time reduction is in direct proportion to the VPS used:

- VPS = 8, scan time = 256/8 = 32 heartbeats
- VPS = 20, scan time = 256/20 = 12 heartbeats

While higher VPS values lead to shorter scan times, one disadvantage of selecting too high a VPS value is that temporal blur may result within the cardiac cycle. Temporal blur is directly proportional to the acquisition

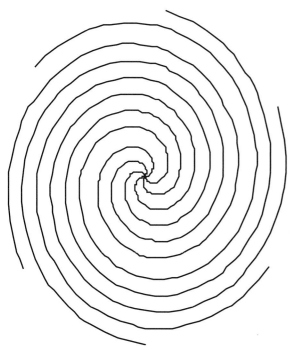

**FIGURE 32-2**   The k-space trajectory of a multiarm spiral scan. This scan utilizes two read gradients, each applied in a sinusoidal manner to produce the curved trajectories in k-space. Coverage of k-space is rapidly achieved. To reconstruct spiral data as an image, it is necessary to regrid the spiral data to a rectangular matrix.

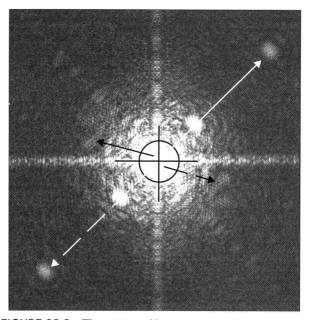

**FIGURE 32-3**   The nature of k-space symmetry is illustrated. For the indicated features, a line reflected through the center of k-space indicates a similar feature at the mirror point. Note that the symmetry is not necessarily left to right, or top to bottom, but rather through the center.

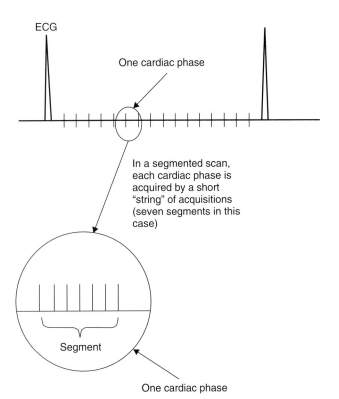

**FIGURE 32-4** The nature of segmented scanning to speed up cardiac gated imaging is illustrated. When a sufficiently rapid imaging sequence is available, a number of lines of k-space (i.e., a segment) can be acquired at each cardiac phase before advancing to acquire data for other cardiac phases. In this way, the scan time is reduced by the views per segment (VPS) factor. ECG, electrocardiogram.

time for each cardiac phase (see Fig. 32-5). For instance, for a scan with a TR of 4 milliseconds, the segment duration time (i.e., time within each cycle over which data are accumulated for each cardiac phase) is directly proportional to the VPS selected:

- VPS = 8, segment time = 32 milliseconds
- VPS = 16, segment time = 56 milliseconds
- VPS = 20, segment time = 80 milliseconds

Therefore, an upper limit to the usable VPS is dictated by the desired temporal resolution sought. For instance, higher temporal resolution is generally required if valvular structures are to be viewed.

## FURTHER REDUCTION OF CARDIAC SCAN TIME

K-space has additional properties that allow further reduction in the scan time for time-resolved images. In the k-space representation, motion of an object manifests as a change of signal phase. The k-space of a moving object visually does not change, and the only feature

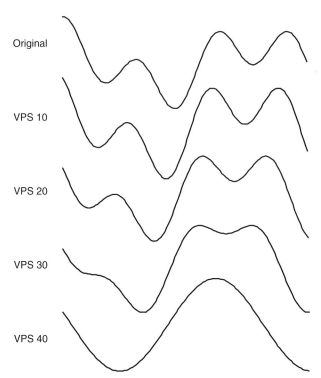

**FIGURE 32-5** The fidelity with which the original waveform is represented is shown for a range of views per segment (VPS). When a low VPS is used, the waveform is represented with good fidelity, but when high VPS values are used, fidelity is lost, and only the broad temporal waveform is seen.

that changes is the phase of the k-space data. Therefore, the temporal behavior of k-space data is quite different from that of the spatial domain images that we commonly look at. Fourier analysis can be used to determine the distribution of phase information (containing temporal information) in a cardiac image series. Simply stacking each k-space data set, and performing a Fourier transform along the time dimension can perform this time series analysis (see Fig. 32-6). The output from this analysis is a series of Fourier coefficient images, labeled from 0 through some maximum number, such as 23. The zeroth coefficient is the average information present in the image series (i.e., static data). The first coefficient is data that varies at a rate of one sinusoidal wave per cardiac cycle (i.e., low frequency variations). The 23rd coefficient is data that varies at a rate of a sinusoidal wave with 23 oscillations per cycle (i.e., high-frequency variations). From the above considerations, it can be appreciated that there is a close interrelationship between the frequency information that can be represented and the VPS selected, which in turn determines the segmentation duration ($T_{segment}$) and the maximum number of frames per cycle that can be realized for a given heart rate. Table 32-1 relates each of these quantities. In the table, it can be appreciated that

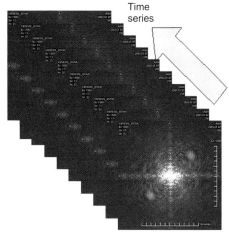

Time series

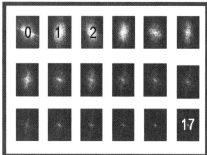

Fourier coefficients

**FIGURE 32-6** To find the distribution of the frequency information in k-space, a temporal series of k-space data are Fourier transformed along the time axis. The resulting series of images is displayed in the right panel. These images are Fourier coefficients, and in this case they are numbered from 0 through 17. Notice that the zeroth coefficient is the most intense and as the series progresses to the last coefficient, the coefficient images lose intensity, which tends to collapse towards the center.

the VPS ultimately determines the maximum frequency information that can be sampled.

From the considerations of temporal blur, we can appreciate that the fidelity with which the frequency information is represented is related to the VPS used; that is, a low VPS allows adequate sampling of high frequency data, and a high VPS (i.e., long segmentation time) is only suitable to sample static or low frequency information (see Fig. 32-7). By examining the distribution of frequency information in the Fourier coefficients, we note that the highest frequency information is concentrated toward the center of k-space, whereas the lower frequency information extends further out toward the periphery of k-space. Therefore, to capture the small amount of high temporal resolution data exacts a high penalty in scan time, because it requires the use of a low VPS applied to the whole of k-space. One solution is to apply a variable sampling rate pattern over k-space and time. By this means it is possible to approximate to an appropriate rate for each region of k-space and thereby acquire data rapidly. The block regional interpolation scheme for k-space (BRISK) is one approach that uses this concept (see Fig. 32-8).

In cardiac imaging, good quality cine images can be obtained using BRISK, utilizing an acceleration factor of

2 to 4 (see Fig. 32-9). Using this it is possible to reduce the scan time, or alternatively obtain multiple slices of cine data in a single breath-hold. Even when employing high VPS values, BRISK allows good scan quality in half the already short scan time. The use of BRISK allows a very short segmentation value to be used to achieve inherently high temporal resolution within the cardiac cycle. This may be useful to view rapidly changing structures such as the valve leaflets.

## RAPID VELOCITY IMAGING

One of the major opportunities in CV MRI is the ability to quantitatively measure blood velocity. However, because of the technical requirements of phase contrast MR there are three features that make the scan time inherently long, and may therefore benefit from rapid scanning sequences:

- Because of imperfections in the system we cannot directly relate phase angle to velocity. Two images are required: velocity compensated and velocity encoded. Phase subtraction of the two data sets is used to undo the effects of phase variations, allowing a flat baseline to be obtained, allowing the velocity data to be measured. Therefore, due to the requirement of comparing two image series to extract velocity information, velocity sensitive imaging takes at least twice as long as conventional cine imaging when encoding velocity in only one direction. To encode velocity in three directions requires a reference and three velocity encoded scans, which further increases the scan time.
- Owing to the requirement to additionally encode velocity information, the time to acquire each line of k-space is increased compared to a non–velocity encoded scan. Therefore, each view of the segment takes longer compared to comparable non–velocity encoded scans, being in the range 7 to 8 milliseconds.

**TABLE 32-1**

Cardiac Views Per Second (VPS) and Frequency

| VPS | Frames (per cycle) | $T_{segment}$ (ms) | Maximum Frequency (Hz) |
|---|---|---|---|
| 4 | 63 | 16 | 31 |
| 8 | 31 | 32 | 15 |
| 12 | 21 | 48 | 10 |
| 16 | 16 | 64 | 8 |
| 20 | 13 | 80 | 6 |
| 24 | 10 | 96 | 5 |

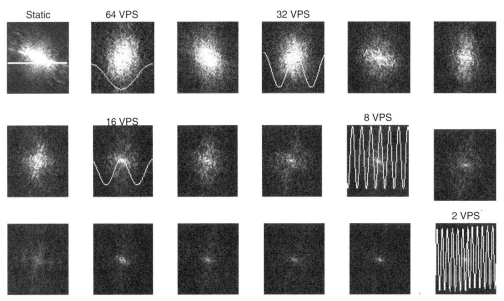

**FIGURE 32-7** The relationship between the Fourier coefficients of Fig. 32-6 and the frequency information is illustrated. The sinusoidal waveforms superimposed on the coefficient images indicate the temporal nature of the data variation. Also indicated above selected coefficients are the views per segment (VPS) that is necessary to sample that frequency of data (with reference to Table 32-1). For instance, the second coefficient indicates that a very slow temporal waveform is represented, and that even a very long VPS (i.e., 64) is capable of capturing that information. Progressively higher frequency data requires progressively lower VPS values to adequately sample that data.

Therefore, to capture adequate temporal information, lower VPS values must be used, which increase scan times.

- To obtain the highest sensitivity to moving blood, a "partial echo" acquisition is commonly used; this reduction of the k-space acquisition is in one direction, and necessitates that k-space is fully sampled in the other direction, that is, NEX = 1, is required which leads to a longer scan time.

Therefore, although phase contrast magnetic resonance (PC-MR) is acknowledged to potentially have high importance, it is rarely used in clinical practice. Although longer scan times can be accommodated, the clinical environment exerts a lot of pressure to perform short scans. One advantage of the BRISK approach is that it can be used with conventional PC-MR to reduce the scan time. Computational fluid dynamics (CFD) has been used to validate BRISK PC-MR. In simulations of BRISK and conventional segmentation scanning, when applied to produce images in uniform scan times, BRISK scans showed higher fidelity (see Fig. 32-10). There are several CV application areas for velocity imaging, including the following:

- Blood flow
- Myocardial tissue velocity mapping
- Inherent contrast for angiography

## REQUIREMENTS FOR REAL-TIME MAGNETIC RESONANCE

To date, application of real-time methods to the CV system has been hampered by the combined challenges presented by cardiac and respiratory motion. The requirements for real-time imaging are as follows:

- High spatial and temporal resolution
- One heartbeat processing time
- High blood/myocardium contrast
- Adequate signal-to-noise

By combining scan features that are currently available, the requirements for real-time imaging can now potentially be met to obtain high spatial and temporal resolution data: for example, a $256^2$ matrix acquired with 50 millisecond temporal resolution through the cardiac cycle. In the following example, moderate acceleration factors for the above-mentioned approaches to rapid imaging are indicated, and the cumulative number of heartbeats (HB) for the acquisition is given:

| VPS 12 | ×12 | 21 HB |
|---|---|---|
| Partial NEX, 0.75 | ×1.3 | 16 HB |
| Parallel imaging, 2 | ×2 | 8 HB |
| BRISK, 4 | ×4 | 2 HB |
| Dual echo EPI, 2 | ×2 | 1 HB |

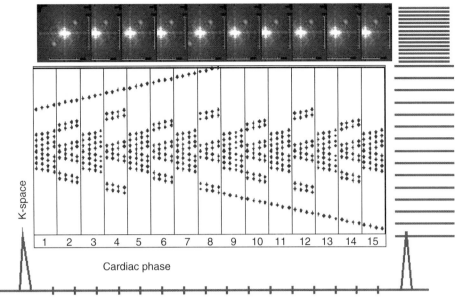

**FIGURE 32-8**   The rapid block regional interpolation scheme for k-space (BRISK) sampling approach is illustrated. Along the top row are indicated a number of k-space data sets representing cardiac phases from the start of the electrocardiogram (ECG) R wave to the end of the cycle. The line to the side indicates that the sampled k-space lines that are acquired at each cardiac phase. In the lower section, the vertical axis represents the full range of k-space sampled, and the horizontal axis represents the cardiac phases at which data are required. Conventionally, k-space lines would be sampled at each cardiac phase. In this sequence, however, only the center of k-space is sampled at a high temporal sampling rate, whereas regions of k-space further from the center are sampled at progressively increasing sparse rates. The data approximates the sampling rate indicated by the Fourier coefficients of Fig. 32-6. After the data has been sampled in this way, it is possible to use data interpolation to fill in the missing data points. After the missing data has been filled in, each cardiac phase is fully represented at a reduced sampling time.

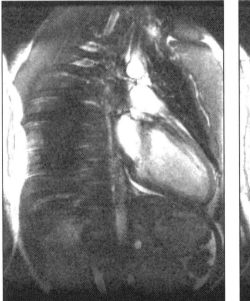 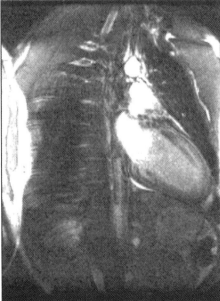

**FIGURE 32-9**   Example of a conventional (left) and a rapid block regional interpolation scheme for k-space (BRISK) (right) scan, each utilizing a high views per second (VPS) parameter. The conventional scan was acquired in 10 seconds, whereas the BRISK scan was acquired in 5 seconds.

**FIGURE 32-10** Example of a conventional (left) and a rapid block regional interpolation scheme for k-space (BRISK) (right) phase contrast velocity scan. The conventional scan was acquired in approximately 1 minute, whereas the BRISK scan was acquired in a breath-hold duration time of 15 seconds.

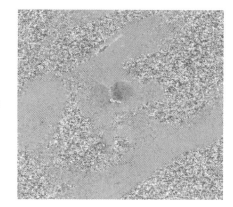 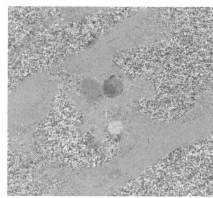

## SUMMARY

Rapid imaging can be accomplished by combining multiple strategies. Improvements are expected in reliability and ease of acquisition for major application areas, including the following:

- Perfusion
- Angiography
- Quantitative flow imaging
- Functional imaging

When real-time CV imaging is realized for MRI, further application areas are expected.

# CHAPTER 33

# Jet Flow Imaging

Mark Doyle

## WHY STUDY JET FLOW?

The presence of jet flow is always associated with pathology. However, simple identification of jet flow is not sufficient to adequately characterize the pathology, including stenotic and regurgitant valves. To be of clinical value, the jet flow must be quantitatively characterized to allow grading or staging the pathology.

## JET FLOW FIELD FACTS

While jet flow velocities can be high (in excess of 5 m per second) the acceleration terms can be extremely high (in the range 10 to 200 m per $s^2$). Although it is not common to characterize jets by their acceleration terms, these terms can have a dramatic impact on the accuracy of phase contrast–magnetic resonance (PC-MR). Close to the jet origin the flow field is not turbulent but has a core of laminar flow. As the jet progresses into the static or counter flowing blood, regions of eddy flow develop, which gradually encroach on the laminar jet core and eventually degrade it into turbulent flow (see Fig. 33-1). Depending on the flow conditions, the transition from laminar to turbulent flow may occur over a relatively short distance or may extend quite far into the vessel or chamber.

## TWO COMPONENTS OF FLOW

While a high velocity jet is an obvious manifestation of pathology and appears distal to it, the convergent flow field is found proximal to the stenotic site. *In vivo*, owing to the confined structures of the heart, the jet may encounter a vessel or chamber wall after traversing a very short distance and therefore the jet may not have an opportunity to develop the flow field characteristic of "free jets". However, just past the stenotic origin, the jet flow will converge, and at this point it is still characterized by laminar flow. The region of maximal convergence is termed the *vena contracta*. A free jet can ideally be characterized by measuring flow in only the direction along the jet.

In the convergent zone proximal to the jet, a complex three-dimensional (3D) distribution of low velocity flow is found. In the convergent zone, we ideally require measurement of all three velocity directions to characterize flow conditions. However, assumptions can be made to reduce the flow problem to a 1D case, but these assumptions are often incorrect, because they may oversimplify the situation. To fully characterize flow in the convergent zone, it is desirable to quantify velocity in all three directions for each plane visualized. These separate flow components can be visualized as individual components, but to get a more comprehensive view, quiver plots can be used to combine the two in-plane components, for example, left-right and vertical, into one intuitive image format. Using quiver plots, eddy currents can be visualized breaking off the tip of the fully develop jet.

## JET ONSET

The onset of jet flow is typically very sudden, and for a jet that develops in <40 milliseconds, it can be appreciated that even with a frame rate of 7 milliseconds (a typical lower limit of scanner performance) only a few frames will capture jet onset. Consider that a temporal resolution of 20 frames per cycle (a more typical performance level) corresponds to 50 milliseconds per frame, and in this instance, onset of jet flow through maturity would be completely missed or blurred into one time frame.

## VELOCITY VERSUS ACCELERATION

While jet velocities can be high (1 to 10 m per second), high velocities do not pose a problem for

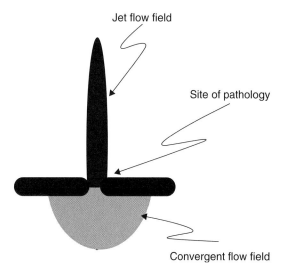

**FIGURE 33-1** At the site of a stenosis, two distinct flow patterns are seen: on the proximal side, flow accelerates toward the orifice while only achieving relatively low velocities, and when passing through the orifice it becomes a high-velocity jet. The vena contracta describes the jet region where the cross-sectional area is minimal and the velocity is maximal, and this typically occurs a few millimetres distal to the orifice.

PC-MR. The problem for PC-MR is the high accelerations that are present in jet flow. In Fig. 33-2, we plot velocity and acceleration on the same graphs to show how they are related to each other for a jet flow waveform. In this example, at peak jet flow, the maximum velocity is approximately 160 cm per second,

whereas at the jet origin the maximum velocity is close at 130 cm per second. However, the maximum acceleration is dramatically different between these two locations, being 80 cm per $s^2$ versus 30 cm per $s^2$, respectively. Acceleration is problematic because its presence violates some of the key assumptions inherent in PC-MR:

- Velocity does not change appreciably over image time for each frame.
- Velocity is uniform within each voxel.

Therefore, to accurately measure velocity in jet flow fields, the acquisition needs to satisfy the following two conditions:

- High frame rates
- High spatial resolution

Conformation to these conditions typically leads to dramatically long scan times.

## PROXIMAL FLOW FIELD

The difficulties in imaging jet flow fields using PC-MR have led to a focus on the convergent flow side. The convergent flow field can be quantified using one of two methods:

- Proximal iso-velocity surface area (PISA)
- Control volume

Examination of the proximal flow field can be used to quantify the amount of blood passing through a

**FIGURE 33-2** Simultaneous plots of velocity and acceleration for jet flow at two distinct positions: top panel, just past the jet origin and lower panel, close to the tip of the fully developed jet. Notice the increase in acceleration at the jet tip, although the velocity does not increase substantially between the two points.

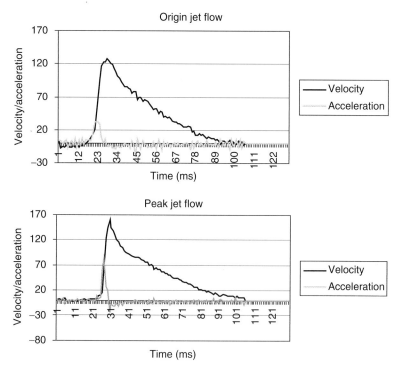

region of interest such as a stenotic valve. Typically, full 3D visualization of convergent flow is not feasible, and in the simplified PISA approach, only the radius of the isovelocity contour in one direction is measured. Alternatively, the control volume approach can be used, but it requires imaging of several slices, with multiple velocity directions encoded in each slice. For these reasons, quantification of jet flow from an examination of the convergent flow field has not gained widespread acceptance in the magnetic resonance (MR) community. The complexities of this problem make direct visualization of the jet attractive.

## DIRECT JET VISUALIZATION

Assuming that the jet flow can be accurately measured using PC-MR, it is possible to capture this information in one to two slices, capturing either through-plane or in-plane flow. Therefore, direct jet imaging using PC-MR is desirable. However, as indicated earlier, acceleration is problematic for PC-MR and it follows that jet imaging may be inherently prone to artifacts, because commonly applied PC-MR approaches have relatively poor spatial and temporal resolution.

The reason for poor temporal resolution is embedded in the PC-MR scan sequence. Velocity is encoded in the phase of the MR signal by applying specially designed gradient waveforms. These gradients take longer to apply than regular imaging gradients, thereby extending the echo time (TE). Typically, acceleration is not explicitly accommodated in the design of the flow encoding gradients because it would take too long to compensate for, which would further extend the TE. Therefore, it is generally assumed that the gradients are applied sufficiently fast to avoid errors due to acceleration. The assumption is generally true for TEs <4 milliseconds. However, the assumptions break down when multiple lines of k-space are acquired over time and assigned to a single cardiac phase.

## ORIGIN OF PROBLEM

In flow imaging, it is common to encode the reference and the flow encoded data within each cardiac cycle. In the presence of high acceleration, the velocity encoded by the reference scan could be higher (or lower) than that encoded by the flow encoded scan. Therefore, owing to the segmentation process, the two scans become systematically shifted in time relative to each other. In Fig. 33-3, the top panel show the velocity curve derived from temporally registered velocity compensated (VC) and velocity encoded (VE) data sets and the lower panel shows the distorted velocity curve that results when the

Temporally registered

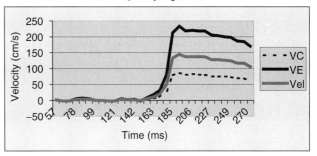

Temporally shifted

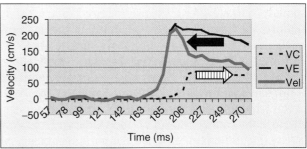

**FIGURE 33-3** A major source of inaccuracy in measuring jet flow using phase contrast–magnetic resonance (PC-MR) is illustrated. The graphs show the velocities that are measured using the velocity compensated (VC) and velocity encoded (VE) scans over time in the cycle. The true velocity (Vel) is obtained by subtracting the two curves (corresponding to the phase subtraction process in PC-MR). In the top panel, we observe a true jet velocity of approximately 150 cm per second in the case when both VC and VE plots are temporally registered. In the lower panel, the effect of temporally displacing the two source data sets (VC and VE) is shown where the displacement direction of the VC and VE plots are in opposite directions as indicated by the *arrows*. In this instance, the relative time shifts are responsible for distorting the velocity curve (Vel), in which the observed velocity exceeds 200 cm per second, whereas the true maximal velocity is only 150 cm per second, as shown in the top panel.

VC and VE data sets are shifted relative to each other. Note, that in this example, jet velocity is overestimated because of the time shift between encoding the VC and VE data sets. Clearly there is a problem in PC-MR related to its sensitivity to acceleration.

## SOLUTION TO PROBLEM

One solution to the problem of acceleration-induced velocity overestimation is to arrange for each frame of the reference scan to be acquired at exactly the same position in the cardiac cycle as the VE scan. This can be achieved by splitting the acquisition of the reference and flow encoded scans over separate heartbeats, instead of interleaving them as is conventionally done. However, flow data encoded in the phase information is very sensitive to small differences in variations that occur between cardiac cycles and splitting the acquisition in this way generally leads to excessive motion-related artifacts.

## JET FLOW IMAGING CONDITIONS

Therefore, we have seen that to accommodate the high acceleration terms, the reference and VE acquisitions must be temporally registered. Additionally, a high number of frames per cycle are required to accurately capture the rapid changes inherent in the jet flow waveform. These two requirements dictate that low data segmentation values should be used, which in turn leads to extended scan times when using conventional approaches, and this still does not address the issue of the temporal alignment of the VC and VE data sets. Owing to the combination of VC and VE data interleaving and segmentation, an effective temporal displacement is introduced, which may lead to signal aliasing in high acceleration jet flow, although the velocity encoding

parameter (VENC) is not truly exceeded. However, one possible solution is to temporally shift the VC and VE data at the post-processing stage, such that temporal alignment is achieved. To a large extent, this process can result in extraction of the true velocity information, and may remove a large amount of the artifactual signal aliasing.

## BLOCK REGIONAL INTERPOLATION SCHEME FOR K-SPACE RAPID IMAGING

The block regional interpolation scheme for k-space (BRISK) rapid sampling scheme can be used to acquire flow data fast, even when employing low data segmentation values (see Fig. 33-4). Further, it has the additional characteristic that the sparsely sampled data are temporally interpolated to fill in the unsampled data points. During this interpolation process it is possible to arrange for data to be additionally temporally aligned. Therefore, BRISK imaging has potential to accurately image jet flow with a short scan time (see Fig. 33-5). In Fig. 33-6, BRISK was successfully applied to image

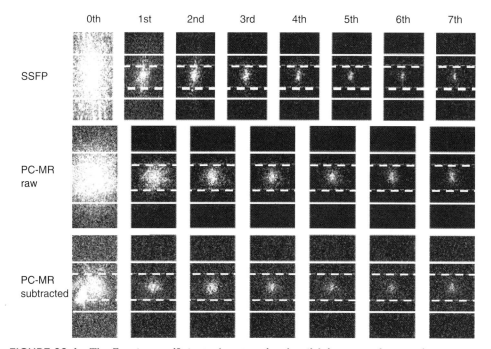

**FIGURE 33-4** The Fourier coefficients (see text for details) for a steady state free precession (SSFP) cine scan (top panel), a phase contrast–magnetic resonance (PC-MR) scan (middle panel), and the subtracted PC-MR data (lower panel) are compared. The *lines drawn on the coefficients* correspond to the distinct regions dynamically sampled in the rapid block regional interpolation scheme for k-space (BRISK) sampling scheme superimposed on the Fourier coefficient images zero through seven. The *solid lines* indicate the extent required to capture cardiac motion, as indicated in the top panel, and the *dotted lines* indicate the lower extent of data required to capture the dynamic velocity data, lower panel. Note, that to obtain velocity data, narrower data bands are sufficient (lower panel), allowing BRISK to be highly efficient when applied to PC-MR imaging.

Free breathing

Breath-hold

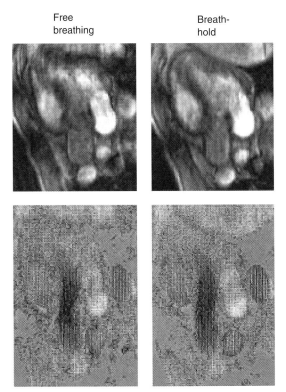

**FIGURE 33-5**  Comparison of free breathing and breath-hold magnitude and velocity vector plot scans. The free breathing scans were obtained using conventional phase contrast–magnetic resonance (PC-MR) and the breath-hold scans were obtained using the rapid block regional interpolation scheme for k-space (BRISK) approach. The magnitude image is shown in the top panel and in the lower panel, blood flow at end-systole is represented. Note in comparison to the conventional scan, the BRISK magnitude and velocity images show sharp edge detail, reflecting that BRISK data were acquired during a breath-hold.

jet flow, whereas images acquired using conventional scanning suffered signal aliasing.

## BLOCK REGIONAL INTERPOLATION SCHEME FOR K-SPACE ADVANTAGE IN JETS

We have seen that temporal alignment performed by BRISK allows accurate representation of jets with high acceleration components. We now approach the issue of how rapidly the PC-MR data can be acquired using BRISK. For functional cardiac imaging, the BRISK scan time is approximately 25% of the full scan time. However, for flow imaging, the BRISK scan time can be reduced to approximately 15% of the full scan. This high reduction factor is possible because, typically, cardiovascular flow patterns result in the velocity data contracting even

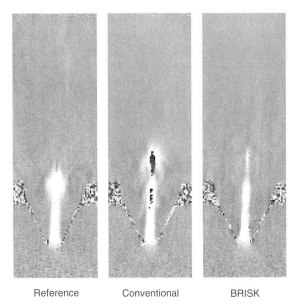

Reference          Conventional          BRISK

**FIGURE 33-6**  Three representative views of jet flow, for (i) a temporally registered phase contrast–magnetic resonance (PC-MR) scan (Reference), (ii) a conventional scan, in which data were acquired in an interleaved manner, and (iii) block regional interpolation scheme for k-space (BRISK), in which data were acquired in a temporally interleaved manner, but were post-processed to temporally align them. Notice that in the conventional scan, artifactual signal aliasing is seen. This is not present in the Reference scan or the temporally aligned BRISK scan.

more rapidly toward the center of the k-space-time axis. In Fig. 33-4, the top row shows the Fourier coefficients for cardiac functional image data obtained using the steady state free precession (SSFP) sequence, where we note the large region of k-space which contains dynamic information. The middle panel shows a raw PC-MR data set and the lower panel shows a subtracted PC-MR data set. Note that the subtracted PC-MR data tends to shrink toward the center of k-space at a faster rate than the SSFP data. This aspect allows further reduction in the region that has to be dynamically sampled using the BRISK approach, while allowing adequate capture of flow information. In part, BRISK can acquire fewer data lines in flow imaging because of the high degree of coherence that exists between pixels in the flow field. This is a reflection of the high degree of coherence that exists between flowing spins.

## BLOCK REGIONAL INTERPOLATION SCHEME FOR K-SPACE AND CONVERGENT FLOW

In the convergent flow region, the maximum velocity is often quite low, typically <20 cm per second, and maximum temporal acceleration is also typically low, being <1 m per s². In this region, BRISK PC-MR data closely matches the reference scan data. While jet flow can be well represented with a single velocity component, convergent flow requires measuring at least two flow components to capture in-plane flow.

## DIRECT JET FLOW IMAGING WITH BLOCK REGIONAL INTERPOLATION SCHEME FOR K-SPACE

In the example of Fig. 33-6, the jet flow maximum velocity was 165 cm per second and the maximum acceleration was 134 m per s². A reference scan was implemented such that all flow compensated and flow encoded lines were acquired at exactly the same temporal position, thereby avoiding any source of error due to temporal misalignment of the VC and VE data. In this case, BRISK imaging was able to closely match the reference scan information. Conversely, a conventional, that is, temporally unregistered scan demonstrated velocity signal aliasing. Jets can be characterized by the rate of progression of the jet front, measured in meters per second, which can be represented as a 3D surface, with height above the surface representing velocity, one axis representing space, and one time (see Fig. 33-7). The BRISK jet progression shows the sudden onset of jet flow, followed by a gradual trailing off of the velocity. Conversely, the temporally unregistered conventional scan shows regions of aliasing in the 3D jet progression.

Note that the aliased regions are associated with the regions of high acceleration, whereas the decaying jet side does not suffer from regions of signal alias due to the generally low accelerations present.

## BLOCK REGIONAL INTERPOLATION SCHEME FOR K-SPACE VERSUS CONVENTIONAL

Overestimation of jet velocity by the conventional unregistered scan is a function of several features including the following:

- Acceleration
- The number of frames per cycle
- The temporal shift between VC and VE data sets

The temporally registered BRISK consistently represents jet flow more closely, independently of these features. After temporally registering the BRISK data, the velocity curve behaves in a predictable manner in that high frame rates will better represent the rapid transient flow conditions, allowing better capture of the peak velocity (see Fig. 33-8).

## JET CROSS-SECTION

Another method used to characterize jet flow is to measure its cross-section at the vena contracta. Together with a measure of velocity at this point, flow

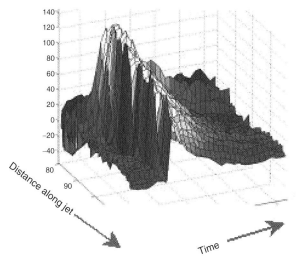
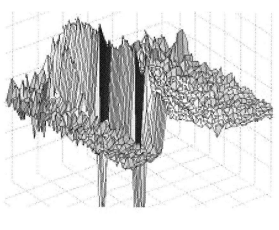

**FIGURE 33-7**  Velocity-distance-time plots for jet flow, for left panel: block regional interpolation scheme for k-space (BRISK) and right panel: conventional data. Height above the plane represents velocity, and in the BRISK data set, the sudden onset of jet flow is seen as the initial steep upslope, and the gradual decay of jet flow is seen as the gentler downsloping feature. The corresponding conventional scan exhibits similar features, but is marred by sudden discontinuities corresponding to regions of signal aliasing.

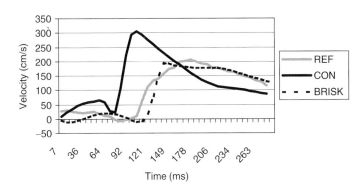

**FIGURE 33-8** The degree to which jet velocity can be overestimated by a conventionally interleaved scan is shown. Compared to the reference or block regional interpolation scheme for k-space (BRISK) velocity-time plots, the conventional data set exhibits a peak velocity which is 150% of the true peak velocity. REF, reference; CON, conventional data set.

volume can be calculated. Figure 33-9 shows flow profiles at a position 2 mm from the jet origin. The BRISK scan with 32 frames per cycle closely represented the profiles from jet onset past peak flow compared to the reference scan (129 frames). The only exception was at the onset of flow, where BRISK underestimated the flow width. When the jet is measured as the full width at half maximum (FWHM), the BRISK data closely matches the reference scan, again, except at the sudden onset of jet flow, which corresponds to the point of maximal acceleration.

## JET LENGTH

Jet theory states that in free jets, the length of the laminar jet core is approximately four times the orifice diameter. Using the 95% level to determine the extent of the laminar core, the jet length can be automatically determined. Analysis of the central jet profile showed that jet length by BRISK with 32 frames per cycle was in close agreement the reference scan with 129 frames per cycle showing only a 3% error. Lower frames per

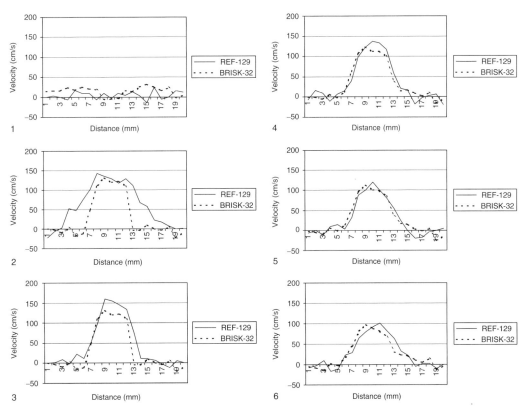

**FIGURE 33-9** Profiles across the jet flow at a distance 2 mm from the jet origin are seen at successive time points, each separated by 30 milliseconds. In frame 2, at the point of jet onset, it can be seen that the BRISK data set, despite describing the correct velocity underestimates the jet width. However, at all other successive time points, the BRISK data closely matches the reference data. REF, reference; BRISK, block regional interpolation scheme for k-space.

cycle measurements tended to overestimate jet length by approximately 15%.

## SUMMARY

Jets are problematic for conventional phase velocity imaging due to the high acceleration terms, and not necessarily because of the high velocity terms. Both conventional data and the rapidly acquired BRISK data can be temporally aligned by performing suitable post-processing, thereby eliminating one important source of error in measuring jet flow. BRISK allows high temporal sampling rates to be achieved in a breath-hold time frame. Using BRISK, three velocity components can be acquired in a breath-hold, which is suitable for non–jet flow, including convergent flow.

# CHAPTER 34

# K-Space Revisited: An Informal View

Mark Doyle

An air of mystery surrounds k-space and treatments of it tend to either require advanced mathematical knowledge or else are too brief in nature. Here we will consider k-space in a relaxed, informal manner to engender familiarity, at the expense of comprehensive coverage. Please be aware that some of the illustrations are intended to be of a light-hearted nature (not strictly factual).

## NON–MAGNETIC RESONANCE IMAGING EXAMPLE

Perhaps the greatest difficulty involves relating k-space to the magnetic resonance imaging (MRI) sequence. However, k-space is not, by any means, exclusive to MRI. Let us consider a picture of some flowers. Every image, from whatever source, can be represented in the k-space format (see Fig. 34-1). For our working definition of k-space, we shall consider it to be the result of performing the mathematical operation of the Fourier transformation (FT) on an image.

## FOURIER THEORY

Fourier theory simply indicates that every signal waveform can be represented as a sum of sine and cosine waves. The conceptual difficulty here often involves relating a photograph, for example, of flowers, to a signal waveform. We can regard the flower picture as a signal, with intensity variations spread over two dimensions. To see this more clearly, we can tip the image over to visualize the intensity of the two-dimensional (2D) signal distribution (see Fig. 34-2). As we keep tipping the image we eventually see it in a side view, clearly showing it to be a signal intensity waveform, although of a complex nature.

When viewed as a normal image, these intensity waveforms are represented as pixel intensities in a photograph or on a monitor screen. Obviously, the signal intensity view is not commonly seen. However, we now have an increased awareness of the relationship between an image and its signal content. Note that "image" features are still discernible in the "signal intensity" representation.

Given that the flower picture is a really a 2D signal waveform, let us concentrate on one line from the picture. Fourier theory says that this line "signal" can be represented by a series of sine and cosine waves. To consider what that means, let us explore a simpler example: a single sine wave. When we describe it, we consider it in terms of amplitude and frequency. In the case of a single sine wave it has parameters of frequency 1 cycle, and amplitude 1 (arbitrary units). The Fourier theory states that this single sine wave can be represented by a sum of sine and cosine waves! This is not such a big conceptual leap, because, by inspection, it already is a sine wave (see Fig. 34-3, top panel). However, let us continue and ask what does the Fourier transform of this sine wave look like? We can describe the Fourier transform signal as a single spike, centered on position 1, with an amplitude of 64. It is hard to imagine, but we are making great progress.

Flushed with this success, let us consider a sine wave with more cycles (see Fig. 34-3, middle panel). As we describe it, we note that it has parameters of frequency 10 cycles, and amplitude 1. Again, we ask what does the Fourier transform look like? As we describe it, it has a single spike at position 10, with amplitude 64. Moving, rapidly ahead, we consider yet another, higher frequency sine wave, that is, one with even more cycles (see Fig. 34-3, lower panel). As we describe it, it has parameters of frequency 20 cycles, and amplitude 1. In this case the Fourier transform is again a single spike, this time centered at position 20, with amplitude 64.

## INTERPRETATION

By these multiple illustrations we see what is happening: a sine wave can be described by the number of

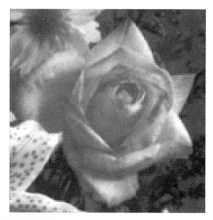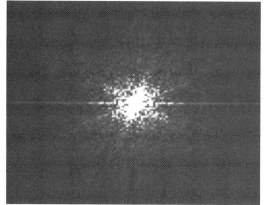

**FIGURE 34-1** An image of a flower and its corresponding k-space representation. K-space is a concept that is not unique to magnetic resonance imaging (MRI). This flower k-space has exactly the same form as a conventional magnetic resonance (MR) image.

cycles (oscillations over its length) and its amplitude. Alternatively, to save us the effort of counting these cycles, we could perform a Fourier transform, which directly tells us how many cycles there were in the original sine wave, which is represented by a

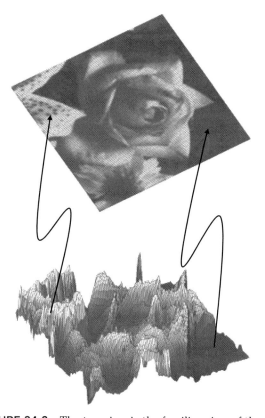

**FIGURE 34-2** The top view is the familiar view of the flower picture, where signal is conventionally represented as bright and dark pixels. By tipping the image on its side, we see the signal intensity variations distributed over the two-dimensional (2D) plane. In this 3D view, it is apparent that the flower picture is really a 2D plot of signal intensity.

spike of signal at the number corresponding to the frequency content. However, we note that a sine wave of amplitude 1 generated a Fourier spike of amplitude 64. This apparent discrepancy is because there is a linear scaling factor that connects the two.

## MULTIPLE SINE WAVES

Now, let us step it up a notch: consider two sine waves: amplitude 1 for each; frequencies 1 and 10 cycles (see Fig. 34-4). In this instance, the Fourier transform has two spikes, one at position 1 and one at position 10. Each of them has amplitude 64. Now consider three sine waves: amplitude 1 for each; with frequencies 1, 10, and 20 cycles. The Fourier transform has three spikes at positions 1, 10, and 20; each with amplitude 64. So as we can imagine, the sine wave signal soon gets too complicated to state by inspection what frequency information is present. However, we now have the Fourier transform to count the cycles for us, and tell us what frequencies were originally present. This can be accomplished, safely, reliably, and repetitively.

## FLOWER IMAGE

We can now return to the line from the flower image, which we now view as a signal waveform. Fourier theory says that this "signal" can be represented by a series of sine and cosine waves. The Fourier transform of the flower signal line shows a series of peaks, some so close together that they merge together, and one dominant peak at frequency position 64 (see Fig. 34-5). The interpretation of this Fourier transform signal is that the intensity line from the flower picture can be represented by sine and cosine waves, the amplitude of which can be read off from the Fourier transform plot. This represents

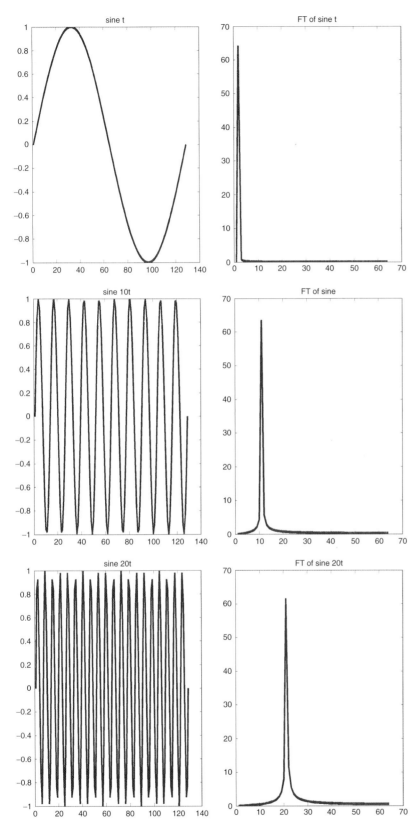

**FIGURE 34-3**   Three sine wave signals and their corresponding Fourier representation. It is apparent that the single sine wave (top) is represented by a single spike in the Fourier plot at position 1. The sine wave with 10 cycles (middle) is represented by a single Fourier spike at position 10, and the sine wave with 20 cycles (lower panel) is represented by a single Fourier spike at position 20. FT, Fourier transform.

**FIGURE 34-4** An example of a more complex waveform and its Fourier representation is shown. The top panel shows two sine waves, one with 1 cycle and one with 20 cycles, which are added to form the more complex waveform shown in the lower left panel. The corresponding Fourier representation immediately shows two spikes, one at position 1 and one at position 20. The Fourier transform (FT) representation efficiently tells us which frequency components were contained in the original (complex) waveform.

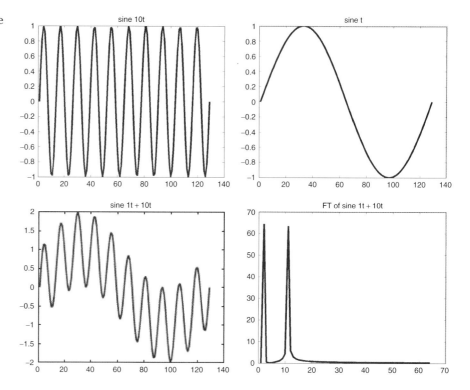

a significant step toward developing an understanding of how k-space relates the signal intensity (which is the flower picture) to a sum of sine and cosine waves (which is the MRI signal).

the flower signal (formally flower image) as a 2D signal distribution. But before this conceptual leap can be appreciated, let us consider a pseudo-historical event of long ago and far away.

## ONE-DIMENSIONAL VERSUS TWO-DIMENSIONAL

Thus far, all the Fourier illustrations have related to 1D, but not to 2D signals. Specifically, in the above-mentioned example of the flower, we extracted one line from the 2D flower image. We will now consider

## FOURIER "HISTORY"

Fourier was made a baron by Napoleon (true). As he roamed Europe, he came to the Swiss Alps, and found a village that he liked to visit (false). However, he wanted to know in advance of his arrival, which villagers were

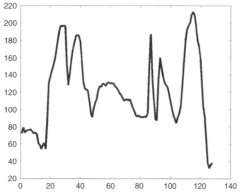
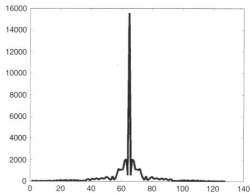

**FIGURE 34-5** A cross-section profile from the flower image is shown along with its corresponding Fourier representation. The Fourier representation shows us the amplitudes of the composite sine and cosine waves that go to make up the original image cross-section profile.

| A |
|---|
| B |
| C |
| D |
| E |
| F |

| A | A | A | A | A | A |
|---|---|---|---|---|---|
| B | B | B | B | B | B |
| C | C | C | C | C | C |
| D | D | D | D | D | D |
| E | E | E | E | E | E |
| F | F | F | F | F | F |

**FIGURE 34-6** Two hypothetical village layouts are shown. One is a simple, single street of houses, and one is a grid of houses, comprised of rows of parallel streets. As indicated in the single street layout, each house was issued with a bell of a specific frequency (e.g., A, B, C, etc.). Each of the rows of houses was issued with the same frequency bell, with the house at the top of each street having an A bell and so on. When only a single street of houses is present, a person with perfect pitch can identify each house that is occupied, by listening to the sound of the bells, even when all the bells are rung at the same time. However, in the more complex grid village, when all the bells are struck at the same time it is not possible to distinguish between houses along each row, because each row has the same frequency bell.

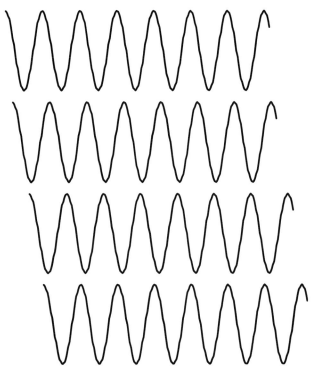

**FIGURE 34-7** Relating to the "grid village" of Fig. 34-6, it is possible to distinguish between rows of houses if the bells are rung with a progressive delay between rows. In this case, the beat pattern formed by the bells with the same frequency provide a person with perfect pitch sufficient data to identify which houses are occupied along each row. However, this occupancy information cannot be determined from a single ringing of the bells, and the bells have to be rung a number of times: the number of times being equal to the number of houses per row, and each time they are rung the delay between them being increased slightly.

in residence. With the villagers' permission, he issued unique bells to each household, and when he appeared on the mountain overlooking the village, they would ring their bells in unison. Using his perfect pitch, Fourier could tell who was at home, because it is possible to distinguish distinct frequencies, even when they are sounded simultaneously (see Fig. 34-6). This worked well as long as the village was essentially only a single street. However, as the village prospered, additional streets were added, such that upon Fourier's next visit it had grown to form a grid. However, bells further up or down the scale, either made them too large to handle, or too small for the sound to carry. Therefore, Fourier was presented with the problem of how to identify which houses were occupied when confined to a limited range of bells. To address this considerable problem he devised the following scheme: The first household of each street was issued with an "A" bell; the second household of each street was issued with a "B" bell, and so on. Fourier instructed the villagers to ring their bells, as many times as there were rows of streets, six in the example shown here (see Fig. 34-6). However, the twist was that each time they rang the bells, successive

streets would introduce a slight and progressive delay to their ringing. The slight delay in ringing the bells between streets introduced a "beat-pattern" (just like tuning a guitar string with a tuning fork) (see Fig. 34-7). In technical terms, the slight delay that was introduced to the bell ringing was equivalent to introducing a phase shift between each bell of the same note. Naturally, Fourier could distinguish these phase shifts using his perfect pitch. But because there were six streets, to uniquely identify the houses by row, he required six different phase shifts to be applied. Still, it was a solution to the problem. Therefore, Fourier solved a very tricky problem, armed with a limited set of bells; he was able to distinguish which houses were occupied in a 2D grid, by introducing a slight delay to cause a progressive beat pattern. Each time the bells were rung, the beat pattern would change due to the progressive time delay introduced and the dependency of the beat pattern on the details of house occupancy.

## APPLICATION TO MAGNETIC RESONANCE IMAGING

In MRI, we apply gradients to the body. These gradients cause spins to precess at unique frequencies. This gives us a signal that allows us to distinguish spins along the direction of the gradient. This would be sufficient if the body was a 1D object. The signal acquired in the presence of a linear magnetic gradient corresponds directly to a sum of sine and cosine waves, each sine wave possessing frequency and amplitude—the frequency being dependent on the position along the gradient and the amplitude being dependent on the number of spins present. In the same manner that Fourier only had so many bells, in MRI we can physically only apply one gradient at a time (e.g., the X gradient). In the direction orthogonal to the gradient, we have to differentiate successive lines by introducing a progressive phase difference (see Fig. 34-8). This is accomplished by successive applications of the phase gradient (e.g., the Y gradient). In this manner, the magnetic resonance (MR) signal comes to us *directly* as a series of sine and cosine waves. Therefore, to identify the intensity of the signal source (i.e., the body) in a 2D manner, we need to Fourier transform the MR signal.

Whereas Fourier did all this processing intuitively in his head (false), we require computers to perform the Fourier transforms (true).

## K-SPACE OF FLOWER PICTURE

Even if it is a flower picture, it still obeys the laws of k-space. Let us look at some of these features. To examine the very center of k-space, we will set all regions around it to zero, (see Fig. 34-9). When we Fourier transform this dramatically reduced k-space signal, it is observed to relate to very low-frequency image information. In other words, the image is dramatically blurred. From this, we can conclude that the center of k-space relates to low-resolution image features, that is, the center of k-space relates to broad contrast features. Now we look at a larger region, still centered on the center of k-space. After performing the Fourier transform, we see that the image formed resembles a low-resolution image. In other words, the regions of k-space close to the center relate to low frequency information in the image. Now, we consider only retaining the outer region of k-space. On performing the Fourier transform, we see that it relates

**FIGURE 34-8** The principle of accumulating k-space data is shown, with the final image formed by performing a Fourier transform (FT) on the k-space data. Here the X gradient corresponds to the different frequency bells in the grid village of Fig. 34-6, and the Y gradient (applied with a series of amplitudes) corresponds to the series of phase offsets achieved by the progressive time delays in ringing the bells.

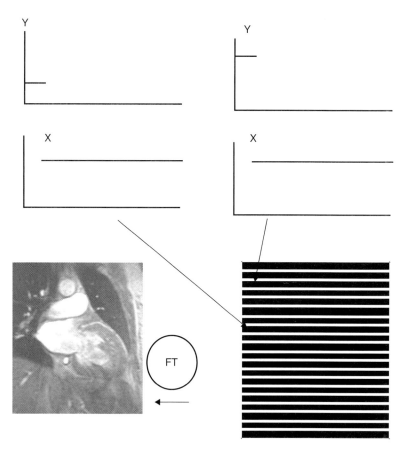

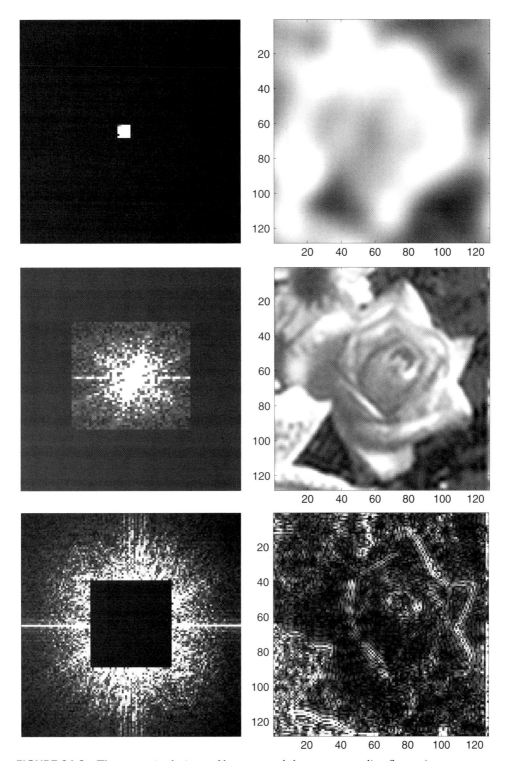

**FIGURE 34-9** Three manipulations of k-space and the corresponding flower image are shown. In the top panel, only the very center of k-space is allowed to contribute (the rest of the k-space data are set to zero). The corresponding flower image is a very blurred representation. In the middle panel, a wider region of k-space is allowed to contribute, and the corresponding flower image has sharper detail, although not as sharp as the original. The lower panel shows the result of only retaining the outer region of k-space (i.e., setting the central data to zero). In this case, only the sharp edge detail of the flower image is represented.

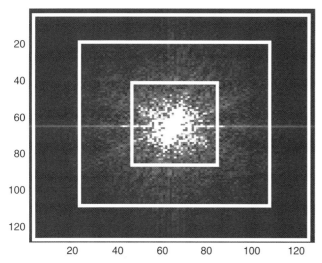

**FIGURE 34-10** Three regions of k-space are outlined. The central data represents low spatial resolution features (i.e., broad contrast), the mid region, represents features with sharper detail, and the outer region represents very high spatial frequency information, corresponding to the crisp edges in the image domain.

only to high-frequency information in the image, that is, edge information. The lesson that we can draw from this is that by sampling progressively larger regions of k-space, we represent first the broad image contrast, then finer details, and finally very fine detailed features (see Fig. 34-10).

## SUMMARY

In summary, we can appreciate that every image, picture, photography, and diagram is really a signal waveform. Signal waveforms can be represented in k-space. In the special case of MRI, gradients are used to encode data in the k-space format directly.

# CHAPTER 35

# Complete Protocol Example

Mark Doyle

## OUTLINE

For the fictitious "XYZ Trial", we will discuss how the required views and features of the cardiovascular magnetic resonance (CMR) protocol should be obtained. In the XYZ Trial, the main information to be obtained concerns cardiac function. We will point out some efficiency notes including features to be aware of and approaches to overcome some commonly encountered difficulties.

## GENERAL CARDIOVASCULAR MAGNETIC RESONANCE REQUIREMENTS AND CARDIAC VIEWS

In the XYZ Trial, CMR data are to be used to evaluate patients for entry into the trial. The CMR data requested may differ substantially from your normal diagnostic protocol, and special attention should be paid to the required elements of each scan. For study completeness, it is essential that views contain the correct landmark information. The fictitious XYZ Trial requires four data sets (see Fig. 35-1), along with blood pressure measurements:

- Long axis two-chamber cine
- Long axis four-chamber cine
- Multislice short axis cine series
- Phase contrast velocity scans of aortic outflow

Some details of the key scans to be obtained are outlined in the Table 35-1.

To obtain the key scans, additional planning scans are also required. Planning scans occupy time, as does the positioning of target scans. This overhead has to be accommodated when budgeting time to perform the protocol, as should activities such as patient preparation, establishing the electrocardiogram (ECG) signal, obtaining blood pressures, and transmission of data.

## PATIENT PREPARATION

After normal patient screening and precautions have been observed, position the patient on the scanner table (typically feet first). Connect ECG leads, respiratory gating device, and blood pressure cuff. The XYZ Trial protocol requires that blood pressure be monitored at the time of the CMR examination. Ideally, this information should be acquired at 2-minute intervals throughout the CMR examination. Manually record the end-systolic, end-diastolic, mean blood pressure and the time at which they were measured. Once the patient is positioned on the scanner table and a strong ECG signal is established, "center" on the midline of the chest, approximately 8 cm (3 in.) above the zyphoid notch.

## PLAN SCAN GUIDELINES

Plan all scans using the end-diastolic cardiac phase to ensure that the heart is seen in its maximally extended condition. Wherever possible, use ECG triggered scans to plan views. If a view does not contain the required features, consider repeating the scan and/or repeating the scout scan from which it was planned. If image quality is suboptimal, consider remedial action before proceeding. Note that ECG and respiratory-related issues are responsible for most quality issues and that problematic scans that are used for planning further views usually compound problems further into the study.

## SCAN PHILOSOPHY

Acquire scans in a progressive order such that planning of the next scan relies on the previously acquired scan. Do not proceed to the next step until you are satisfied

**FIGURE 35-1** The four key views to be obtained for the fictitious XYZ Trial are shown (top-left and clockwise): two-chamber cine, four-chamber cine, phase contrast cine, and short axis cine.

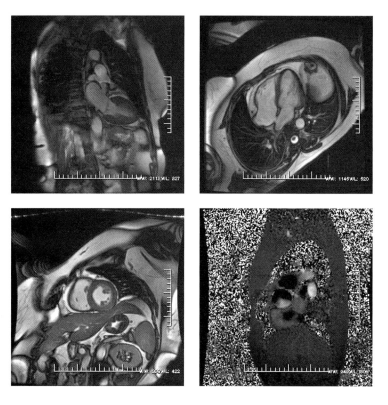

that the previous scan data has been adequately acquired.

## SCOUT IMAGING

Obtain a non–cardiac triggered scout image-set. A typical set consists of three sets of orthogonal scans:

- Seven slices transverse
- Seven slices sagittal
- Seven slices coronal

Non–ECG triggered scouts are generally of too low a quality to allow for detailed planning purposes. For this reason, acquire an ECG triggered set of scout images. Typical parameters are:

- 256 × 128 matrix

**TABLE 35-1**

Key scan details

| Scan | Type | No. of slices | Plan time | Scan time/scan wait |
|------|------|------|------|------|
| Two chamber | Cine | 3 | 4 | 15 s/20 s × 3 |
| Four chamber | Cine | 3 | 1 | 15 s/20 s × 3 |
| Short axis | Cine | ~15 | 1 | 15 s/20 s × 15 |
| Velocity | Cine | 1 | 3 | 4 min |

- Gradient echo, repetition time (TR)/echo time (TE)/ flip 10/3/20
- Steady state free precession (SSFP) sequence, TR/TE/ flip 4/2/60

Plan a set of approximately eight transverse slices centered through the heart from a coronal scan. Perform the scans under breath-hold conditions, or conditions similar to those to be used for the cine images to be obtained later.

## BREATH-HOLDING GUIDELINES

During breath-holding, it is important to note that the heart may be in a different position compared to normal breathing. When planning breath-hold scans, more reproducible results are achieved when planning them using scans obtained under the same breath-hold strategy. For consistency in breath-hold position and to maximize compliance, the following instructions may be given to the patient after all "prep" scan procedures are complete and the scan is ready to proceed:

- "Take a deep breath in"
- "Leave it out half way"
- "Do not breathe" (start scan)

Upon scan completion, instruct patient to breathe. If a patient experiences difficulty in performing breath-holding, consider administering oxygen:

- 2 L per minute
- Titrating O$_2$ saturation up to 90%

## CARDIOVASCULAR MAGNETIC RESONANCE CINE FEATURES

All of the key scans to be obtained are cines, that is, cardiac triggered, showing movie information throughout the cardiac cycle. Exact details of performing cine scans will typically vary from site to site. In the XYZ Trial, general guidelines are given describing details of the cine imaging technique. All cine scans should be cardiac triggered. If possible, perform cine scanning using a breath-hold method. If breath-holding is not feasible, use respiratory compensation and/or respiratory gating/triggering. The SSFP sequence should be used to obtain all cine scans. Common acronyms for the SSFP sequence are as follows:

- True fast imaging with steady precession (FISP)
- Fast imaging employing steady-state acquisition (FIESTA)
- Balanced fast field echo (FFE)

The cine sequences should be acquired with a field of view (FOV) set to avoid signal fold over. Typical parameters are as follows:

- FOV 30 cm × 30 cm
- Matrix 224 × 224
- Slice thickness 8 mm
- Slice gap 0 mm
- Views per segment 16
- Cardiac phases 20 (alternatively, cardiac phase interval 35 milliseconds)

## PLAN TWO-CHAMBER VIEW

Using the triggered transverse scout sets, select the slice in which the left ventricle (LV) is seen in its largest view (see Fig. 35-2). Plan three slices with zero gap between them and with the central slice passing through the apex and base of the LV. The slice is typically positioned to be parallel to septum. After following these guidelines, the central slice acquired should be the desired two-chamber view. Commonly although one of the slices on either side may be the required view. Review all three slices to decide which is the best two-chamber view. Important points to note in the two-chamber view are that the left atria are seen throughout cardiac cycle and the apex of LV seen clearly. Features to avoid are the LV obscured by the septal wall and obtaining a truncated view of the atria (see Fig. 35-3).

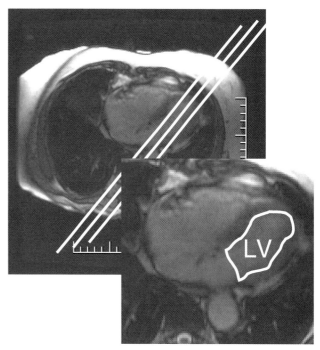

**FIGURE 35-2** The plan scan to obtain a two-chamber view form a transverse scout. There are three slices planned through the left ventricle (LV) that are parallel to the septum (shown in the insert). Ideally, the center slice should be the required two-chamber view, but normal variation and nonreproducibility in breath-hold position may result in one of the outer slices producing a better two-chamber view.

## PLAN FOUR-CHAMBER VIEW

From the two-chamber view, plan the four-chamber view (see Fig. 35-4), with three slices planned under the expectation that the central slice will be the required view, conforming to the following conditions:

- Image plane passes through LV apex
- Image plane bisects the valve plane at the base

Ideally, the central slice acquired should be the desired four-chamber view. Commonly although one of the slices on either side may be the required view, review all three slices to decide which is the best four-chamber view. Important points to note in four-chamber view are as follows:

- Left and right atria seen throughout cardiac cycle
- Apex of LV and right ventricle (RV) seen clearly
- Ideally, the RV and LV apex should come to one point

## SHORT AXIS IMAGING

Short axis images are to be obtained in a series of parallel slices oriented perpendicular to the septum.

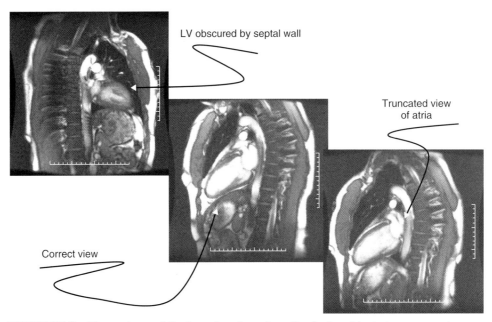

**FIGURE 35-3** Three views of the two-chamber view, the first and last views are not acceptable because of being obscured by the septal wall or truncation of the atria, respectively. The middle view is acceptable because it shows the left ventricular and atrial cavities in full cross-section.

The gap between slices should be set to zero. Using the end diastolic 4-chamber view, plan short axis slices to extend beyond the valve plane (see Fig. 35-5). To ensure that the heart is fully imaged, it is important that the most apical slice does not contain any myocardium. The most basal slice should be positioned to be above the level of the mitral valve plane at end-diastole (see Fig. 35-6). These precautions ensure that the whole heart has been imaged. If the short axis scans are completed and the apex is seen in the last slice, *the whole scan set may have to be repeated.* To avoid this happening, if your scanner permits, plan approximately four more apical slices than you anticipate needing. Then, when starting at the most basal slice, proceed to scan through the apex. When no myocardium is seen in any frame near the apex, terminate the scan, assuming that the data acquired already is not lost by this action.

## AORTIC VELOCITY CINE IMAGING

The final required image set is a phase velocity encoded cine series of the ascending aorta (AA). The scan can be planned from a sagittal view. The cine scan requires setting velocity encoding parameters:

- Velocity encoding direction set to through-plane
- Velocity sensitivity set to ±1 m per second (100 cm per second)
- Set phase method to "difference" or "quantitative" (manufacturer dependent).

**FIGURE 35-4** The plan scan (left panel) and four-chamber view (right panel) are shown. As for the two-chamber view, three views are planned on a two-chamber view. The middle slice should be the ideal one, because it bisects the apex and the valvular plane. The features to observe in the four-chamber view are common apex of left and right ventricles, and full cross-sectional views of the atria. RV, right ventricle; LV, left ventricle, RA, right atrium; LA, left atrium.

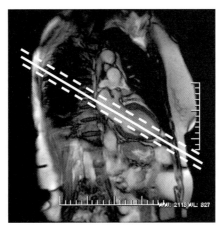
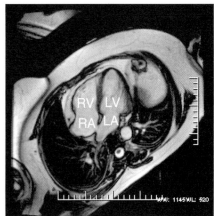

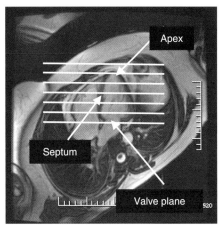

**FIGURE 35-5** The plan scan setup for the short axis view is shown. The slices are planned from a four-chamber view in the end-diastolic phase, parallel to the base and perpendicular to the septum. Note that slices are planned starting above the base and extending below the apex.

The scan may take several minutes to perform and cannot typically be performed during a breath-hold. If available, use respiratory compensation or respiratory gating. If respiratory gating is not available, obtain multiple averages (e.g., 2 number of excitations [NEXs]). Plan the aortic cross-section view from a sagittal scout. Obtain a gated sagittal scout planned off a transverse scout scan that best identifies the LV and descending aorta (DA). Plan up to eight sagittal slices centered

slightly to the right of the patient's DA and obtain a triggered gradient echo series. Of the sagittal scouts, one plane should contain the AA and pulmonary artery (PA) in a single view. Using this view, either draw or imagine, a line originating at the aortic valve and following the initial direction of blood flow (see Fig. 35-7). The scan plane is positioned to cut this line at right angles and also bisect the circular PA. The aim of this is to see the aorta in circular cross-section (see Fig. 35-8). Perform the velocity cine scan using respiratory gating/triggering as discussed earlier. Two data sets are generated:

- Magnitude images
- Phase/velocity images

Since this will typically be the last examination performed, examine the data before study termination. The most common problem will be "aliasing" seen in the phase images. Aliasing is caused by the velocity encoding limits being set too low. If this occurs, repeat the scan with the velocity limit increased, say, by 50%.

## TIPS AND EFFICIENCY NOTES

Spend time up-front to obtain a good ECG signal. If the signal is weak or otherwise poor take remedial action:

- Shave off hair.
- Abrade the skin.

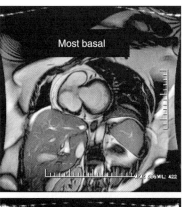
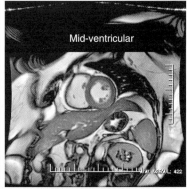
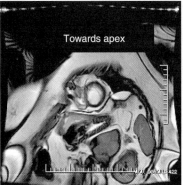
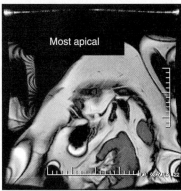

**FIGURE 35-6** Four representative short axis cine views are shown, the first being the most basal, clearly positioned above the valve plane, and the last slice clearly positioned below the apex of the heart, because no myocardial features are visible in this slice. The remaining slices are thereby guaranteed to span the full extent of the left ventricle (LV).

**FIGURE 35-7** A sagittal scout scan, in which the ascending aorta (AA) and pulmonary artery (PA) are seen, is used to plan the scan through the AA. The planed view bisects the PA and is perpendicular to the line defining the major axis of the AA, as indicated in the second panel.

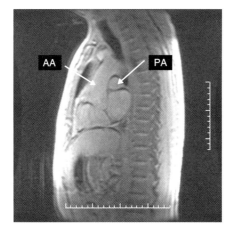
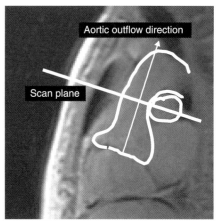

**FIGURE 35-8** Representative frames from the phase contrast cine scan through the ascending aorta. The moving blood shows up as bright and dark features against the mid-level gray of static tissue.

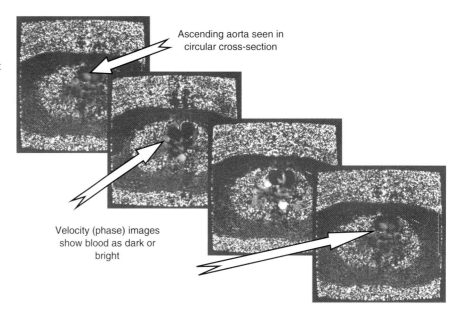

Ascending aorta seen in circular cross-section

Velocity (phase) images show blood as dark or bright

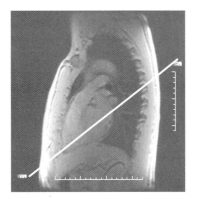
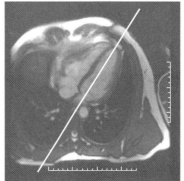
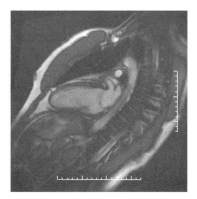

**FIGURE 35-9** An alternate means to obtain the two-chamber view is shown. The first frame shows a sagittal scout in which the view is planned to pass through the LV apex and bisect the base. The resulting view resembles a four-chamber view (middle panel), and using this plane, the two-chamber view is planned using a slice that passes through the apex and that bisects the base. The resulting view should be a two-chamber view (last panel).

- Change the reference lead.
- Reposition the leads.

For scans performed under breath-hold conditions, if the patient cannot sustain the breath-hold consider the following actions:

- Reduce the scan time by increasing the "views per segment" or "looks" or "turbo factor" for cardiac triggered scans.
- Allow more time between breath-holds.
- Induce a state of mild hyperventilation by rapidly having the patient breath in and out before suddenly holding the breath.
- Decrease the scan matrix in the phase encoding direction.
- Use a partial matrix (e.g., NEX. 75).

After obtaining the four-chamber view consider planning a second two-chamber view. Generally this "double oblique" two-chamber view is better than the original "single oblique" view. Plan a view from a sagittal scout, through LV apex and left atria (see Fig. 35-9). The view obtained is similar to the four-chamber view. Plan the two-chamber view by bisecting the base and apex from this four-chamber view.

As the XYZ Trial progresses, it is likely that scanner performance will improve. Always use the current "best practice" methodology to obtain the required cardiac views. If a patient has a bad study, consider rescheduling (possibly later the same day). Review data, with special attention to key features before the patient leaves the scanner. Usually the Trial sponsor will provide example images. Observe these and note key features that must be included to obtain valid data. Remember, omission of one key data set or feature may invalidate the whole data set!

## SUMMARY

Strive for the highest image quality.

- Ensure good patient compliance
- Ensure that correct views are obtained
- Ensure that each image has required features
- Employ current "best practice" to obtain cine images
- Repeat scans if necessary for highest quality
- Note blood pressures throughout scan

# CHAPTER 36

# Artifacts

Mark Doyle

## OVERVIEW

Successful identification of artifacts is crucial to allow correct interpretation of image features. Because image formation is dependent on numerous acquisition and patient features, there are consequently multiple manifestations of image artifacts. Major sources include the following:

- Motion
- Blood flow
- Susceptibility
- Fat and water resonance differences
- Incorrect imaging parameters

## MOTION

To encode each k-space line requires application of two separate gradients:

- Frequency encoding (X)
- Phase encoding (Y)

The imaging gradients relate the frequency of spins at each location to position within the image. When the signal is sampled, the main feature of the spins that determines their position in the image is how the signal phase progresses throughout the two-dimensional (2D) k-space domain. K-space has the property that motion of an object is efficiently represented as a change of phase in the k-space signal. For instance, the k-space representation of a ball bouncing around the magnetic resonance imaging (MRI) scanner visually looks the same for each position of the ball (see Fig. 36-1). For each frame, the phase of the k-space signal is different. To appreciate the origin of this, consider a spin moving along a magnetic field gradient: it experiences a progressively increasing precessional frequency as it moves into a progressively increasing magnetic field. In this way, a moving spin will accumulate phase at a different rate compared to a static spin. Therefore, following a gradient echo operation, a moving spin will accumulate a net phase that is due in part to its position and its motion. However, because phase information is used in k-space to encode position, it follows that moving spins will appear at irregular positions within the image and that these positions do not merely reflect the new position that they moved to. Spin motion results in artifacts because the Fourier transform does not have enough information to correctly assign the spins to one position within the image. The type of motion that takes place determines the form of the motion artifact:

- Cyclic motion—cyclic repeating artifact
- Irregular motion—random, dispersed signal artifact
- Slow motion—confined, localized blurring of object

### Breathing Artifact

When performing rapid imaging, the motion of the diaphragm can be appreciated because the diaphragm moves approximately 5 cm during regular breathing. The cyclic respiratory motion is typically regular and this property usually causes respiratory artifacts to reinforce as regions of displaced signal within the image (see Fig. 36-2). Not surprisingly, moving features such as internal organs and the chest wall generate signals that propagate throughout the image. Their regular motion tends to make these moving features appear as if they were in two positions on average and produce a displaced "ghost image." In images acquired under free breathing conditions, a strong respiratory motion artifact is typically seen as a "ghost," that is, a displaced image chest wall and lung cavity. Other, possibly fainter, features are typically present also. Scout images are widely regarded as "throw away images," and are usually acquired under free breathing and possibly noncardiac triggered conditions. Naturally, unless some form of respiratory compensation is used, these images

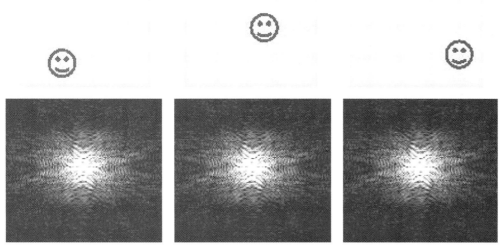

**FIGURE 36-1** The top panel shows a ball bouncing around inside the magnetic resonance imaging (MRI) scanner, three snapshots are shown. The corresponding k-space maps are shown below the images. Visually, there is nothing to distinguish one k-space map from another. This illustrates that motion of a real object (i.e., the ball) is represented in the phase of the k-space signal. To visualize phase, as opposed to magnitude, requires additional image processing.

will be of lower quality, have less distinct boundaries, and be contaminated by artifact. Commonly, breath-hold imaging is employed to reduce or eliminate respiratory artifacts. Table 36-1 summarizes some features that differentiate images acquired under breath-hold and free breathing conditions.

## Respiratory Gating

An alternative to breath-holding is to employ respiratory gating. Respiratory gating requires some means of monitoring the diaphragm position within the respiratory cycle and adjusting the scan acquisition accordingly. Strategies of adjusting data acquisition include the following:

- Not acquiring data during periods of high motion
- Tracking the mobile feature and applying real-time adjustment of the imaging slice
- Acquiring regions of k-space that have higher or lower sensitivity to motion in a manner that is dependent on the details of motion

## Pulsatile Blood Flow

A noncardiac triggered scan tends to represent pulsatile blood vessels as regularly repeating patterns. This form of artifact is especially problematic for time of flight (TOF) 2D angiographic imaging, because the frequency of the pulsatile blood flow is highly organized relative

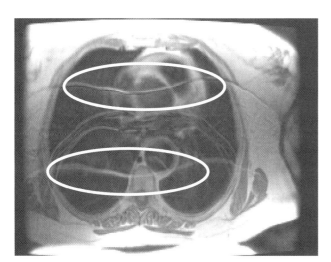

**FIGURE 36-2** This image was acquired under free breathing conditions and displays common breathing artifacts. Coherent ghost images of the chest wall are seen repeating through the image (*circled*).

**TABLE 36-1**

Features of Images Acquired Under Breath-Hold and Free Breathing Conditions

| Breath-Hold | Free Breathing |
| --- | --- |
| Sharp clear edges | Blurred features |
| Vessels look clear and free of anomalies | Vessels look as if dissected |
| Motion is smooth and continuous | Motion is choppy and sudden |

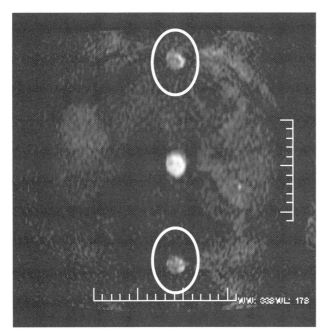

**FIGURE 36-3** Pulsatile flow artifacts are shown (*circled*). This image was taken as part of a time of flight scan. The scan time was rapid relative to the pulsatile blood cycle, and hence the spacing of the ghost images of the vessel are seen relatively widely spaced.

to the acquisition and imposes a definite pattern in the phase information over successive k-space lines. The repeating ghost vessels tend to be very prominent (see Fig. 36-3).

## Direction of Motion Artifact

Motion artifact exhibits a preferential direction within the image and occurs in the phase encoding direction. Consider that the measurement gradient is applied for only a short time duration relative to most motion features whereas the phase encoding gradient is applied at multiple times throughout the motion cycle. Therefore, the phase encoding process is more highly disrupted by motion. For this reason, motion artifacts predominantly occur as displacements along the direction of the phase encoding gradient (see Fig. 36-4).

## Rapid Scout Imaging

There are three features that are problematic when using nontriggered, non–breath-hold scout images:

- Respiratory artifact
- Cardiac motion artifact
- Incorrect position for planning future breath-hold images

Apart from the more obvious disruption of image features resulting from respiratory and cardiac motion

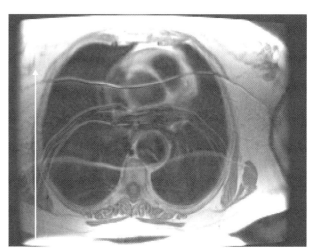

**FIGURE 36-4** The direction of the ghost artifacts takes place in the direction of phase encoding gradient (*arrow*). The phase encoding process is highly disrupted due to the relatively long intervals between application of each phase encoding gradient, during which time, the body has moved to a new configuration.

artifacts, which can often be "read through," the feature that is possibly the most disruptive occurs when using the image to plan another view. Typically, the planned view will be acquired under breath-hold conditions. In this case, there is a strong possibility that the planned view will be misaligned due to the difference in mean position of imaged features.

## FLOW

Flow is a special type of motion that has many unique features due to the fluid properties of blood. Under normal physiologic conditions, flow within the body is laminar, and no turbulence is present. However, many disease states result in formation of flow jets, which have their own special considerations. The presence of jet flow is indicative of pathology.

### Jet Flow

Jet flow is often associated with high velocities, and more importantly high-velocity gradients. The velocity gradient causes spin dephasing within a voxel. Often this spin dephasing is so severe that signal loss results. Turbulent flow also results in spin dephasing, which in turn results in signal loss. Jet flow signal loss is technically an artifact, although it is a useful clinical sign of pathology. In gradient echo imaging, signal appearance is dominated by the TOF effect, which generally makes flowing blood appear bright. However, in the region beyond a vascular stenosis, there may be a region of signal loss associated with a combination of features including jet flow, high flow gradients, and turbulence. This extended region of signal loss, occurring beyond the site of stenoses, can be erroneously interpreted as an extended stenotic region. Therefore, the extent and severity of vascular plaque can be overestimated when looking for regions of low or zero signals in flow sensitive images.

## Flow Signal Loss

In TOF angiographic images, signal loss may occur in vessel segments that lie predominantly in an in-plane orientation due to the slow passage of blood through the slice. Also, because 2D TOF images are acquired as a series of individual slices, it is possible that slice misregistration artifacts can occur within the series. These are sometimes more apparent in rotation views of the vasculature, and appear as sudden discontinuities.

## Phase Velocity Imaging

In phase velocity imaging, if the velocity exceeds the velocity sensitivity that was set, aliasing will occur. Aliasing is distinguishable from normal flow by the sudden appearance of white on black or black on white signal. Aliasing is caused when the velocity encoding limits are set too low. Unless there is access to sophisticated unaliasing software, the only solution is to repeat the scan with the velocity limit increased, say, by 50%. However, if a flow pattern gradually transitions from black to white (or *vice versa*) this is probably not aliasing, but represents a complex flow pattern involving bidirectional flow.

## SUSCEPTIBILITY ARTIFACTS

A magnetic field passing through a material with a uniform consistency is affected by that material in a manner that is dependent on its magnetic susceptibility, $\chi$. Whenever a boundary is encountered between materials with a distinctly different susceptibility, the magnetic flux lines become distorted (see Fig. 36-5). Metals have a very high susceptibility, and consequently flux lines are strongly attracted to metals. As the name implies, susceptibility expresses the affinity that a material has for magnetic flux. A high susceptibility material diverts flux lines from surrounding tissue into and through the high susceptibility material. Because flux lines cannot be broken and because they are continuous they are observed to bend toward the high susceptibility material. Consequently, if a high susceptibility material diverts flux lines, then it necessarily sets up complex magnetic gradients in the surrounding tissue. The gradients thereby formed can be so severe that the spin

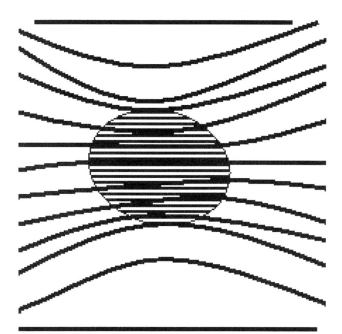

**FIGURE 36-5** When a material such as a metal is placed in a uniform magnetic field, lines of magnetic flux bend in space to preferentially pass through the metal. This bending of flux lines results in the susceptibility artifact. The static magnetic gradient caused by the material is responsible for rapidly dephasing the spin signal in the surrounding body.

signal is rapidly dephased, and therefore shows up as a signal void on images. Susceptibility artifacts are often observed in features such as sternal wires, which cause a relatively large signal void compared to the diameter of wire (see Fig. 36-6). Vascular stents can result in susceptibility artifacts that can mimic a high-grade stenosis. Stent material is designed to have a low susceptibility:

- Nitinol
- Nickel
- Titanium

Even stents that are made of low susceptibility material can "shield" the vessel from the radiofrequency (RF) signal, preventing the RF pulse fully penetrating the stent, and thereby contributing a low signal. Coronary stents are particularly problematic for myocardial perfusion imaging. Their presence has to be noted, and their effect on perfusion carefully interpreted. Another special consideration for myocardial perfusion imaging is the susceptibility artifact set up by the gadolinium contrast agent. Gadolinium in high concentration can cause a susceptibility signal void. To distinguish this from a signal void associated with low perfusion, one must evaluate the homogeneity and the timing with which the myocardium enhances as the paramagnetic agent enters the myocardium. Typically, as the gadolinium passes through the right ventricle, it may set up a

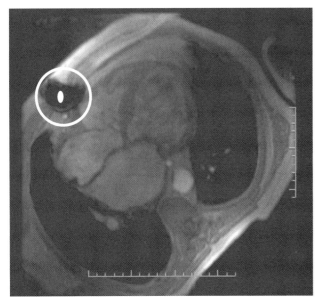

**FIGURE 36-6** A large susceptibility artifact (*circle*) was caused by the relatively small cross section sternal wire (*dot*).

susceptibility gradient that causes signal dropout in the septum in patients without significant coronary artery disease. Accordingly, if this territory is the only one with a "defect" one should not necessarily assume abnormal perfusion, but rather suspect an artifact of the MR method. Susceptibility artifacts depend on several features:

- Shape and orientation
  - A sphere is the worst shape
- Material
  - Each material has a susceptibility rating, $\chi$
  - Metals have a high susceptibility
- Field strength
  - Higher fields have bigger effects
  - Higher density of flux lines

## FAT EFFECTS

Fat and water each contribute a strong signal in the proton resonance. The fat resonance frequency is separated from water by 1.5 parts per million (ppm). At 1.5 T, this evaluates to 224 Hz (64 MHz $\times$ 1.5 $\times$ $10^{-6}$). Note that in encoding k-space, the measurement gradient is applied for several milliseconds. During this time fat accumulates additional phase relative to water (due to the increased resonance frequency). Because the imaging gradients relate the frequency of spins to position within the image, fat features are consequently displaced relative to water features. The direction along which the fat–water displacement occurs in is parallel to the measurement gradient. The fat–water shift artifact is often called the *chemical shift artifact*. For most conventional

imaging sequences, this manifests as a thin bright line when fat shifts onto a water region or a dark line when fat signal shifts away from a water region. However for imaging sequences with long signal readout periods, such as spiral and echo planar imaging, the fat–water shift can be several pixels in distance; consequently, these techniques commonly employ fat suppression techniques.

## IMAGING PARAMETERS

Sometimes, the imaging parameters that we choose generate the artifact, or alternatively, the scanner, may incorrectly set a parameter. The latter error often occurs during the "prescan" adjustments that the scanner goes through before acquisition of each image series commences.

### Gibbs Ringing

Ideally, the amplitude of the sampled k-space region should gradually (asymptotically) approach zero toward the edge of k-space, that is, the signal should blend into the noise background. If this condition is met, k-space is described as, mathematically speaking, a well-behaved function. However, if we only sample k-space up to a boundary where it still has appreciable signal, then there is a sudden termination of high signal at the edges of k-space. This is particularly the case for low-resolution imaging, where this sudden termination of signal leads to "Gibbs ringing," that is, lines of repeating edges in images (see Fig. 36-7). In low-resolution cardiac images, Gibbs ringing is typically seen as a repetition of sharp, high contrast features, such as the ventricular free wall and the left ventricular (LV) septum. In high-resolution cardiac images, Gibbs ringing is almost completely absent at normal intensities. Gibbs ringing is most prominent for regions of sharp contrast.

### Steady State Free Precession Resonance

In steady state free precession (SSFP) imaging a steady state is established, requiring exacting control of the signal phase. Consequently, the SSFP sequence is highly sensitive to setting the correct resonance frequency, which is typically carried out before initiating each scan series, that is, it is set during the prescan. However, because of inhomogeneities in the magnetic field there are typically some regions of the body which are at off resonance frequencies. The SSFP resonance from these regions manifests as a region of low signal, typically forming a band or stripe (see Fig. 36-8). This off-resonance artifact can be corrected by restarting the scan with an altered resonance frequency (possibly adjusting it manually). However, unless the magnetic field homogeneity is not corrected, this procedure only

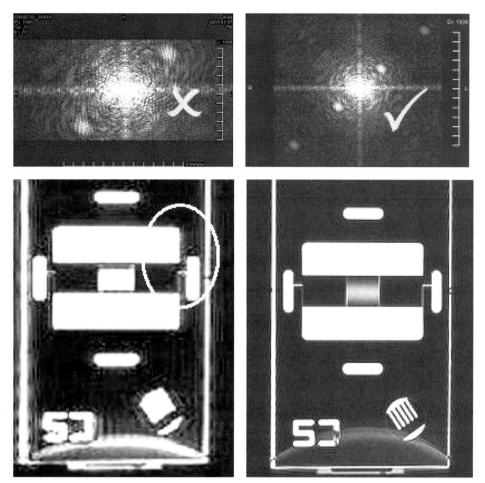

**FIGURE 36-7** Examples of Gibbs ringing are shown. The upper panel shows two examples of k-space coverage; the *cross* indicates the example where k-space is not well sampled because the signal has high intensity right up to the edge of k-space. The example with a *check mark* indicates that k-space was adequately sampled, because the signal mostly blends into the noise level at the edges of the region. The corresponding images are shown in the lower panel: in the left panel, Gibbs ringing is very apparent (*circled*) emanating from high contrast edges; in the right panel, little evidence of Gibbs ringing is seen, although even here it is not absent.

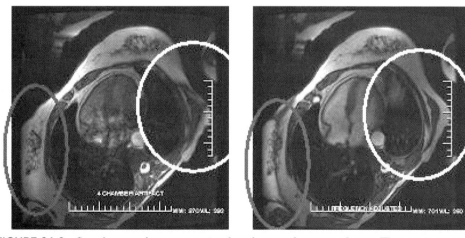

**FIGURE 36-8** Steady state free precession banding artifacts are shown. These two images were each taken with the resonance frequency adjusted by a few tens of Hertz between each acquisition. Corresponding regions are *circled*, to show either the presence or absence of the off-resonance banding artifact in each image. It can be appreciated that the artifact has merely changed location between each image.

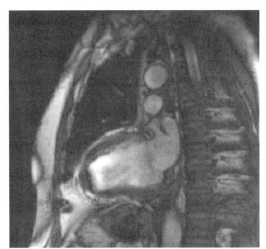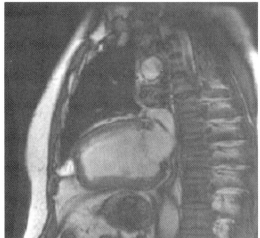

**FIGURE 36-9** Example of steady state free precession (SSFP) off-resonance artifact due to the presence of thrombus. Thrombus is seen in the apex of the ventricle in this two-chamber long axis view. In the left panel, the thrombus extent is overestimated. After adjusting the resonance frequency and repeating the image acquisition, the extent of the thrombus can be better appreciated in the right panel.

results in shifting the banding artifact from one region to another. If the signal-banding artifact falls over a region with flow, then an obtrusive and large flow artifact often is seen. Note, as is common to motion-related artifacts, the flow artifact occurs in the direction of the phase encoding gradient. It can be appreciated that in general there is no one correct frequency, and if the artifact is obtrusive, adjustments to resonance frequency and homogeneity have to be made, largely on a trial-and-error basis (see Fig. 36-8). Regions of thrombus are particularly problematic to off-resonance artifacts. Thrombus, due to susceptibility differences, naturally causes localized field inhomogeneities, which result in off-resonance artifacts in SSFP images (see Fig. 36-9).

## SUMMARY

Awareness of the various sources of signal artifact can help avoid misinterpretation, which can lead to over calling or misdiagnosing disease. Major sources of artifact include the following:

- Motion
- Susceptibility
- Fat and water resonances
- Incorrect imaging parameters

Although improvements in scanner performance and specifications are continually being made, it is unlikely that artifacts will completely be eliminated from the system, and indeed, as increasingly sophisticated sequences are introduced, they may bring with them increased sources of artifact. As a general rule, if an incorrect assumption is made concerning prevailing conditions, then artifacts will result.

# CHAPTER 37

# Patient Safety in Cardiovascular Magnetic Resonance Imaging

Mark Doyle

Safety, as with any diagnostic medical technique, is a critical issue, and safety procedures and rules should, at a minimum, be familiar to the physicians responsible for the scan and to the technician performing the scan. Major sources of safety concern are as follows:

- The potential of the magnetic field to move or dislodge an object or device
- The possibility that the radiofrequency (RF) field will heat a conductor such as a pacemaker electrode
- The potential for inducing electric currents in a conductor, again such as a pacing electrode
- The misinterpretation of artifacts that can confound diagnoses

## PACEMAKERS

The most common implanted devices that generally excludes the patient from having a magnetic resonance imaging (MRI) study are:

- Pacemakers
  - Permanent
  - Temporary
- Automated implantable cardiovascular defibrillators
- At least six deaths have occurred in patients with pacemakers, thought to be related to an MRI procedure

However, exclusion of patients with pacemakers is not absolutely prohibited, and a careful risk–benefit analysis should be performed before allowing a patient with a pacemaker into the scanner. First, the patient should not be pacemaker dependant, the pacemaker should be put into the synchronous mode, and sequences with low specific absorption rate (SAR) should be used. As a precaution, allow extra time between individual scans to permit heat that might be generated to dissipate.

## PROSTHETIC HEART VALVES

Prosthetic heart valves are generally magnetic resonance (MR) compatible. A possible exception is the pre-6,000 series Starr-Edwards valve (a caged ball device used clinically several decades ago). To our knowledge there has never been a report of an untoward incident involving a heart valve prosthesis.

## NONHAZARDOUS IMPLANTS

Nonhazardous implants include the following (when designated as MR compatible):

- Sternal wires
- Bypass graft clips
- Properly installed intravascular coils
- Stents
- Filters

However, all of these may result in an MR signal artifact.

## HAZARDOUS IMPLANTS

Hazardous implants include the following:

- Intracranial aneurysm clips
- Ocular prostheses
- Cochlear prostheses
- Penile prostheses

## EXTRANEOUS METAL DEVICES AND OBJECTS

Technicians, especially, must also be aware of the potential danger associated with metallic devices that may accompany the patient, including the following:

- Wheelchairs
- IV poles

- Oxygen tanks
- Iron shot filled hemostatic "sandbags"
- Pens
- Beepers
- Cell phones
- Hairpins (bobby pins)
- Shoes
- Badge tags

These, and other devices, may become dangerous projectiles in the vicinity of an MR system (see Fig. 37-1). The most dangerous time is when the patient is in the scanner bore and another person is in the room. It is imperative that all extraneous objects (that could contain metal) be removed from personnel entering the scanner room. It is important to note that just because something is marked "MR compatible" it does not mean that it truly is.

- It may have been refurbished with noncompatible parts.

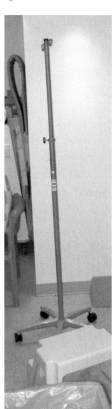 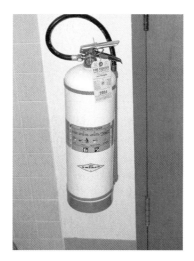 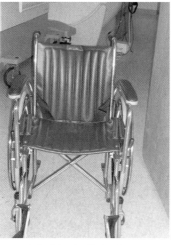

**FIGURE 37-1** Extraneous metal objects that, at some time, may find their way into the scanner room should be magnetic resonance imaging (MRI) compatible and clearly labeled as such.

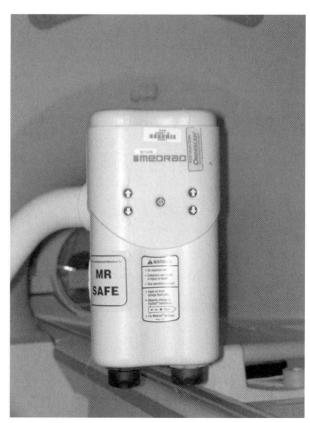

**FIGURE 37-2** Power injectors are required to administer contrast agent and saline flush, and should be of a special design to make them magnetic resonance (MR) safe. As always, a safety label should be prominently placed on all apparatus allowed in the scanner room.

- It may have been mislabeled.
- It may be attached to something which is not MR safe.

It is advised to test everything that claims to be MR safe yourself when no one is in the magnet, and beware of changes and updates made to these objects (see Fig. 37-2).

## RESOURCE

A useful resource is the web site that lists current devices and their degree of MR compatibility:

- http://www.MRIsafety.com/

The list is constantly being updated.

## STATIC MAGNETIC FIELD ZONES

It has been proposed that the following three zones be established around the scanner:

- Public access restricted by reception area
- Patient and care workers restricted to outside of the 5-G line

- The scanner area restricted by locked doors (preferably key controlled)
- Access to the scanner room controlled by the scanning technician and/or physician

We advocate the use of metal detectors placed in the path to the scanner. These give an audible warning, which gives the technician extra time to react to an intruder. Further, it may alert the intruder to the potential for danger and they may stop on their own accord.

## GRADIENT FIELDS

The rapidly changing magnetic gradients that are required for imaging produce a rate of change of magnetic field (dB/dt), which can induce strong currents in conducting objects that may result in burn injury, including the following:

- Wires
- Electrocardiogram (ECG) cables

The combination of strength and speed of switching gradients is summarized in the slew rate parameter (see Fig. 37-3). Slew rate incorporates the gradient strength and time of switching the gradient. It is measured in milli Tesla per meter per millisecond. Over time the slew rate available in commercial systems has increased exponentially. However, there is a physiologic limit of slew rate imposed because of neuromuscular stimulation. A slew rate of approximately 200 mT/m/milliseconds causes significant neuromuscular stimulation whereby a voltage is induced in the body that can result in muscular twitching. The strong dB/dt associated with gradients depends on the following three factors:

- Switching speed (~200 μs)
- Gradient strength (~40 mT per m, 400 G per cm)

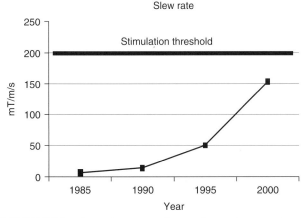

FIGURE 37-3    Over the years, the gradient slew rate has exponentially increased in commercial scanners. There is a physiologic threshold at approximately 200 mT/m/second above which patients may experience muscular twitching.

- Distance over which the gradient is applied (gradient is dB/dx)

For this reason, peripheral regions of the body are exposed to higher rates of change of gradient per unit time compared to more central regions.

## RADIOFREQUENCY FIELDS

RF fields can induce electrical currents to flow and may thereby heat up a conductor, resulting in burn injury. An RF circuit can be established in two ways:

- Loop paths
- Resonant standing waves

### Radiofrequency Loops

Larger loop paths have increased danger of causing RF heating. This is due to the greater amount of flux lines passing through the loop. External devices that may form loops include the following:

- Pulse oximetry cables
- ECG cables

MR-compatible cables, that is, those designed to reduce the incidence of heating or induced currents are

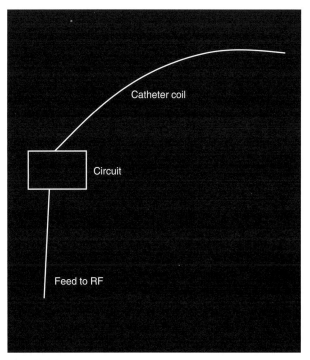

FIGURE 37-4    If a catheter is to be used or left in place during a magnetic resonance imaging (MRI) scan it should have circuitry attached to "detune" it and prevent it resonating with the scanner. If it did resonate, it could heat up to the point where it would melt and cause internal injury to the patient. RF, radiofrequency.

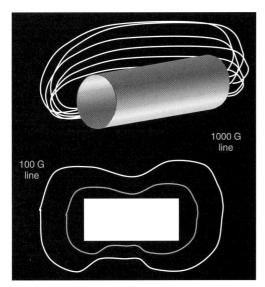

**FIGURE 37-5**  Lines of magnetic flux are represented threading through the scanner system. Below are shown the 1,000 Gauss and 100 Gauss lines. Note that as the scanner is approached, the magnetic field increases rapidly, and carries the danger that a metallic object may be accelerated into the scanner before the individual has time to react.

available and must be used in an MR facility. All non–MRI compatible metal cables and detection devices must be removed from the patient before entering the scanner. Even in the absence of extraneous devices, RF burns have been reported by loops forming between contact

**FIGURE 37-6**  The falloff of magnetic field strength with distance from the scanner is represented in the top figure, and in the lower figures an even steeper curve describes the rate of change of field with distance from the scanner. The rate of change of field ultimately determines the attractive force experienced by an object. Therefore, as the magnet is approached, the attractive forces increase rapidly.

between the hand and the leg. To minimize the danger of formation of this type of RF loop it is advisable to avoid skin-to-skin contact by careful placement of arms or inserting a cloth between the hand and other body regions.

## Radiofrequency Standing Waves

Any conductor that approaches the dimensions of the RF wavelength presents a danger to formation of standing waves:

- Frequency = 1/wavelength

Catheters are close to one fourth the wavelength of RF in use in clinical systems and have been reported to have melted in the scanner. To prevent catheters from heating up the patient, special circuitry is introduced to electrically detune the catheter such that it no longer resonates in the system (see Fig. 37-4). Naturally, these catheters are of a special design, and all other catheters should be regarded as MR incompatible.

## MAGNETIC FIELDS

Magnetic fields do not move things, magnetic gradients do. The flux lines are very dense at the opening to the magnet and this represents a region of high gradient (see Fig. 37-5). Because the field falls off with an inverse cube variation, the gradients become very strong very rapidly as the magnet is approached. One

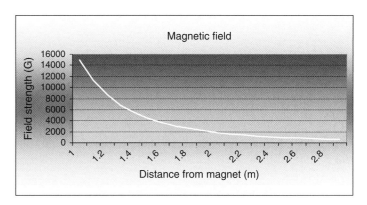

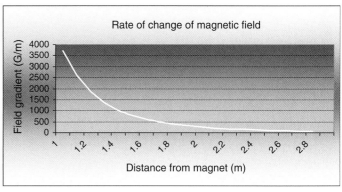

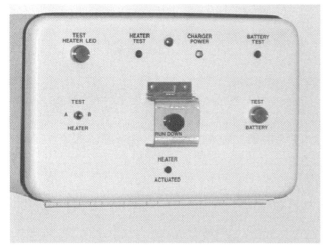

**FIGURE 37-7**    The quench button for the scanner is usually protected by a flip-up covering to prevent accidental activation. The location of the quench button should be known to all regular users of the scanner.

danger here is that a device being "tested" for magnetic interaction may suddenly be pulled into the magnet with an unstoppable force because the rate of change of field at the magnet opening demonstrates a very steep curve (see Fig. 37-6).

## SCANNER ROOM SAFETY

A metal object of approximately 2-lb weight, could require the strength of four people to pull it out of the magnet. If someone's body or limb is trapped by a metal object, quench the magnet immediately. Do not equivocate, DO IT! The location of the quench button

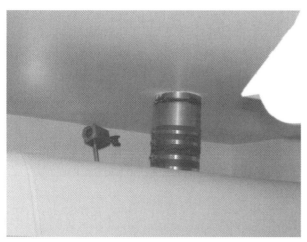

**FIGURE 37-8**    The pipe through which quench gases escape is typically located at the top of the scanner and is usually vented to the outside.

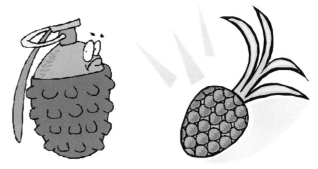

**FIGURE 37-9**    Distinguishing between artifacts and diagnostic features is a safety issue, primarily for physicians, but may also affect how a scan is performed by the technician. (Images reproduced from Hemera, The big Box of Art.)

should be known to all scanner room personnel (see Fig. 37-7).

## QUENCHING

When the magnet quenches, the superconducting wires suddenly become resistive. The hundreds of amps that are present instantly heat up the helium in the system. Helium expands by a factor of approximately 20,000, and to allow for this rapid expansion the helium gas exits the magnet through a bursting valve and escapes into the atmosphere (see Fig. 37-8). If the valve becomes blocked or malfunctions, the scanner room can instantly become filled with helium. The pressure generated is such that walls, windows, and doors may burst outward. If the room is not vented, the oxygen in the room will be displaced, and suffocation may ensue.

## MISINTERPRETATION

Artifacts, if not recognized, can be interpreted as clinical features and erroneously reported. Knowledge of artifacts therefore becomes a safety issue (see Fig. 37-9).

## SUMMARY

MRI has a culture of safety:

- It is integral to every action, rule, regulation, and procedure.
- The potential for danger is very real, and could cost loss of life or limb.
- The adoption of MRI "universal precautions" should be followed for every scan.

**$^1/_4$ Wavelength**    See Resonant Standing Wave.

**1-1 Pulse**    Describes the RF pulse sequence in which two RF pulses are applied separated by a short time interval with both RF pulses of equal amplitude. This type of pulse is used in tagging. The 1-1 pulse is the first pulse combination in a binomial expansion.

**1-3-1 Pulse**    Describes the RF pulse sequence in which three RF pulses are applied, each separated by a short time interval, with the first and last RF pulses of equal amplitude and the middle pulse being three times as powerful. This type of pulse is used in tagging. The 1-3-1 pulse is the second pulse combination in a binomial expansion.

**2D**    Two Dimensional.

**3D**    Three Dimensional.

**AA**    Ascending Aorta.

**Absolute Signal**    See Magnitude Signal.

**Active Shielding**    See Actively Shielded Magnet.

**Actively Shielded Magnet**    This type of magnet has a low fringe field. Actively shielded magnets are designed with a counter wound magnet surrounding the primary magnet. The counter wound magnet suppressed the field outside the system although not dramatically affecting the internal field.

**Aliasing**    Aliasing is the general term for artifacts created when the encoded feature exceeds the encoded dynamic range. When applied to imaging, the phenomena describes the effect of an image feature within the sensitivity range of the receiver coils but outside the range determined by the field of view. Aliased image features appear to be at the opposite end of the image in the phase encoding direction. When this term is applied to velocity imaging, it describes the condition where the velocity sensitivity is set too low, and high velocities appear as low velocities, and vice versa.

**Aligned**    Spins that are aligned with the main magnetic field direction are said to be in the low energy state. For a spin $^1/_2$ system, there are two energy states, low and high, that is, aligned and antialigned. This configuration is governed by quantum mechanical laws of energy state occupancy.

**Antialigned**    Spins that are antialigned with the main magnetic field direction are said to be in the high-energy state. For a spin-half system, there are two energy states, low and high, that is, aligned and antialigned. This configuration is governed by quantum mechanical laws of energy state occupancy.

**Artifact**    An image feature that is erroneously represented in the image is an artifact. Typically, the artificial feature is the result of motion or some distortion of the magnetic fields necessary to produce the image.

**ASSET**    Commercial name for parallel imaging.

**AV**    Aortic Valve.

**$B_0$**    (Commonly, B zero, alternately B naught). The universally accepted symbol for the main magnetic field is $B_0$. $B_0$ is a vector quantity, describing the strength of the magnetic field and its direction. Conventionally, $B_0$ is aligned along the Z direction of the system.

**$B_1$ Field**    (B one). The $B_1$ field is a magnetic field applied in the transverse plane, which rotates at a radiofrequency precessional rate. The $B_1$ field is applied to excite or rephase spins.

**Back Projection Reconstruction**    This describes the process of generating an image from a series of projections. Typically, the projection data comprises an evenly distributed series of projections through the object, covering the range zero through 180 degrees. Effectively, each projection is filtered and the intensity smeared across the image plane in the direction corresponding to the projection angle. After this process is performed for all projections, a conventional image is seen.

**Balanced FFE**    This is a commercial acronym for the steady state free precession sequence: Balanced (gradient) Fast Field Echo.

**Bandwidth**    This describes the frequency response of a time domain operation such as applying an RF pulse or temporally sampling data. An inverse relationship exists such that a short RF pulse or sample interval corresponds to a wide bandwidth. Bandwidth is a convenient means of describing the ultimate effect in the frequency domain. Bandwidth is measured in Hertz (Hz).

**Biot-Savart Law**    This expresses the magnetic field generated at a distance from a current carrying element. It is the basis of electromagnetic coil design.

**Bipolar Gradient**    Describes the condition of applying a gradient, initially with one polarity (e.g., positive) and followed in time by the opposite polarity (e.g., negative). The gradient is said to have two poles or lobes. Each lobe describes the section of gradient with a uniform polarity.

**Birdcage Coil**    This is a phased array coil that is formed into a continuous loop, resembling a birdcage. It allows quadrature detection. Each "leg" of the birdcage is tuned such that the phase of the cyclic magnetic field progresses in a stepped manner from leg to leg.

**Black Blood Sequence**    This describes any imaging sequence in which moving blood does not contribute to the signal. Typically, spin echo and spin echo variants are black blood sequences, because to contribute to the signal, blood has to experience both RF pulses. If the two RF pulses are slice selective, then moving blood will not refocus.

**Blood Pool Agent** This is a contrast agent that is confined to the blood pool. Typically, it has a high molecular weight (70,000 to 100,000).

**Blood Pool Normalization** This is a signal processing operation performed to analyze myocardial perfusion data. It takes into account the rate of delivery of the contrast agent to the myocardium. Typically the normalizing function is assessed by measuring the upslope of the ventricular blood pool signal. This slope is then used to divide the upslope of the myocardial perfusion data. This operation effectively accommodates differences purely due to the input function. More sophisticated processing is possible using this basic input data.

**Body Coil** This is a large RF coil that is sensitive to rotating magnetic fields over the complete sensitive region of the scanner. The coil is generally configured to allow RF transmission and RF signal reception. Generally, the body coil performs relatively poorly as a receiver coil, because it is optimized for uniform excitation.

**Boil Off** This describes the process whereby helium is lost from the scanner Dewar. Typically, the boiled off helium gas is collected, reliquefied, and reintroduced to the system.

**Boltzman's Distribution** The population of the two energy states of the spin system in the presence of a magnetic field is governed by Boltzman's distribution. This is the thermodynamic derived curve describing occupancy of each energy level. At normal temperatures, the occupancy of each energy state is almost equal.

**Bolus Following** Describes the process of imaging separate body sections for a single administration of a contrast agent. The body regions are imaged in succession, following the passage of the agent through the body, such as from the iliac vessels to the feet.

**BRISK** Block Regional Interpolation Scheme for K-Space. This is a sparse sampling scheme that acquires dynamic data rapidly. The sparse sampling pattern ensures that data near the center of k-space is sampled at higher rates than data towards the periphery. Data that are not directly acquired are filled in by interpolation.

**Burster Valve** The burster valve is a large valve at the top of the scanner, typically vented to the outside. When the system quenches, the helium rapidly expands and boils off. This occurs rapidly, and the burster valve detaches in an explosive manner, rapidly venting the magnet to the atmosphere.

**BW** See Bandwidth.

**CCD** See Charged Coupled Device.

**Centric (Encoding)** Describes the manner in which k-space is filled. In this case the central region of k-space is sampled at the start of the imaging sequence. Importantly, the spin conditions that pertain at the time of sampling the central lines of k-space largely determine contrast in the final image.

**CFR** See Coronary Flow Reserve.

**Channel** A channel describes the combination of a coil element (of a phased array receiver coil) and the sampling electronics in the scanner hardware. To realize the optimal utility of a phased array receiver system, ideally each coil element should have its own receiver electronics. Ultimately, the number of channels available in the system limits the performance of parallel imaging.

**Charged Coupled Device** This describes solid-state circuitry that can function in a high magnetic field environment. Video monitoring is typically accomplished by using charged coupled devices.

**Chelating** This is the chemical process of surrounding an element with a "molecular cage" to isolate it from its surroundings. Typically, chelation is performed to protect the body from a toxic agent.

**Chemical Shift** Describes the displacement of the fat signal relative to the water signal as a result of differences in frequency between the two materials.

**Cine** An image series, typically representing successive time periods through the cardiac cycle. Historically, "cine" refers to time-resolved gradient echo imaging.

**CMR** Cardiovascular Magnetic Resonance.

**CNR** See Contrast-to-Noise Ratio.

**Coil Element** An individual coil of a composite set forming a phased array coil. Each coil element exhibits high sensitivity to the body region that it is closest to.

**Common K-Space** This is a grid tagging approach that exploits the observation that the center of k-space is identical in the horizontal stripe tag set and the vertical stripe tag set. In this acquisition approach, only one set of tag patterns is excited for any given cardiac cycle, depending on which region of k-space is being acquired. Because only one tag set is excited at a time, there is no interaction between the two tag sets. The end result is that tags persist longer into the cardiac cycle, and the acquisition time is not extended beyond that of a conventional tag sequence.

**Contiguous Slices** Describes the condition of acquiring parallel slices with no gap between each slice in a multislice acquisition.

**Contrast Angiography** Describes the processes of obtaining angiographic contrast by the administration of a contrast agent.

**Contrast-to-Noise Ratio** This is a dimensionless quantity that describes how strong the image signal of one tissue type (e.g., myocardium) is relative to another tissue type (e.g., fat) when normalized by the image noise. A CNR of 1:1 indicates no net contrast, whereas a CNR of 5:1 is considered excellent.

**Control Volume** This describes the principle of conservation of material whereby the net flow traversing an arbitrarily shaped surface (i.e., the control volume) that completely encompasses an orifice will equal the flow through the orifice.

**Convective Acceleration** Describes the component of flow acceleration that is related to its spatial position: for example, consider steady flow converging on a stenotic orifice; as the orifice is approached, the velocity increases even in the presence of steady flow.

**Convergent Flow Field**  This describes flow accelerating towards a stenotic orifice. Typically, the convergent zone has a complex 3D flow field. Under certain simplifying circumstances, the convergent flow field is characterized by a series of concentric hemispherical shells of uniform flow. In this case, the convergent flow field is characterized by the radius of any one of the velocity shells.

**Convolution**  This is a mathematical operation describing the combining of two (or more) signals. A multiplication operation in k-space is equivalent to a convolution operation in the (inverse) image space. For instance, a truncated k-space matrix is equivalent to multiplying a full k-space matrix by a function with value 1 in the center and 0 at the edges. The Fourier transform of this "square function" is a sinc function (i.e., a decaying sine wave). In the image space, each pixel is convoluted with a sinc function, that is, each pixel effectively spreads out to resemble the sinc function.

**Core Lab**  A centralized site or laboratory that performs standardized measurements on data taken in a trial.

**Coronary Flow Reserve**  This describes the relative change in coronary flow between resting conditions and conditions of vasodilatation.

**C-SPAMM**  A dual sequence variation on spatial amplitude modulation method for producing cardiac tagging. In this version, two tagged images are obtained with opposite spin phases, such that on combination, tag fade is traded for progressive loss of signal-to-noise.

**DA**  Descending Aorta.

**dB/dt**  (D B by D T). Describes the rate of change of magnetic field. Many processes in magnetism are sensitive to the rate of change of magnetic flux lines as opposed to the absolute concentration of flux lines. The rate of change of magnetic field is measured in milli Tesla per second (mT/second).

**Deconvolution**  This is a mathematical operation for separating two (or more) distinct signals. Typically, the signals are overlapped because of some shortcut in sampling k-space. There is a simple relationship between k-space and convolution (see convolution), whereby multiplication in one space is equivalent to convolution in the inverse space. Despite this simple relationship, the process of deconvolution is inherently noisy.

**DENSE**  Displacement ENcoding with Stimulated Echo is a tissue tracking acquisition that overcomes some of the limitations of tagging. The DENSE acquisition allows myocardial displacement to be tracked on a pixel basis, and permits direct visualization of myocardial displacement. The approach is based on encoding displacement during a stimulated echo acquisition.

**Dewar**  This describes the vacuum chamber or flask that thermally isolates the helium-filled section containing the magnetic windings from the room temperature components.

**DIR**  See Double Inversion Recovery.

**Dixon Method**  This describes a spin echo sequence that exploits the in and out-of-phase signals of fat and water and is used to produce a separate fat and water image.

The sequence requires the acquisition of two images, each separated by a slight delay in echo time such that in one image the fat and water signals are in phase, and in the second image the fat and water signals are out of phase.

**Double Inversion Recovery**  This describes the process of obtaining contrast based on the inversion recovery processes. In this case, a second inversion pulse is applied at the time of the null point of the short T1 component (typically fat). The spin system is imaged after a further delay. The end result is that both short and long T1 components contribute a strong signal.

**ECG**  See electrocardiogram.

**Echo**  Describes the process of recalling a signal such that spins come into phase and form a high signal. Following attainment of the signal peak, referred to as the *echo peak*, the spins dephase relative to each other and the echo signal decays. The time from the midpoint of slice excitation to the echo peak is referred to as the *echo time*, TE.

**Echo Planar Imaging**  This is a rapid gradient echo imaging sequence. Essentially echo planar imaging recalls a series of gradient echo signals in rapid succession. Each gradient echo signal encodes a line of k-space, and sufficient data are generated to compile a complete k-space matrix in approximately 50 milliseconds.

**Echo Train Length**  Describes the number of echoes in a series of echoes recalled from a single excitation of the spin system. A gradient echo or spin echo sequence that has been adapted to recall a series of echoes to speed up the acquisition can be characterized by the echo train length.

**Eddy Current Compensation**  This describes the combination of hardware and software that are used to reduce eddy currents. Strategies involve employing self-shielded gradients, applying special waveforms to the gradient transitions, and isolating the gradients form the rest of the system.

**Eddy Currents**  These are transitory currents set up in response to changing magnetic flux lines. Eddy currents generate eddy fields.

**Eddy Fields**  These are transitory magnetic fields set up by eddy currents. Eddy fields disrupt image formation.

**EKG**  See electrocardiogram.

**Electrocardiogram**  The electrocardiogram signal describes the recording or monitoring of the electrical signal associated with electrical synchronization of the heart cycle.

**Electromotive Force**  This describes the voltage generated in response to changing magnetic lines of flux. Because it is generated in response to changes, the electromotive force is usually transitory in nature.

**EMF**  See Electromotive Force.

**EPI**  See Echo Planar Imaging.

**Equilibrium Signal**  This describes the signal attained following a series of RF pulses such that successive pulses produce a constant level signal.

**Ernst Angle**  This describes the optimal RF flip angle that can be applied at a given repetition time (TR), for a tissue with a given T1, to produce the largest steady state signal. Following a single RF pulse, a large amount of signal may be seen. However, after applying a train of RF pulses, a lower signal is seen, due to the competing processes of T1 relaxation, which repopulates the longitudinal spin component, and the result of bringing spins into the transverse plane by applying the RF flip angle. The Ernst angle is given by the formula: Arc cosine (exp [−TR/T1]).

**ETL** See Echo Train Length.

**Faraday Cage** The scanner is housed in a Faraday Cage that shields it from external RF signals. Essentially the Faraday cage is a copper-lined room that attenuates RF signals from the outside world.

**Fast Fourier Transform** This refers to a particularly efficient algorithm for performing the signal processing operation of the Fourier transform. Ideally, this routine requires that the matrix have dimensions of a power of 2, such as 256.

**Fast Spin Echo** The fast spin echo sequence is effectively an extended spin echo sequence. Instead of terminating the sequence after applying the basic excitation and refocusing pulses, the sequence is extended to apply a series of refocusing pulses. Each refocused echo is used to form a separate line of k-space. In this mode, k-space is complied rapidly, with the speed up factor being determined by the number of echoes sampled.

**FFT** See Fast Fourier Transform.

**FID** See Free Induction Decay.

**Field of View** This describes the physical dimensions of the section of the body being imaged. If the image is to be a 2D view, then the field of view will only have two dimensions. Typically, the field of view dimensions are given in millimeters or sometimes centimeters.

**FIESTA** This is a commercial acronym for the steady state free precession sequence: Fast Imaging Employing Steady-State Acquisition.

**Filter** A mathematical operation to restrict or enhance some aspect of a signal. Typically, filters are applied in one domain to achieve certain effects in the inverse (or Fourier) domain. For instance, applying filter to accentuate the central region of k-space boosts the low spatial frequencies in the image domain. In this case, the image appears to be smoother and have less noise.

**Filtered Back Projection** See Back Projection Reconstruction.

**First Moment** Describes the mathematical product of the gradient strength and the time of application. This is an integral operation, and positive and negative gradients can be applied to zero out the first moment. The significance of the first moment is that it describes the sensitivity of the gradient sequence to uniform velocity. By nulling the first moment, the effects of uniform velocity are removed, independent of the systems velocity.

**Flow** This is technically the flow rate, and describes the amount of fluid passing a point per unit time. When integrated over time and space it can be used to calculate the flow volume.

**Flux Lines** This term describes the density of magnetic field lines. Flux lines travel from the north pole to the south pole. Flux lines cannot be broken, but can be distorted (i.e., bent in space) from their ideal path depending on the surrounding materials.

**Fold-Over Artifact** This describes the excess signal seen when the physical dimensions of the body exceed the field of view set for the phase encoding direction. The artifact is referred to as *fold-over* because the excess body signal is effectively folded over on the opposite edge of the image. Fold-over only occurs in the phase-encoded direction. When 2D imaging is employed, there is only one phase encoding direction. When 3D imaging is used, there are two phase encoding directions for fold-over to occur in. Also, see Aliasing.

**Four-Chamber View** See Horizontal Long Axis.

**Fourier Coefficients** These are the individual points in the Fourier domain signal, that is, the result of applying a Fourier transform to a function generates a series of Fourier coefficients in the transform domain. The Fourier coefficients represent the amplitude of the respective sine and cosine waves that contribute to the original function. For instance, the zeroth Fourier coefficient (the first one generated) corresponds to the constant background level; the first Fourier coefficient corresponds to the amplitude of the sine or cosine waves that undergo one complete oscillation over the original function, etc. up to the last Fourier coefficient which represents the amplitude of the highest frequency sine or cosine wave contained in the original function. See Fourier Theory.

**Fourier Domain** This describes the signal resulting from applying a Fourier transform to the original signal. The Fourier domain has the dimension of the inverse of the original signal domain. For instance, if the original signal is a function of time, then the Fourier domain signal is the inverse of time, which is frequency.

**Fourier Theory** Fourier theory states that all signal waveforms can be decomposed into (or described by) a series of sine and cosine waveforms.

**Fourier Transform** A signal processing algorithm performed in the computer that converts data from one domain into the inverse domain. For instance, the k-space data is time domain data, and the image is produced by Fourier transforming k-space data. In this example, the image is in the frequency domain. It can be appreciated that the frequency domain signal corresponds to image information, because the applied imaging gradients imposed a frequency distribution over the sample.

**FOV** See Field of View.

**Free Induction Decay** Describes the signal following tipping the spins into the transverse plane. In the transverse plane, the spins freely precess, and the signal is detected by electromagnetic induction. Further, the signal decays due to spin relaxation, hence the highly succinct and descriptive name given to the signal.

**Frequency (Encoding) Gradient** The gradient applied as data are rapidly sampled, forming one line of k-space. In most imaging sequences, the frequency encoding gradient is applied in an identical manner for each application of the pulse sequence. This reflects the property that the frequency encoding gradient traverses k-space from one edge to the opposite edge, irrespective of which line of k-space is being sampled.

**Fringe Field** Describes the residual magnetic field that exists outside the targeted region. For instance, the main magnetic field is targeted to the center of the imaging system, but the magnetic field that is felt outside the magnet is the fringe field.

**FT** See Fourier Transform.

**Gad** See Gadolinium.

**Gadolinium** This is a heavy metal, which is used as a contrast agent because of its property of being highly paramagnetic.

**Gauss** The Gauss is a unit of magnetic field strength. There are 10,000 Gauss (G) in one Tesla (T). A field strength of 5 G is generally considered to be a universally safe magnetic field that should not ordinarily interfere with the operation of pacemakers and surgical implants.

**G-Factor** See Goodness Factor.

**Ghost (Image, or Feature)** A ghost is a special type of artifact that results in a typically, faint rendition of a complete image feature such as a blood vessel represented at a displaced position. Usually, the original image feature and the ghost are both distinctly seen.

**Gibbs Ringing** This is a series of repeating lines in an image. It is related to acquiring an image with low resolution, and reflects the fact that acquisition of k-space was terminated while there was significant signal at one or more boundaries of k-space. Effectively, Gibbs ringing is a convolution related artifact. See Convolution.

**Golay Coil** This is an electromagnetic coil that generates a magnetic gradient in the X (or Y) direction in a cylindrical geometry scanner system. Conceptually, the Golay coil is a split Helmholts coil, with the split section forming the basis of generating the vertical (or horizontal gradient).

**Goodness Factor** With respect to parallel imaging, the degree to which coils of a phased array set overlap in sensitivity determines how noise propagates as a result of the de-convolution process. Ideally, coil sensitivities should only minimally overlap. The degree to which they conform to this ideal is captured in the "goodness-factor" or "g-factor". A g-factor of 1 is ideal, and values higher than this reflect the additional noise that parallel imaging produces. Therefore, high goodness factors reflect a poorly performing system.

**Gradient** This describes the variation in magnetic field over a spatial direction, and is necessary for achieving conditions for slice selection and imaging. Without application of a gradient, there would be no feature to differentiate spins from one part of the body to another. The gradient exists over three dimensions, in that the field produced is always directed along the main field direction, but the variation in field only occurs along one spatial direction. In a typical imaging system, there are three gradient systems, corresponding to the orthogonal X, Y, and Z Cartesian axes.

**Gradient Echo** Describes the process of forming an echo by initially applying a gradient of one polarity to dephase spins followed by applying the gradient in reverse polarity to rephase spins. Imaging sequences based on the gradient echo process are sometimes referred to as *black blood* or *cine sequences*.

**GRE** Gradient Recalled Echo.

**Gyromagnetic Ratio** Described by the symbol, $\gamma$, it is the constant of proportionality describing the frequency of spin precession relative to the magnetic field strength. The gyromagnetic ratio is unique for each spin series such as muscle.

**Helmholtz Coil** This is an electromagnetic coil comprised of two circular loops separated by a distance of one coil's diameter. Ideally the magnetic field between the two coils approximates to a uniform magnetic field. When current is driven through the Helmholtz coil a uniform magnetic field is generated. Conversely, when the spins precess in the volume between the two coils, they generate a magnetic field that is uniformly detected as a voltage generated in the Helmholtz coil.

**Helmholtz Coil Pair** This describes a pair of circular coils of the same diameter, and separated by a distance of one coil's diameter, aligned to be on axis with each other. The field generated between the two coils approximates to a uniform field.

**Horizontal Long Axis** Describes the view of the heart in which the four main cardiac chambers are seen: left and right atria, and left and right ventricles.

**Imaging Station** Describes the section of the body that is imaged using a 3D contrast angiographic sequence. Each station, or region, generally requires repositioning the patient for each acquisition.

**In-Phase (Signal)** When two signals, such as fat and water, differ slightly in frequency, the two signals will form a beat pattern. When the beat pattern is at its maximum, the two signals are said to be in phase with each other. Phase conditions at the each peak reflect the phase conditions of the entire image. Therefore, if the two signals are in phase at the echo peak, the image is said to be an in-phase image. When spins are in phase, they contribute an overall high signal.

**Inductance** This is the property of a coil that dominates its impedance, that is, resistance to electrical current. Unlike resistors, the impedance only opposes currents that are changing. Inductance has the symbol, L, and is measured in Henries. High inductance is associated with coils encompassing a large volume and coils with higher numbers of turns. Physically, inductance is related to the volume of magnetic flux lines generated by a coil per unit current.

**Interpolation** Describes the image or signal processing process of filling in data in between sampled points. For instance, in a time resolved series only 10 data points may have been acquired, and after interpolation, 15 points may be used to represent the same span of time. Interpolation can be performed by zero filling in the Fourier domain.

**Interrupt Panel** An interrupt panel allows electrical cables to enter and leave the scan room without introducing a path for RF interference. The interrupt panel has attachments for cables and circuitry to filter out inadvertent RF signal.

**Inversion Recovery** This describes the signal preparation process of inverting the spin system by application of a 180 degree RF pulse. The inverted spins relax back to equilibrium through the T1 process. During this recovery time, some spins may relax faster than others, and by imaging the system before full recovery, contrast is achieved based on differences in T1 relaxation times.

**IR** See Inversion Recovery.

**Isocenter** Describes the location that is the effective magnetic center of the scanner. At the isocenter, all the gradients cross the zero point (i.e., they cross from positive to negative polarity at this point).

**Jet Length** Describes the length of a jet of flow. The theory of free jets (i.e., jets that do not impinge on chamber walls) indicates that the laminar part of a jet has a length of four times the stenotic orifice through which the jet is traveling. In the jet proper, flow is laminar, and when the flow velocity falls below 5% of the sustained level, the jet is said to have terminated. At the peak of jet flow (i.e., for a fully developed jet) the distance from the jet origin to the point where velocity falls to 95% of the peak velocity defines the jet length. Beyond the region defining the jet length the jet disintegrates into turbulent flow. Equivalently, the jet length is defined as the distance from the stenotic orifice to the point of the vena contracta (i.e., the narrowest portion of the jet). This definition accommodates the condition when the jet is not necessarily free, but may be advancing into counter flow.

**K-Space** This is a central feature of CMR, and describes the signal space in which each image is acquired. To convert the k-space signal into an image requires application of a Fourier transform. The k-space signal is some times referred to as *phase space*. Imaging gradients have to be applied to formulate data into k-space. The k-space data arrays, or matrices, are complied internally in the computer system. K-space data have an inverse relationship to the image, that is,. if the image represents the distribution of frequency information; k-space represents the distribution of time information (frequency has units of inverse time).

**LA** Left Atrium.

**Laminar Flow** Describes a flow field in which velocity varies relatively slowly across it.

**Lamor Equation** This describes the relationship between a spin's precessional frequency and the magnetic field experienced by that spin. The constant of proportionality connecting frequency and field strength is unique for each spin series, and is given by the gyromagnetic ratio, or equivalently the magnetogyric ratio.

**Lattice** Describes the environment in which spins exist. Any physical interaction that is not described by spin–spin interactions is said to be a spin–lattice interaction. The lattice then is a catchall phrase that describes the thermodynamic environment in which the spin system has its existence.

**Left Ventricular Outflow Tract** Describes the view of the heart in which the left ventricle, aortic valve, and outflow tract are seen.

**LV** Left Ventricle.

**LVOT** See Left Ventricular Outflow Tract.

**Magnetic Attraction** Objects that are attracted to magnets are really moving into regions of increasing flux density. Under conditions of uniform flux lines there is no preferred direction of motion. Therefore, a metallic object outside of the magnet is attracted towards the center of the magnet where the density of flux lines is highest, and the metallic object comes to rest at the center.

**Magnetic Gradient** See Gradient.

**Magnetogyric Ratio** See Gyromagnetic Ratio.

**Magnetohydrodynamic Effect** See T-Wave Elevation.

**Magnitude Signal** This describes the feature of visualizing only the magnitude component of the vector signal. In a magnitude signal there is no influence of signal phase. A magnitude signal cannot distinguish between positive and negative signals. Conventional images are of the magnitude format.

**Matrix** The k-space data set.

**Maximum Intensity Projection** This is an image rendering routine that projects the maximum intensity onto a viewing plane. The end result is an angiographic view similar to a conventional angiogram.

**Maxwell Coil** This is a gradient coil that generates a gradient along the Z-axis for a cylindrical geometry system. The gradient is designed with two equal diameter circular coils on axis with each other, and separated by $\sqrt{3}$ times the radius. The current in each coil is driven in opposing directions to establish the gradient.

**Measurement Gradient** See Frequency Encoding Gradient.

**MIP** See Maximum Intensity Projection.

**$M_0$** (M Zero). This describes the net magnetization of the body when placed in a magnetic field.

**Motion Sensitivity** An artifact that is due to motion of the imaged object.

**MOTSA** Multiple Overlapping Slabs For TOF Angiography. This is a 3D angiographic sequence that employs multiple overlapping slabs. Each slab is fairly narrow and therefore incurs relatively little signal loss due to flow saturation.

**Multishot** This describes the process of obtaining multiple lines of k-space using a basic imaging sequence applied in rapid succession.

**Mutual Inductance** This describes the ability of one coil to sense the presence of another coil. Coils interact by the amount of flux lines that are generated by one coil and pass through the other coil. When the net amount of flux lines is zero (e.g., there are as many positive as negative flux lines) the mutual inductance is said to be zero.

**MV**  Mitral Valve.

**Nanoparticles**  In CMR these usually describe contrast agents that have dimensions in the nanometer range.

**Neuromuscular Stimulation**  This describes the phenomena of applying a magnetic field with a high slew rate to induce electrical signals in the body such that muscular twitching results. A slew rate of approximately 200 mT/m/second is sufficient to induce neuromuscular stimulation.

**NEX**  See Number of Excitations.

**No Phase Wrap**  This is a parameter, that, when activated, limits the influence of fold-over artifacts. The parameter activates a combination of partial NEX and field of view options to reduce or eliminate the fold-over artifact.

**Null Point**  This describes conditions in inversion recovery imaging when the inverted spin system for one T1 type tissue has relaxed such that there are as many positive spins as there are negative spins. Under this condition there will be no net signal seen when an imaging sequence is applied. This special time is said to be the null point.

**Number of Excitations**  This is a parameter that describes how many signals are acquired for a k-space matrix. If NEX>1, it describes the condition of performing signal averaging (e.g., 2, 4 averages). If NEX<1, the k-space matrix is acquired such that only one half is fully sampled, and the other half is sampled in a partial amount. The unsampled portion of k-space is filled in at the post-processing stage, exploiting the symmetry inherent in k-space. At the end of a partial NEX acquisition, because k-space data are fully generated (from a combination of acquired and generated data), the resulting image has resolution equivalent to a full k-space matrix acquisition. In a partial NEX acquisition, the signal-to-noise ratio is reduced compared to a full acquisition.

**Nyquist (Sampling Rate)**  This describes minimum data sampling conditions in the time domain that are necessary to correctly represent the frequency content of the signal. In essence, the Nyquist condition dictates that at least two sample points should be acquired per wavelength for the highest frequency signal present. This is fully characterized by the interval between sampled time points. See Bandwidth.

**Occupancy**  This describes the spin population of each of the allowed energy states, aligned or antialigned. Under normal conditions, occupancy of each state is approximately equal.

**Off-Resonance**  Describes any signal that is not in synchronization with the reference frequency of the scanner.

**Off-Resonance Artifact**  An artifact generally associated with the steady state free precession sequence. Signals that are off resonance will appear as regions of dark and bright banding in the image.

**Out-of-Phase (Signal)**  When two signals, such as fat and water, differ slightly in frequency, the two signals will form a beat pattern. When the beat pattern is at its minimum, the two signals are said to be out of phase with each other. Phase conditions at the echo peak reflect the phase conditions of the entire image. Therefore, if the two signals are out of phase at the echo peak, the image is said to be out of phase. When spins within an individual voxel are out of phase with each other, they contribute an overall lower signal.

**Over-Contiguous Slices**  Describes the condition whereby parallel slices are acquired in an overlapping manner.

**PA**  Pulmonary Artery.

**Parallel Imaging**  This is a means of reducing the imaging time by exploiting differences in signal sensitivity between distinct coil elements of a phased array coil set. In parallel imaging, a sparse sampling factor is applied to reduce the number of lines of k-space sampled. In this mode, acquired lines are more widely spaced than required for a full field of view scan. If the missed lines were not replaced, the resulting image would suffer dramatic fold over artifacts, because the field of view is effectively reduced by this process. The missing data are filled in at the post-processing stage, using information derived from the sensitivity of each separate coil element. Effectively, the coil elements provide several simultaneous views of the field of view, mathematically generating a set of simultaneous equations that can be solved.

**Paramagnetism**  This describes the phenomena of a contrast agent that increases the local magnetic field. Generally, the agents that have this property, if suitably free, will tumble and rotate at frequencies in the RF range. These agents effectively reduce the T1 of tissues that they come in contact with.

**Parasagittal Aorta**  Describes the view of the aorta showing the aorta as a "candy cane".

**Para-axial Aorta**  Describes the view of the aorta showing the cusps of the aortic valve.

**Partial Echo**  This describes the condition under which only a truncated section of an echo is captured. This is often done to reduce the echo time (TE). A partial echo is realized in a gradient echo sequence by truncating the initial dephasing lobe of the gradient. In this case, the echo signal is not fully dephased, and the echo formed will first be seen as a partially rephased signal, that is, an incomplete, or partial echo. Generally, the trailing portion of the echo is fully sampled.

**Partial Inversion**  This is a spin preparation condition achieved by applying an RF flip angle >90 degrees and <180 degrees. It is used when less than a full inversion is required, typically due to time constraints.

**Partial Phase Field of View**  This describes the condition that the matrix dimension corresponding to the phase encoding direction is reduced compared to a square matrix. The reduction factor is described by the partial phase field of view parameter. For example if the partial phase field of view parameter is set at 0.75, and the full scan matrix is $256 \times 256$, then the acquired matrix will be reduced to $256 \times 192$.

**PC–MR**    See Phase Contrast–MR.

**Phase (Encoding) Gradient**    Describes the gradient applied to prepare the signal before measuring a k-space line. On each successive application of the imaging sequence, the phase encoding gradient is applied at a different amplitude, corresponding the individual line of k-space to be acquired during that pass of the imaging sequence.

**Phase Correction**    When a special property of an image is encoded in the signal phase, it is usually necessary to compare this property against the phase of a reference image. The process of comparing the phase is referred to as *phase correction*.

**Phase Field of View**    This parameter describes preferentially reducing the field of view in the phase encoding direction. A value of 0.75 will reduce the field of view in the phase encoding direction by 25%.

**Phase Gradient Artifact**    This describes an artifact in phase contrast–MR, where velocity is represented as signal phase. Ideally, the static background features should have zero phase. When a gradient is present in the background static regions, this is referred to as a *phase gradient*. It is possible to correct the measured velocity for the linear phase gradient by subtracting or adding velocity based on the additional amount related to the gradient.

**Phase Image**    This describes the condition of viewing (as an image) the phase of the spin system. The phase is restricted to the range 0 to 360 degrees, and therefore the image may have a flat appearance compared to the high dynamic range of the magnitude image.

**Phase Roll Artifact**    This is an artifact that has its origin in the off-resonance sensitivity of steady state free precession imaging. In this sequence, spins that are not exactly on resonance will experience phase differences that lead to signal attenuation. These regions of off-resonance spins usually follow the gradual roll-off of field inhomogeneities, leading to bands of bright and dark signal regions. When a band falls over a region of motion, severe disruption can ensue.

**Phase Sensitive Detection**    This describes the process of detecting a precessing signal such that the two orthogonal components of the spin system are detected simultaneously. This is accomplished in the receiver electronics by comparing the detected signal against an internal frequency signal (the resonance frequency of the system). Phase sensitive detection allows separation of higher and lower frequencies.

**Phase Velocity Mapping**    See Phase Contrast–MR.

**Phase Contrast–MR**    Refers to velocity sensitive imaging using the phase of the MR signal. Velocity is directly encoded into the signal phase.

**Phased Array Coil**    A phased array coil is a configuration of RF receiver coils that exhibit high sensitivity on a regional basis. Each coil element is associated with a unique receiver channel. An individual coil element is highly sensitive to a relatively small volume. When channels are combined, the resulting image has overall good SNR in all regions.

**PISA**    Proximal Iso-velocity Surface Area. This describes flow conditions in the convergent zone. In this region, flow ideally converges on the orifice in hemispherical shells. This is only strictly true for a circular orifice with small dimensions (i.e., a pin-prick). Velocity is assumed to be perpendicular to each hemispherical shell, and thereby the flow through the shell can be calculated based on simple geometric calculations.

**Pixel**    Picture Element. This describes the smallest section of an image. An image is composed of many pixels.

**Plan Scan**    Describes the process of obtaining a scan for the express purpose of planning a further view. Usually, the result of plan scanning is to obtain multiple oblique views.

**Plug Flow**    Describes a flow field in which the flow profile seen in cross section is relatively flat.

**Point Spread Function**    This describes the manner in which one pixel spills into other pixels. Ideally, each pixel should be self-contained and not interfere with other pixels. However, depending on the imaging encoding method and how consistent the signal data are, the effective point spread function may be such that pixels spill over considerably into other pixels, which are usually, but not necessarily, adjacent.

**PPM**    Parts Per Million.

**PR**    See Back Projection Reconstruction.

**Prepulse**    See Preparation Pulse.

**Prescan**    This describes the actions that the scanner performs to optimize the upcoming acquisition. The features optimized include: determination of the correct RF power level, adjustment of the receiver signal gain, and determination of the correct resonance frequency. Generally, prescanning is performed automatically; however, the operations can be manually overridden.

**Precession**    This describes the wobbling action of spins that are tipped from alignment with the main magnetic field. The precession frequency is relatively slow compared to the spin frequency. Precession occurs due to interaction between the spin's angular momentum and the restoring force exerted by the magnet. The interaction of the two causes the spins to precess instead of realign.

**Preparation Pulse**    This describes a combination of RF and gradients that are applied before acquiring an image. The preparation pulse is designed to bring about some spin condition that produces contrast. Examples include inversion recovery pulses and T2 preparation pulses.

**Projection**    This describes the process of summing spins along a line from a series of parallel lines that are perpendicular to a line through the sample. Such a view represents a projection (similar to a shadow) of the object being studied. The significance of projections is that they can be generated by applying a single imaging gradient. Of further significance is that the k-space representation of a projection corresponds to a line passing through the center of k-space.

**Projection Reconstruction**  See Back Projection Reconstruction.

**Proximal Flow Field**  See Convergent Flow Field.

**PSF**  See Point Spread Function.

**PVM**  Phase Velocity Mapping, see Phase-Contrast MR.

**Q Factor**  See Quality Factor.

**QA**  Quality Assurance.

**Quadrature Detection**  This describes the ability to simultaneously detect both components of the transverse precessing spin system. Quadrature detection allows the SNR to improve by $\sqrt{2}$.

**Quality Factor**  This describes the "lossyness" of the RF system. The coil quality factor, Q, is frequency dependant and is related to the ratio of energy stored to power lost. Generally, a coil with a high Q value produces images with a good SNR.

**Quench**  Describes the process of suddenly stopping a superconducting magnet from operating. A quench is brought about by heating of one section of the superconducting coils. When this occurs, the whole of the system flips from superconductive mode to resistive mode. When this happens, the energy is dumped into heating up the liquid helium. This causes the helium to rapidly boil off. The magnetic field collapses over a matter of milliseconds. This is referred to as *quenching the system*. Quenches can occur by accident (sometimes for no apparent reason), and sometimes they are initiated by hitting the quench button.

**R Value**  See Relaxivity.

**RA**  Right Atrium.

**Rare Sampling**  See Sparse Sampling.

**Read Gradient**  See Frequency (Encoding) Gradient.

**Real Time**  This describes the operation of the scanner such that it allows acquisition and display of images as the action is taking place. The ability to use real-time scanning for patient monitoring and assessment is crucial for diagnostic tests that involve stress testing. Generally, real-time images are of lower quality compared to conventional diagnostic scans.

**Receive RF Coil**  This describes an electromagnetic coil configuration that is sensitive to the $B_1$ field produced by precessing spins. The $B_1$ field is directed in the transverse plane. Note that from the spin perspective, the transverse plane does not correspond to the geometric transverse plane, but indicates that the spins are tipped perpendicular to the $B_0$ direction. Receiver coils are generally optimized for sensitivity as opposed to uniformity.

**Rectangular Field of View**  See Phase Field of View.

**Reduced Field of View Imaging**  See Parallel Imaging.

**Reference Image**  When a special property of an image is required, such as signal phase, it is usually necessary to compare this property against a reference image. The comparison reference image is usually acquired under similar conditions to the target image, with the exception of the encoded property. Because phase information is usually highly disrupted, to visualize any feature encoded in the phase (such as velocity or signal sign) requires comparison against a reference image.

**Refocusing Gradient**  This describes a gradient that is applied to bring spins back into phase coherence with each other. A linear gradient is required to refocus spins that are dephased by a linear process.

**Regridding**  This describes the process of applying post-processing to position k-space points on a regular, rectangular or square grid. This process is necessary for k-space data points not acquired in the exact order required for image generation by using a Fourier transform.

**Relaxation**  This describes the process whereby a perturbed spin system gradually returns to its natural state. On an individual level, each spin can only occupy one of two energy levels, high or low, and the effects of relaxation are immediately implemented when a spin relaxes from its high energy state to the low energy state. However, when considered as a group, the return to normal conditions is governed by exponential curves due to the high number of spins involved.

**Relaxivity**  This describes the effect of reducing T1 by introducing a contrast agent. The inverse of the T1 produced by the contrast agent is captured in the relaxivity value. Ideally, the relaxivity is proportional to the concentration of the contrast agent.

**Resonant Standing Wave**  This describes the phenomena of establishing a nontraveling RF wave. Typically, the conductor may be a straight wire, which, if it is of a length close to one fourth of the RF wavelength, is in danger of establishing a standing wave. This standing wave will rapidly and dramatically heat up the wire, burning any body region in contact with it. At 1.5-3T, the resonant lengths are close to the dimensions of the body.

**Respiratory Gating**  This describes the means of synchronizing an acquisition with respiratory motion. Respiration may be monitored using a physical device such as belt and bellows, attached around the waist of the patient, or through image tracking using navigator pulses. Typically, the acquisition is triggered to the time at end-expiration.

**RF**  Radiofrequency.

**RF Loop**  This describes a conductive closed loop in which RF waves can be induced. In general, when a higher number of flux lines pass through the loop, there is more interaction with RF energy. The RF energy can heat up any material in contact with the loop. The orientation and area of the loop are important determinants of how external RF fields interact with it.

**Right Ventricular Outflow Tract**  Describes the view of the heart showing the pulmonary artery, valve, and right ventricle.

**Rotating Reference Frame**  This describes the signal detection process, whereby signal at the resonance frequency is detected as a static (DC) level. This is effectively accomplished by comparing the detected signal to an internal reference signal. By this means, the signal is detected as the net difference from the reference frequency.

**RR Interval** This describes the length of the cardiac cycle, that is, the interval between one ECG R wave and the next ECG R wave. The formula to calculate the RR interval based on heart rate (HR) is RR = 60,000/HR

**RV** Right Ventricle.

**RVOT** See Right Ventricular Outflow Tract.

**Saline Flush** This describes the action of following an injection of medication or contrast with a bolus of saline solution. The purpose of the saline flush is to force the remaining medication or contrast agent through the tubing and into the patients' vein.

**Sampling Density** This describes the number of lines or points that are sampled per unit length, for example, sample points per millisecond, or number of lines per unit of k-space. Features in the sampling (time) domain have consequences in the inverse (frequency) domain. The sampling density of k-space relates to the physical property of field of view, that is, a high sampling density in k-space relates to a large field of view.

**Sampling Rate** See Nyquist.

**SAR** See Specific Absorption Rate.

**Saturated Signal** This describes the condition when all the spins are tipped into the transverse plane. In this case, higher or lower RF pulse tip angles will not increase the signal, and the signal is therefore said to be saturated. This corresponds to a 90 degree RF pulse.

**Scout Image** This describes an image acquired with the express purpose of permitting planning of further views. Typically, scout images are obtained along the three primary axes: transverse, sagittal, and coronal.

**SE** See Spin Echo.

**Segmentation** This describes the process of acquiring a segment of k-space (i.e., a number of lines) using either repeated application of a basic imaging sequence, or acquiring multiple lines by recalling a number of echoes. Segmentation is a means to produce time resolved images in a rapid manner.

**Selective Excitation** This describes the process of targeting a very narrow band of frequencies to selectively experience the excitation RF flip angle. Typically, the selected band corresponds either to the water frequency or the fat frequency of the proton resonance.

**Selective Saturation** This describes the process of targeting a very narrow band of frequencies to selectively undergo a 90 degree flip angle. Typically, the selected band of frequencies corresponds either to the water resonance or the fat resonance.

**Self-Shielded Gradients** These are gradients that are magnetically isolated from the rest of the system by incorporating a counter-wound gradient outside of the main gradient system.

**SENSE** Commercial name for parallel imaging.

**Sensitivity Map** This describes a, typically, rapidly acquired image of a large field of view obtained in order to get a low resolution view of the body. This view is used to measure the sensitivity of each element of the phased array coil, and this information may be used in operations such as parallel imaging.

**Shim Coils** These are a collection of several magnetic coils that are applied in a static manner to make the main magnetic field more uniform.

**Shim Gradients** These are static, low level, gradients applied to correct for inhomogeneities in the main $B_0$ field. Dynamic shimming can be performed to correct for gross inhomogeneities before each scan. Most of the shim gradients are not adjustable at run time.

**Shimming** This describes the process of applying small correctional gradients to make the main magnetic field more uniform.

**Short Axis** Describes the view of the heart in which the left ventricle is seen in circular cross section. In this view, the right ventricle is often seen as a "half-moon" view.

**Signal Decay** This describes the process whereby the spins become progressively in and out of phase and lose coherence. The loss of coherence in phase results in signal decay. The T2 parameter describes the half-life of spin coherence due to natural spin–spin interactions.

**Signal-to-Noise Ratio** The signal-to-noise ratio is a dimensionless quantity that describes how strong the image signal is relative to the image noise. An SNR of 1:1 is unintelligible, whereas an SNR of 100:1 is considered excellent.

**Sinc Function** This describes a shape resembling a decaying sine wave. It is significant in that the Fourier transform of a sinc function is a square or "top-hat" function.

**Slab Saturation** See Venous Suppression.

**Slab Selection** This describes the combination of RF and gradients required to select a thick slice.

**Slew Rate** The combination of magnetic gradient strength and switching speed is encapsulated in its slew rate. Slew rate is measured in milli Tesla per meter per second (mT/m/second). Typically, gradients in commercial scanner systems have slew rates in the range 100 to 200 mT/m/second.

**Slice Gap** This describes the distance in millimeters between parallel slices in a multislice acquisition.

**Slice Profile** This describes the cross-sectional shape of the imaged slice. Ideally, the slice profile (i.e., the shape from one edge to the other) should be flat, that is, a square function. In practice, the slice profile typically has a more curved shape, with lower angles at the edge compared to the middle of the slice.

**Slice Selection** This describes the combination of RF and gradients required to select a thin slice.

**SMASH** Commercial name for parallel imaging.

**SNR** See signal-to-noise ratio.

**Solenoid** This describes an electromagnetic coil wound in a cylindrical shape. This coil design very efficiently generates a magnetic field when current is passed through the coil.

**Source Image** This describes the image data in its most direct format. Typically, angiographic data may be presented using substantial post-processing algorithms. The source images will have undergone minimal processing and typically correspond to transverse views through the body.

**SPAMM** See Spatial Amplitude Modulation Method.

**Sparse Sampling** When k-space is not fully sampled, it is said to be sparsely sampled. Typically, the missing lines are to be filled in by use of some post-processing algorithm. The sparsely sampled k-space data can be acquired in a more rapid time compared to a full k-space matrix. The time reduction factor is given by the product of the sparsity factor and the full acquisition time.

**Spatial Amplitude Modulation Method** This describes the method of applying line or grid tags to an image by the interleaved application of RF pulses and gradients. The RF pulses invert the spin system, and the gradient refocus spins in a pattern that varies in a sinusoidal manner across the field of view.

**Spatial Frequency** This describes the rate of change of intensity from one pixel to another. For instance, if a series of adjacent pixels had an intensity of 0 and 1 repeating, this is said to be a high spatial frequency pattern. However, a series of pixels with very similar or uniform intensity are said to have a low spatial frequency pattern. In terms of k-space, low spatial frequency information is represented in the central region of k-space, whereas the highest spatial frequency information is represented in the extreme periphery of k-space.

**Specific Absorption Rate** This describes the measure of how much RF power is deposited in the body. Power is the rate of doing (or equivalently absorbing) work. Sequences with high SAR levels may cause unsafe heating of the body.

**Spin $1/2$ System** Describes the spin system applicable to protons. Spin values are either $+1/2$ or $-1/2$, describing alignment or antialignment with the magnet, respectively.

**Spin Dephasing** The spin system is composed of many (trillions) of individual spins. When the spins are initially knocked into the transverse plane they are in phase with each other, and contribute a high signal. As imaging gradients are applied, some spins advance in phase, whereas others lag in phase. The net result is referred to as *spin dephasing*. When the spins are completely dephased, for every positive spin (e.g., along positive X axis) there is a negative spin (e.g., along negative X axis). Under these conditions the spins cancel each other out, and no signal is seen. This corresponds to a state of complete spin dephasing.

**Spin Echo** This describes the process of recalling an echo by applying a second "refocusing" RF pulse. The refocusing pulse is optimally of value 180 degrees. The refocusing pulse essentially flips the dephased spin system like a pancake, such that under the influence of constant gradients, spins come back into focus. Consequently,

the spin echo sequence can refocus spin dephasing due to the natural inhomogeneities of the main magnetic field.

**Spin System** This describes the environment and physical properties of the spins. In terms of thermodynamics, each spin exchanges energy with other spins (characterized by the T2 time) and with the lattice (characterized by the T1 time).

**Spin–Lattice Interaction** See T1.

**Spin–Spin Interaction** See T2.

**SPIO** See Superparamagnetic Iron Oxide.

**Spiral Scanning** This describes an imaging sequence that uses a spiral trajectory in k-space. Spiral scanning accomplishes this by use of gradients that vary as a sinusoidal waveform with gradually increasing amplitude. One feature of spiral scanning is that it does not require sharp gradient transitions. Also, spiral scanning data requires re-girding such that the acquired spiral data are shifted and modified to fit on a regular rectangular grid that is suitable for Fourier processing.

**SSFP** See Steady State Free Precession.

**Standing Wave** See Resonant Standing Wave.

**Star Artifact** This is a common artifact seen in projection reconstruction images emanating from bright features. Technically, it reflects the distribution of the point-spread-function of a projection reconstruction pixel.

**Static Tissue Suppression** Describes the process of suppressing static tissue by applying a series of RF pulses. Typically, the pulses are applied at a high flip angle (higher than the Ernst angle), and the equilibrium signal has a low value.

**STE** See Stimulated Echo.

**Steady State Free Precession** This is an efficient imaging sequence which essentially combines all three echo types: gradient echo, spin echo, and stimulated echo. The essential features of the sequence are that by combining all three echoes, the signal-to-noise ratio is inherently high. To combine all three echoes for each signal readout requires that the sequence attain a steady state. This is achieved by running the sequence at a regular TR, until the same signal is achieved on application of each RF pulse.

**Sternal Wires** These are wires left in the chest following a surgical procedure. They typically result in a localized artifact but are not generally hazardous.

**Stimulated Echo** This describes the process of recalling an echo by application of three RF pulses. The optimal performance of the stimulated echo sequence is if each RF pulse has a value of 90 degrees. Essentially, the first RF pulse tips spins into the transverse plane. The combination of the second and third RF pulses performs a refocusing operation similar to a spin echo sequence. The major difference between a stimulated echo and the spin echo is that in the stimulated echo, the action of the second RF pulse generally only operates on 50% of the spins, and therefore the sequence is inherently signal poor.

**Super Conductivity** This describes the condition whereby electricity will flow even in the absence of an applied voltage. This can be achieved for certain materials if they are cooled to very low temperatures. Liquid helium is very close to absolute zero Kelvin (K) and is used to produce the conditions required for superconductivity. A superconducting magnet, once powered, does not require additional energizing.

**Superconducting Magnet**  In a superconducting magnet current flows in the windings without being connected to an external voltage supply. This condition is referred to as *superconductivity*. Certain materials become superconducting at low temperatures, such as achieved when immersed in liquid helium. Under normal circumstances the magnet is active at all times.

**Superparamagnetic Iron Oxide**  This is a nanoparticle with a very high paramagnetic effect. It has to be used with more caution because it never clears the body. It has a size of approximately 50 nm.

**Surface Rendering**  This describes a means of viewing 3D angiographic data. The surface of a vessel lumen is identified by a combination of intensity thresholding and editing out competing structures and this surface data is represented in a 3D manner.

**Susceptibility, $\chi$**  This is the property that materials have that describe the affinity of that material for magnetic flux lines. Metals have high susceptibility values, and thereby attract flux lines from a large surrounding area.

**T-Wave Elevation**  The electrocardiograph signal generally is used to detect the R wave. However, the T wave sometimes competes in amplitude with the R wave. The reason for this is that the T wave corresponds to a point in the cardiac cycle when blood is rapidly ejected from the heart. Because blood is an electrically conductive tissue, as it moves through the magnetic field, it generates its own electrical signal. This additional electrical signal is seen as an elevation of the T wave.

**T1**  (T One). T1 relaxation time. The T1 relaxation time describes the rate at which spins relax back to alignment with the main magnetic field. The T1 time constant describes the exponential half-life of the process.

**T1 Weighting**  (T One Weighting). A T1 weighted image produces contrast due to the T1 properties of the tissue being imaged. In this case, using a relatively short repetition time and high RF flip angle, or alternatively, using some form of spin preparation, such as applying of an inversion recovery pulse is required to effectively image spins under short TR conditions. When imaging under effective short TR conditions and employing a relatively high RF flip angle, spins with a short T1 value will relax rapidly, and contribute a bright signal, whereas spins with a long T1 value will only have relaxed slightly and contribute a low signal. Such an image is said to be T1 weighted.

**T2**  (T Two). T2 relaxation time. The T2 relaxation time describes the rate at which spins lose coherence with each other. To experience T2 relaxation, spins must have a component in the transverse plane. The time constant describes the exponential half-life of the signal.

**T2 Blurring**  (T Two Blurring). This describes the process of loosing signal due to a long signal readout, as occurs in sequences such as EPI and spirals. As the long signal read-out proceeds, signal decays due to the T2 relaxation process. The loss of signal manifests in the image as a blurring of features. Tissues with shorter T2 values will be more highly blurred.

**T2 Weighting**  (T Two Weighting). A T2 weighted image produces contrast due to the T2 properties of the tissue being imaged. In this case, a relatively long echo time is required, or alternatively, some form of spin preparation is required, to effectively image spins under long TE conditions. When imaging under effective long TE conditions, spins with a short T2 value will have decayed appreciably, whereas spins with a long T2 value will contribute a bright signal. Such an image is said to be T2 weighted.

**T2***  (T Two Star). This describes the effective T2 that is measured in practice. Typically, the measured T2 is lower than the ideal due to contamination and is referred to as *T2\**.

**Tagging**  Describes the process of laying down a series of bright and dark signal stripes on a rectangular grid, typically at the start of the ECG R wave. The signal pattern deforms with the image, allowing detection of relative motion of dynamic features.

**TE**  Time to Echo peak.

**Temporal Blur**  This describes the loss of clarity of dynamic features due to effectively sampling data for too long in each frame of a time series. In general, this is a problem for segmented sequences, when the segmentation duration exceeds a "reasonable value". The term *reasonable value* is dependant on the speed of the movement to be captured.

**Tesla, T**  Tesla is the SI unit of magnetic field strength. Common field strengths for MR systems include 1.5 T and 3 T.

**Three-Chamber View**  Describes the view of the heart showing the aortic valve, mitral valve, and right and left ventricles.

**Time of Flight**  This describes the contrast that is due to physical motion of blood. Because blood refreshes an imaging slice or volume, it has no history of spin excitation pulses. Therefore, as the spins enter the region, they yield a relatively bright signal compared to the static tissue.

**Timing Sequence**  This describes an imaging sequence applied before a scan that requires synchronization of contrast agent administration and acquisition. The timing sequence is applied to a representative region at a rapid rate. A small injection of contrast is administered and the time for the contrast to arrive in the region of interest is determined by counting frames.

**TIR**  See Triple Inversion Recovery.

**Tissue Contamination**  This is a term used in 3D contrast angiography to describe the condition whereby the contrast agent enters the musculature and thereby elevates the signal background against which vessels are visualized.

**TOF**    See Time of Flight.

**TR**    Time of Repetition of the pulse sequence.

**Transmitter RF Coil**    This is the electromagnetic coil that is designed to transmit the RF magnetic field that results in spin excitation. Generally, the transmit coil generates a uniform magnetic field such that spins at all locations undergo the same tip angle. The transmit coil generates the rotating $B_1$ field.

**Transverse Component**    This describes the component of the net magnetization spin vector, $M_0$, that lies in the transverse plane (i.e., orthogonal to the main magnetic field, $B_0$). In any imaging sequence, only the transverse component of the spin system contributes to the signal.

**Transverse Plane**    The transverse plane, is described by the Cartesian co-ordinates of X and Y. These describe the plane perpendicular to the main magnetic field, $B_0$. To be detected, spins must be tipped into the transverse plane. In this plane, they are at an angle to $B_0$ and therefore precess.

**TRICKS**    Time Resolved Intensity Contrast KineticS. This is a sparse sampling approach designed to obtain time-resolved 3D contrast angiographic data.

**Triple Inversion Recovery**    This describes the process of obtaining contrast, based on the inversion recovery processes. In this case, a second inversion pulse is applied at the time of the null point of the short T1 component, and a third pulse is applied when both spin systems are almost fully relaxed. The spin system is imaged after a further delay. The end result is that the short T1 component is typically suppressed and the long T1 component is visualized.

**True FISP**    This is a commercial acronym for the steady state free precession sequence: True Fast Imaging with Steady Precession.

**Turbo Factor**    Equivalent term to performing a segmented scan, with the aim of speeding up the acquisition.

**Turbulence**    Turbulence in the flow field results in extreme dephasing of the spin system. In this case, signal is lost from turbulent regions.

**T-Wave Elevation**    This describes the interaction of rapidly moving blood during systolic ejection and the magnetic field. Blood is an electrically conducting fluid, and as it moves through the magnetic field, it generates its own electrical signal. This phenomena is referred to as the *magnetohydrodynamic effect*. This electrical signal is responsible for elevation of the ECG T wave.

**Two-Chamber View**    See Vertical Long Axis.

**Vector Electrocardiogram**    A vector electrocardiogram utilizes advanced signal processing to detect and display the maximal vector of the electrocardiographic signal. Sensitivity to the vector generally makes detection of the electrocardiogram R wave more robust.

**Vena Contracta**    This describes the region of maximal convergence in jet flow. The vena contracta is the narrowest point of jet flow, and typically occurs a few millimeters past the stenotic orifice.

**VENC**    Describes the Velocity Encoding parameter. This sets the upper and lower aliasing limits in velocity imaging.

**Venous Suppression**    This describes the process of suppressing the venous signal, typically for angiographic imaging. Venous suppression is accomplished by applying a signal suppression slab to the venous side of the imaging region. The suppression slab has a relatively wide width and a high flip angle.

**Vertical Long Axis**    Describes the view of the heart in which only the left atria and left ventricle are seen.

**View Sharing**    Describes the process of generating intermediate images to those that were directly acquired in a time-resolved image series. The intermediate images are generated by effectively "sharing" k-space lines between two successive acquisitions.

**Views Per Segment**    This is the parameter that describes how many lines contribute to a segmented scan.

**Virtual Reality**    Typically, a term applied to viewing 3D angiographic data. A view from within the vessel can be obtained using virtual reality "fly through". The vessel is opacified by image processing and the path through the vessel is determined by user interaction

**Volume Rendering**    A means of viewing 3D angiographic data. Volume rendering is a hybrid between surface rendering and maximum intensity projection viewing. Depth and brightness affect the ultimate rendering in the image. 3D rotation of the rendered image is imperative to appreciate the depth and relative position of vessels.

**Voxel**    Volume Element. Describes the 3D volume of the smallest region imaged in the body. The image counterpart of a voxel (which is corporeal) is the pixel (which is digital).

**VPS**    See Views Per Segment.

**Wave-Guide**    The wave-guide is a metal tube approximately 2 ft long, passing through the Faraday cage and connecting the scan room with the outside world. Although this is an opening that allows limited access for IV lines etc., it attenuates RF signal as it travels along the wave-guide.

**X or Y Gradient**    See Golay Coil.

**Z Gradient**    See Maxwell Coil.

**Zero Filling**    Describes the process of interpolating data by performing zero filling in the Fourier domain. In this treatment, the Fourier representation of the signal is "padded out" by preceding and followed it with zeros. By extending the data in the Fourier domain, it has the effect, when inverse Fourier transformation is performed, of representing the data at interpolated time points.

**Zeroth Moment**    In terms of gradients, this describes the mathematical residual of the positive gradient area versus the negative gradient area. For instance, a bipolar gradient with equal positive and negative gradient lobes will produce a null value for the zeroth order moment.

**ZIP**    See Zero Filling.

Page numbers in italics indicate figures.